Patrick Holford BSc, DipION, FBANT, NTCRP is a leading spokesman on nutrition in the media. He is the author of over 30 books, translated into over 20 languages and selling over a million copies worldwide, including *The Optimum Nutrition Bible*, *The Low GL-Diet Bible*, *Optimum Nutrition for the Mind* and *The 10 Secrets of 100% Healthy People*.

Patrick started his academic career in the field of psychology. In 1984 he founded the Institute for Optimum Nutrition (ION), an independent educational charity, and was involved in groundbreaking research showing that multivitamins can increase children's IQ scores – research that was published in the *Lancet* and was the subject of a BBC *Horizon* documentary in the 1980s. He was one of the first promoters of the importance of zinc, antioxidants, essential fats, a low-GL diet and homocysteine-lowering B vitamins such as folic acid and B_{12}. In the 1990s he campaigned against HRT due to its associated risks with breast cancer.

Patrick is director of the Food for the Brain Foundation, a charity focusing on the link between mental health and nutrition, and director of the Brain Bio Centre, the Foundation's treatment centre. He is an honorary fellow of the British Association of Nutritional Therapy, as well as a registered practitioner of the Nutrition Therapy Council.

By the same author

patrick
HOLFORD

BALANCE
YOUR
HORMONES

THE SIMPLE DRUG-FREE
WAY TO SOLVE WOMEN'S
HEALTH PROBLEMS

piatkus

PIATKUS

First published in Great Britain in 1998 by Piatkus Books as
Balancing Hormones Naturally

Reprinted 1998, 1999 (twice), 2000, 2001, 2002 (twice), 2003 (twice),
2004, 2006, 2007, 2008, 2009, 2010

This updated and expanded edition published as *Balance Your Hormones* in 2011
Copyright © Patrick Holford 1998, 2011

A CIP catalogue record for this book
is available from the British Library.

ISBN 978-0-7499-5339-3

Typeset in Berkeley by Phoenix Photosetting, Chatham, Kent
Printed and bound in Great Britain by CPI Mackays, Chatham ME5 8TD

Piatkus
An imprint of
Little, Brown Book Group
100 Victoria Embankment
London EC4Y 0DY

An Hachette UK Company
www.hachette.co.uk

www.piatkus.co.uk

Contents

Acknowledgements

This book is very much the result of teamwork. In rewriting this book I am deeply grateful for the generous help of Kate Neil, who worked on the original edition, and the meticulous research of Liz Efiong. Also, a big thanks to Dian Mills, who contributed Chapter 19 on endometriosis, and for her advice based on her vast experience treating women's health issues; to Erica White for her help with Chapter 16 on *Candida*; to Dr Tony Coope for his generous help with Chapter 24 on bio-identical hormones, as well as Chapter 12 highlighting the problems caused after pregnancy as a result of hormone imbalances; to Jerome Burne who also helped with material on bio-identical hormones; and to my publishers and editorial team – Gill Bailey, Jillian Stewart, Claudia Dyer and Jan Cutler – who do so much more than dot the i's and cross the t's, and whose support is invaluable. I would also like to deeply thank the late Dr John Lee, a true pioneer, who helped identify the widespread problem of oestrogen dominance, as well as Dr Shirley Bond and Dr Marion Gluck for their help and clinical insights into the use of bio-identical hormones. I am also indebted to the many female clients I have worked with who bear testimony to the approaches included in this book.

Guide to Abbreviations and Measures

1 gram (g) = 1,000 milligrams (mg) = 1,000,000 micrograms (mcg, also written as μg).

Most vitamins are measured in milligrams or micrograms. Vitamins A, D and E are also measured in International Units (iu), a measurement designed to standardise the different forms of these vitamins, which have different potencies.

1mcg of retinol (1mcgRE) = 3.3iu of vitamin A

1mcgRE of beta-carotene = 6mcg of beta-carotene

100iu of vitamin D = 2.5mcg

100iu of vitamin E = 67mg

1 pound (lb) = 16 ounces (oz)

2.2lb = 1 kilogram (kg)

1 pint = 0.6 litres

1.76 pints = 1 litre

In this book 'calories' means kilocalories (kcal)

References and Further Sources of Information

Hundreds of references from respected scientific literature have been used in writing this book. Details of specific studies referred to are listed on pages 358–77. More details on most of these studies can be found on the Internet for those wishing to dig deeper. On page 343, you will find a list of recommended books if you would like to read more about the topics covered.

Disclaimer

Although all the nutrients and dietary changes referred to in this book have been proven safe, those seeking help for specific medical conditions are advised to consult a qualified nutrition therapist, clinical nutritionist, doctor or equivalent health professional. The recommendations given in this book are intended as educational and information and should not be taken as medical advice. Neither the author nor the publisher accept liability for readers who choose to self-prescribe.

All supplements should be kept out of reach of infants and young children.

Introduction

This book examines female health issues connected to hormonal imbalances. Although the female hormones are specifically studied, the role played by other hormones in the body is also discussed in detail, giving you an overall picture of the effects imbalances have on your health and well-being and what you can do to correct them.

The first edition of this book, written in the 1990s, fundamentally challenged the standard treatment of women's health issues, largely founded on using hormone replacement therapy (HRT) and high-dose contraceptive pills, which both contained synthetic hormone-like drugs. It predicted a massive rise in breast cancer and other hormone-related health problems. Many of my cautions, radical at the time, have sadly been proven to be justified and, thankfully, the use of synthetic HRT is now very much on the decline.

When I first wrote this book, hormonal health issues, such as endometriosis and polycystic ovaries, were rather rare. Now they are commonplace. Virtually everyone knows a woman who has been diagnosed with breast cancer. Hormonal health problems are getting worse.

This edition has been substantially rewritten. It seeks to identify the main underlying causes of women's ever-increasing hormonal health problems, such as polycystic ovaries, endometriosis, breast cancer and osteoporosis. Furthermore, it aims to provide solutions to problems such as PMS, menopausal symptoms and post-pregnancy blues using highly effective and safe *natural* medicine. This is based on diet, supplements, lifestyle changes and the judicial use of low-dose bio-identical hormones – the exact same hormones in similar quantities as those produced naturally by your body.

It is only now, 60 years after synthetic hormones were first used, that the real long-term effects of millions of women taking them have become fully realised. The legacy of these drugs includes breast cancer, which is diagnosed in around 50,000 women each year in the UK alone – equating to 125 women every day – and it represents more than a 50 per cent increase in incidence over the past 25 years. However, when you add up all the other totally unnecessary female hormonal health issues that have escalated in the 21st century it becomes clear that few women go through life without encountering some hormonally related health problems.

Without any doubt, pharmaceutical companies have had a lot to gain financially from the widespread prescription of synthetic hormones, and women of all ages are potential customers. Synthetic hormones not only act as contraceptives, but are also widely used in infertility programmes, and were regularly recommended in the form of hormone replacement therapy (HRT) to alleviate the symptoms of menopause. But there are safer alternatives, such as testing for genuine hormonal deficiencies and supplementing low-dose natural, or bio-identical, hormones such as progesterone. Because they were and continue to be unpatentable – and hence much less profitable – I believe that, as a consequence, they remain sadly under-researched.

Pharmaceutical drugs and synthetic hormones are neither the whole reason we are in a mess nor clearly the way out. Research in the last decade has highlighted endemic changes in our 21st-century diet and lifestyle that are unwittingly tipping us out of hormonal balance. A complex web of factors are just as much part of the problem: from our widespread exposure to hormone-disrupting chemicals – the result of environmental pollution, agro-chemicals and our vastly chemicalised world – coupled with eating too much sugar and carbo-hydrates, and too much dairy products, to a lack of nutrients.

The book is designed to help you understand that complex web. It is divided into five parts:

Part 1: The Role of Hormones

This part introduces you to the two female hormones, oestrogen and progesterone, and their important role in the female life cycle, from puberty until after the menopause. I also explain the hormonal problems that women are increasingly encountering and the threats to hormonal balance posed by chemicals and stress. Only by under-standing the complexity of the influences that lead to hormonal imbalances does it become possible to truly rebalance the system and effect positive and non-toxic solutions to a plethora of health issues.

This is called a 'systems-based' approach to medicine: looking at the whole system, the big picture – in this case, the female body – and the fundamental factors that determine a woman's state of health. In truth, these health issues are more often than not the result of a kind of inner 'global warming'.

The simple, yet still dominant, approach of looking for the single most effective treatment, or drug for hormonal conditions, has no chance of success when the root cause is complex. As I will explain later in the book, improving your overall basic health is the key to protecting yourself against a number of female-related illnesses, because this underpins hormonal balance.

Part 2: Staying Hormonally Healthy

The second part of the book starts by focusing on how you can tune up your body's support systems, starting with your digestion and blood sugar. I then explore specific problems experienced by mil-lions of women throughout their lives – from PMS to menopausal problems – and I provide effective natural solutions based on decades of clinical experience.

Part 3: Staying Free From Hormone-related Diseases

The third part focuses on other hormonal problems, including the more serious debilitating issues such as endometriosis, polycystic ovaries, fibroids, osteoporosis, candidiasis and cystitis, as well as life-threatening problems such as breast cancer.

Within Parts 2 and 3 you will find effective solutions for the majority of hormonally related health issues, from depression to migraines and hot sweats, which include making changes to your diet and lifestyle, taking supplements and, in some cases, the judicial use of low-dose bio-identical hormones to help reset the system.

Part 4: Balancing Your Hormones Naturally

In the first edition of this book, I explained that doses of bio-identical hormones that were consistent with a woman's natural production could be taken when she found she was deficient. Since then millions of women have experienced profound benefits through taking them. However, there continues to be widespread mainstream medical ignorance about this subject.

In the 1990s, I teamed up with the late Dr John Lee, author of *What Your Doctor May Not Tell You About the Menopause* and *What Your Doctor May Not Tell You About Breast Cancer* (among others). Dr Lee defined a new syndrome, 'oestrogen dominance', to explain many of these common female conditions. His theory was that many women are suffering from the effects of too much oestrogen, and he backed this up with two decades of clinical experience in the field of female health, as well as published research. He believed that stress, nutritional deficiencies, oestrogenic substances from the environment and taking synthetic oestrogens, combined with a deficiency of progesterone, are all likely contributory factors in the creation of oestrogen dominance. Much of what he said has been proven correct in the last decade of research, but still the use of bio-identical hormones remains much under-researched and undermined. I explain this in Part 4.

Part 5: Your Action Plan for Hormonal Health

It is only in the last few decades that the importance of nutrition has been realised. In fact, the future health and survival of the whole human race depends very much upon sound nutrition. In this part I explain the nuts and bolts of a healthy diet as the basis of hormonal health, as well as describing other natural hormone helpers.

Many women today want to find out more about what is happening to their own bodies and to take responsibility for their health. They want to live a life that is in harmony with their natural design, but they also want to tackle hormonal health issues and stand up against the ineffective, and often dangerous, approaches that are still widespread and which hinge on using profitable synthetic hormones.

Adolescence, pregnancy and the menopause are not diseases that need medicalisation, but there are times when women suffer mentally or physically. Understanding how your body works, and living according to its design, will help you to avoid the problems that many women experience because their hormones are out of balance.

Making simple and beneficial changes to your diet and lifestyle are the first important steps towards balanced hormones and better health. Bio-identical hormonal preparations can also help and are available on prescription. When combined with adjustments in lifestyle and diet, plus the appropriate nutrient and phytonutrient supplementation, these preparations can help to restore the natural hormonal balance in your body and return you to a state of good, natural health.

Part 5 explains how to do this by building your own action plan for hormonal health. I will also introduce you to the many well-qualified practitioners, doctors and nutritional therapists who can help you return to health if you are suffering from a more complex condition that requires testing and treatment, and explain what kind of testing is available (as home-test kits or otherwise).

If you are unsure where to start, either because you have vague symptoms or you have a number of problems, I suggest you read Part 1 and then turn to the Hormonal Health Questionnaire in Appendix 1, as it can help you identify the underlying factors that can contribute to symptoms you might associate with hormonal imbalances. Even if you know only too well what your condition is, I suggest you read Part 1, take the questionnaire and turn to any relevant chapters in Part 2 that your questionnaire answers point to, *before* tackling any specific problems you may have. As I've previously pointed out, hormonal imbalances can be caused by a complex web of factors so it helps to be aware of the big picture.

I hope this book will help you to feel empowered to make changes to your health, avoiding the pitfalls that occur when your hormones are out of balance and opening the way to a happier and healthier life.

Wishing you the best of health and happiness,

Patrick Holford

PART 1

THE ROLE OF HORMONES

In this part I'll explain how two female hormones, specifically, are designed to work to keep the female body in good health through-out a woman's life, and why hormonal health problems have become so prevalent. I'll also explore how diet, coupled with environmental exposure to hormone-disrupting chemicals and stressful lifestyle changes have contributed to widespread hormonal imbalances.

CHAPTER 1

The Female Life Cycle

Two hormones play an essential role in all stages of the female health cycle: progesterone and oestrogen. In this chapter I'll be explaining the basics about what they do and their importance throughout a woman's life, from puberty until after the menopause. The hormones regulate a natural monthly rhythm during the reproductive years and continue to protect the body after the menopause, but their role is greater than this, as this book will explain.

The female hormones: oestrogen and progesterone

To begin with we need a basic understanding of the two hormones – oestrogen and progesterone – and what they do.

Oestrogen is primarily produced by the ovaries. When a girl enters puberty, oestrogen encourages the growth and development of the breasts, uterus, female body hair distribution, and the fat that contributes to the typical female body shape. It also stimulates the lining of the vagina and the production of vaginal secretions, making sexual intercourse more comfortable and protecting and cleansing the vagina. As I'll be explaining on page 7, it also has an essential role in the menstrual cycle, stimulating the release of an egg and the monthly bleed that follows if the egg is not fertilised.

Oestrogen also prompts the body to lay down fat stores during pregnancy so that the mother can use this as an energy reserve after the birth. Later in life it helps to ease the body through the transition to menopause.

Progesterone literally means 'for pregnancy' (pro-gestation). It is the only hormone in the body that is produced in relatively large quantities, usually around 15–20mg a day. All the other hormones are produced in nanogram amounts. By the last three months of pregnancy the mother's body is producing up to 30 times more progesterone than it did in its non-pregnant state. Progesterone also has other biological effects, including helping the body to burn fat for energy and reducing anxiety, as well a lifting the mood by acting as a natural antidepressant.

I explain the roles of oestrogen and progesterone in more detail in Chapter 22.

There are three main hormonal phases in a woman's life: menstruation, pregnancy and menopause. The female body has developed a natural monthly rhythm in which its hormone levels ebb and flow. This is as nature planned it, and provided a woman's diet, environment and lifestyle conform to its natural design, no part of the female life cycle needs to be thought of as an illness or a disabling condition. The aim of this book is to build an understanding of the process and to address particular issues that women experience so that you will be better able to take control and make clear decisions about what steps you can take to enjoy good health.

Women's bodies – no longer a mystery

Until relatively recently, the bodies of men and women were considered structurally similar. In the 4th century the Bishop of Emesa in Syria wrote, 'Women have the same genitalia as men except that theirs are inside the body and not outside it.' It was not until 1890 that medical science began to investigate the workings of the human menstrual cycle.

Medicine was once dominated by men, and the current understanding of the female cycle and female problems is still based on a male perspective, even though there are many more women working in medicine today. The language that medical and scientific men once used to describe the processes that occur throughout the female life cycle still colours our understanding and attitudes even now.

In previous centuries it was extremely rare to find accounts of women's views on how they understood their bodies worked. Because of this, women learned about their bodies largely through men; however, by the 1950s, women started to want to know more about their bodies and to have more control of their reproductive lives. As a result, the natural childbirth and women's rights movements began to develop.

Attempts to control fertility must be as old as childbirth itself. What changed in the second half of the 20th century, however, was the method of control. For the first time in human history, drugs were used widely for the purpose of birth control. Although it was known that these drugs would control fertility, the full implications of their effects on health were not fully realised. Now we have a much better understanding of the effects of these drugs, and of the intricate synchrony of events that control the monthly cycle.

Nature's design

The female anatomy has been designed to ensure the survival of the species, right down to the design of the pelvis. It contains the womb, which under the influence of a fine balance of hormones, prepares for itself every month a special lining in case of pregnancy. If pregnancy does not occur, this lining is shed and the process of building up a new one starts again. The uterus is normally smaller than a fist but can accommodate a baby larger than a football. It contains muscles like

cont ▶

no others found in the body: through regular uterine contraction and retraction they can successfully deliver a baby and yet return to normal size within only six weeks. The ovaries are responsible for producing eggs and are enclosed in sacs that are well protected, deep within the pelvic cavity.

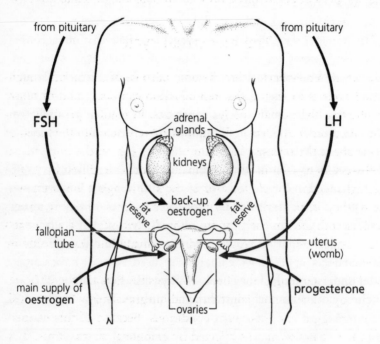

from pituitary

from pituitary

FSH

LH

adrenal
glands

kidneys

fat reserve

back-up
oestrogen

fat reserve

fallopian
tube

uterus
(womb)

main supply of
oestrogen

progesterone

ovaries

The female reproductive system

The female life cycle

The female hormones, oestrogen and progesterone, remain dormant in girls until about the age of 12 or 13. Around then, the hypothalamus, a small gland at the base of the brain, makes a master hormone. This instructs the pituitary gland connected to it to release into the blood two powerful hormones, follicle stimulating hormone (FSH)

The hypothalamus gland senses that the levels of oestrogen and progesterone are low and it releases the first master hormone, which causes the pituitary gland to release FSH. As the name implies, follicle stimulating hormone works on the eggs within the ovaries, ripening one for release and fertilisation. It also stimulates the production of oestrogen by the ovary. Levels of this hormone gradually rise over the first half of the cycle, thickening the growth of the lining of the womb and the breast tissue. The process lasts about ten days and is sometimes known as the 'proliferative stage' of the cycle. It sets the scene for the reception of a fertilised egg.

Follicles are ripened and prepared in both ovaries. Oestrogen levels peak at around day 12 of the cycle, and this gives a signal to the hypothalamus gland to release LH. On day 14 of a normal cycle, a surge of LH brings about ovulation: the release of a mature egg from one of the ovaries. The egg is now free to enter and move down the fallopian tube attached to the uterus. Helped by specialised hair-like tissue, the egg passes down the tube to meet the sperm.

From ovulation to menstruation (days 14–28)

The space that is left behind in the ovary after the egg has been released fills with blood and specialised cells, and builds up into a dense mass known as the corpus luteum. The corpus luteum now becomes the manufacturing site for both oestrogen and progesterone during the second half of the cycle. High levels of both hormones are required to support fertilisation should it occur.

The rise of progesterone just after ovulation increases the body temperature by at least 0.2°C.

If the egg is not fertilised, the corpus luteum breaks down. The blood vessels supplying the womb lining go into spasm and the lining is shed, forming the menstrual flow. The loss of the corpus luteum causes a rapid fall in the levels of oestrogen and progesterone. This low level of oestrogen and progesterone acts as a signal to the hypothalamus gland to release its master hormone and the process starts all over again (see the illustration opposite).

and luteinising hormone (LH). These two hormones are responsible for the development and release of an egg from the ovary. When a girl is approaching the onset of her menstrual cycle, the cells of the pituitary gland and ovary are laden with receptors, which become super-sensitive to these stimulating hormones. It takes about three years for the menstrual cycle to become fully established from the time of the first period. Of the millions of potentially mature eggs that are present before birth, only about 300,000 are left at puberty.

The menstrual cycle

It is worth remembering that the only purpose of the monthly menstrual cycle is to ensure that reproduction can occur and therefore ensure that the human species continues. In regular, precisely synchronised order, the female hormones are released into the blood to bring about the release of a mature healthy egg, in the hope that it will meet an equally healthy sperm and become fertilised by it. The average menstrual cycle lasts for 28 days, although it is not uncommon for cycles to vary between three and six weeks. The cycle repeats itself month after month for the reproductive years of a woman' life – usually about 40 years – and is normally interrupted only ! pregnancy.

The master of this hormonal activity is the hypothalamus. It like a control centre, which shares and integrates many biocher immunological and emotional conditions. Because of this co tion, menstruation can be affected by emotional states, stre other hormones, illness and drugs.

From menstruation to ovulation (days 1–14)

At the beginning of a menstrual cycle the levels of th oestrogen and progesterone are very low because the pared womb lining containing them has been shed. when a fully mature egg is not fertilised by a sperm a pregnancy has taken place. This is known as the m period.

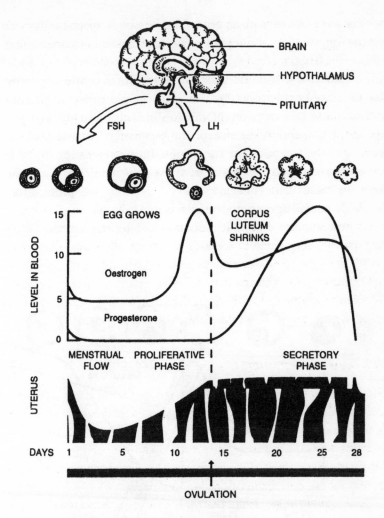

Normal menstrual cycle

Pregnancy

If the egg is fertilised, the corpus luteum continues to produce oestrogen and progesterone in large quantities for the next 12–14 weeks, and in small quantities throughout the pregnancy. Once the fertilised egg has become embedded in the womb, special cells made by the egg produce another hormone called human chorionic gonadotrophin (HCG).

This hormone stimulates the corpus luteum to continue growing for the next 12–14 weeks. By this time, the placenta is sufficiently developed to take over the production of both oestrogen and progesterone to support the rest of the pregnancy. Because levels of oestrogen and progesterone are so high during pregnancy, the brain does not receive any messages from the egg-stimulating hormone, FSH, or the ovulation hormone, LH. Oestrogen and progesterone levels do not fall again until the baby is due to be born.

Hormonal signals, about nine months after the first day of the last period, start labour. Towards the time of labour, the womb

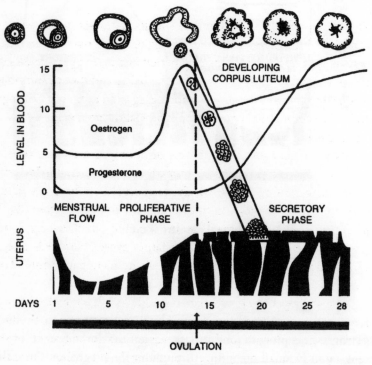

The first stage of pregnancy

becomes increasingly sensitive to oxytocin, a hormone whose action is stimulated by the pituitary gland. Oxytocin stimulates the uterus to contract and begins and maintains the process of the delivery of the baby. Contractions increase under the influence of oxytocin until the baby is born.

After delivery, levels of oestrogen and progesterone rapidly fall. Oestrogen remains low, and there is no rise in progesterone while a new mother is breastfeeding. Progesterone is not produced in any significant amount because the mother is not ovulating. Breastfeeding is known to be a natural contraceptive, although it cannot be fully relied upon and it becomes more unreliable as feeding progresses over the months ahead.

Menopause

The menopause is a process that usually takes about ten years to complete. Sometimes called the 'change of life', it refers to the phase that leads up to the last menstrual period and more or less marks the end of a woman's reproductive life. The balance of the sex hormones is affected: the ovaries stop producing eggs and making oestrogen and progesterone. This process normally starts around the age of 45 and is usually complete by 55.

At the menopause, lower levels of oestrogen are made because they are no longer needed to prepare the womb lining for pregnancy. As oestrogen levels fall, the menstrual flow becomes lighter and often quite irregular, until eventually it stops altogether. As the menopause progresses, many cycles occur in which an egg is not released. These are known as anovulatory cycles. Hundreds of eggs vanish each month, and by the time of the menopause only about 1,000 are left.

The menopause should occur gradually, allowing the body to adapt to its new condition with ease. Because a woman ceases to ovulate, she no longer produces progesterone, so the body compensates by sending a message to the pituitary gland to release increased quantities of FSH and LH. The onset of the menopause is commonly confirmed by a rise in the levels of these two hormones in the blood (see the illustration below).

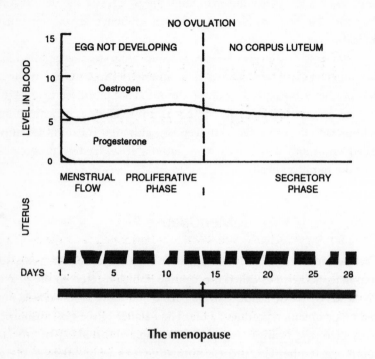

The menopause

As you will have seen, hormones play a continuing and essential role in a woman's life, but in today's world women are increasingly suffering from hormone-related health problems. Chapter 2 asks why this is happening.

The Rise of Hormonal Health Problems

Something is seriously amiss with our hormones. Over the last 50 years there's been an undeniable escalation of hormone-related health problems in men as well as women. The incidence of infertility, fibroids, endometriosis and polycystic ovaries and breasts, as well as ovarian, cervical and breast cancer, have increased steadily and quite dramatically. Even more worryingly, many hormone-related diseases are occurring earlier in life. Complaints like endometriosis, fibroids and ovarian cysts used to be extremely rare in teenage girls but they are now quite common and sometimes result in irreversible infertility.

The reality of the hormonal havoc we now face, especially in the Western world, becomes vividly clear when we look at cancer statistics. Although some non-hormone-related cancers are not greatly increasing in incidence (lung cancer, for example, is on the decline) the hormone-related cancers are very much on the increase.

Breast cancer incidence, for example, has more than doubled over the last 50 years. It now affects one in eight women in Britain at some time in their life, compared to one in 22 in the 1940s. According to the Office of National Statistics, breast cancer is the most common cancer in England. The number of women diagnosed with it is gradually increasing year on year with about a thousand additional cases each year.

Furthermore, hormonal problems don't just relate to women. Although breast cancer rates in men are much lower, rates of breast, testicular and, particularly, prostate cancer are growing year on year. Over the last 30 years, rates of prostate cancer have almost tripled, and this disease now affects around one in ten men at some point in their life with a new diagnosis every 15 minutes.

I am going to show you why these diseases are on the increase and what you can do to virtually eliminate your chances of having them.

The early signs of hormonal havoc

Although hormonal cancers may be seen as the end result of sub-stantial and probably long-term changes in hormonal health, the early warning signs are undeniable. The number of boys born with genital defects or undescended testes has doubled. More girls than ever before are now reaching maturity at the age of nine. Research by Dr Marcia Herman-Giddens of the University of North Carolina found that 48 per cent of black girls and 15 per cent of white girls were developing breasts and pubic hair before their tenth birthdays. 'All of us in paediatric practice had a sense that girls were developing earlier, but we were still surprised at how young many of them were.'[1] Puberty onset has dropped to an average of 11 compared with an average of 13 in the 1970s and 17 in the Victorian age.

Research by Dr Imogen Rogers at the University of Brighton has linked the early onset of puberty with diet. Girls aged 3–7 who ate large amounts of meat and 7-year-old girls who ate more than 12 serv-ings of meat each week were more likely to have reached puberty by the age of 12½.[2] These changes are particularly concerning because early onset of puberty is associated with an increased risk of breast cancer and menopausal problems.

PMS – monthly misery

Women's suffering hasn't always been taken that seriously in medical history, and there is no better example of this than premenstrual syndrome (PMS), the symptoms of which include breast tenderness, fatigue, bloating, headaches, mood swings, depression and irritability. These are symptoms of a hormonal imbalance that affect two in three women. Two surveys by the Women's Nutritional Advisory Service – one in 1985, the other in 1996 – show that the severity of PMS is increasing.[3] In the 1996 survey, mood swings, depression, anxiety and aggressive feelings were experienced by 80 per cent of sufferers premenstrually, and 52 per cent had contemplated suicide in their premenstrual phase. My own 100% Health Survey of over 45,000 women found that 63 per cent of women often suffer from PMS.[4]

In my opinion, and that of Dr Marion Stewart from the Women's Nutritional Advisory Service, PMS (at least on the scale that it is now experienced) is the result of poor nutrition and increased levels of stress due to the changing role of women in modern society. These symptoms completely disappear in 90 per cent of women within four months of changing their diet, taking some exercise and finding effective ways of dealing with stress. (See Chapter 8 if this is something you suffer from.)

Endometriosis – the hidden epidemic

The condition endometriosis occurs when cells like those lining the womb begin to grow on other organs of the body where they do not belong. It is being diagnosed in more and more women in their teens and twenties. Endometriosis can also result in fibroids, growths in the womb that can cause irregular, heavy and painful periods. One in ten women from the ages of 11 to 60, is affected.[5] Symptoms vary but may include severe period pain, heavy bleeding, pain on menstruation or pain with intercourse. The pain can be so severe as to be totally debilitating, affecting a woman's ability to lead a normal, fulfilling life. Loss of fertility is investigated in at least half of those with endometriosis because 30–40 per cent of sufferers cannot conceive; it is a major cause of infertility and is present in up to 43 per cent of infertile women. Although endometriosis is not a new condition, and statistics can vary widely, evidence suggests that it too is very much on the increase. For more information, see Chapter 19.

Beware those lumps

Much more common than breast cancer is the occurrence of breast lumps. These are often fibrocystic lumps known as fibrocystic breast disease. Some women also get cysts in their breasts. In about 85 per cent of cases these lumps are not malignant (cancer-producing); however, the risk of developing breast cancer tends to be higher in those with a history of breast lumps (see Chapter 20).

Polycystic ovaries

Cysts in the ovaries are also an increasingly common problem, especially among younger women, and are strongly associated with blood sugar problems and insulin resistance. (More on this in Chapter 18.)

A good sperm is hard to find

In case you're thinking that women have a raw deal, men have hormonal problems too. Although they may not have to worry about PMS, men do have a menopause with very similar symptoms to women. According to male hormone expert Dr Malcolm Carruthers, the symptoms of the male menopause (known as the andropause) include fatigue, depression, irritability, rapid ageing, aches and pains, sweating and flushing, as well as decreased sexual performance. Having treated thousands of men,

cont ▶

Dr Carruthers, author of *The Male Menopause*, is convinced that the andropause is real and rapidly on the increase.[6] Those most at risk, according to his research, are farmers, possibly due to their frequent exposure to organophosphate in sheep dip, pesticides and other agrochemicals, including hormones used in intensive animal rearing.

However, according to Dr Niels Skakkebaek, a reproductive scientist for the World Health Organization, many symptom-free men are showing signs of hormonal and sexual imbalance. After analysing the data from over 60 scientific studies in the last 50 years, involving almost 15,000 men, he concludes that the average sperm count has dropped by 50 per cent in five decades.[7] It wasn't just the quantity, either, the quality had also fallen, with a lower percentage of healthy sperm able to fertilise an egg. Not everyone agrees that the fall in the sperm count is quite so dramatic, but there is little doubt that an increasing number of men aren't firing on all cylinders.

Men are also facing more and more prostate problems. A highly hormone-sensitive organ, the prostate lies under the bladder and surrounds the top of the urethra (urine duct) in men. Its job is to secrete a slightly acidic fluid that contributes to seminal fluid and improves the motility and viability of sperm. If it is enlarged (a condition known as benign prostatic hyperplasia, or BPH) or affected by benign or malignant tumours, it can act like a clamp and impede the flow of urine. BPH develops after the age of 40 and affects about one-third of all men over the age of 60 – that's about two million men in the UK, resulting in 40,000 prostate operations in the UK every year.

Although there appears to be no direct correlation, both BPH and prostate cancer are very much on the increase. Prostate cancer is the fastest growing cancer and will soon affect as many men as breast cancer affects women.

One in seven couples is infertile

The average sperm count fell from 113 million per ml in 1940 to 66 million in 1990. More recent figures from Denmark show a further decline up to 2006 with over two-thirds of Danish men having a sperm count below 40 million, which is considered the point below which increased infertility can be expected.[8] The National Institutes of Health (NIH) analysed data collected from 1938 to 1990 indicating that sperm densities in the US have exhibited an average annual decrease of 1.5 million sperm per millilitre of collected sample, or about 1.5 per cent per year. The NIH said in a statement. 'Those in European countries have declined at about twice that rate (3.1 percent per year).'

Dr Skakkebaek and others have found that an increasing number of men have these low levels of viable sperm. Professor Louis Guillette, a respected reproductive expert, concluded, 'Today's man is half the man his grandfather was.' Although men account for an estimated 40 per cent of cases of infertility, it is likely that increasing hormonal problems in both men and women are responsible for the gradual decline in overall fertility; so much so, that about one in seven couples is currently infertile. If the fall in sperm count continues, one might expect rates of infertility to escalate rapidly when sperm counts reach half their current average, posing a hitherto unthought-of threat to the human race.

When you put all the pieces of the puzzle together, it is hard to deny that we are having trouble keeping our hormones balanced. The question is why? Are these problems connected or not? And what are the solutions? The next chapter shows how modern living is a recipe for hormonal problems and how simple diet and lifestyle changes can help bring your hormones back into balance.

CHAPTER 3

Hormonal Overload

Our modern chemical world is very different from that of our ancestors. There are now 100,000 synthetic chemicals on the international market, including 15,000 chlorinated compounds such as PCBs. Some of these are put directly into food, others are added indirectly, in the form of pesticide residues or accumulation up the food chain from non-biodegradable industrial contaminants. Some creep into food from packaging and processing. Some we take as medicine. Many of these act like hormones, or interfere with the normal action of our body's hormones.

These hormone-disrupting chemicals include:

- **Organochlorine pesticides** DDT, heptachlor, chlordane, aldrin, dieldrin, mirex.

- **Plastic compounds** Alkylphenols, such as nonylphenol and octylphenol; biphenolic compounds, such as bisphenol-A; phthalates, found in soft plastics such as the lining of cans and original cling film.

- **Industrial compounds** Some PCBs, dioxin; plus those listed for plastics. Dioxins and PCBs accumulate up the food chain so the greatest exposure comes from eating meat and dairy products. Dioxins are also formed from the incineration of waste, thus from the inhalation of polluted air.

- **Pharmaceutical drugs** Synthetic oestrogens and progestogens (called estrogens and progestins in the US).

The sea of oestrogens

Most of the chemicals listed above mimic the role of oestrogenic hormones in our bodies, stimulating the growth of hormone-sensitive tissue. They are classified as xenoestrogens (meaning oestrogenic compounds from outside, as opposed to inside, our bodies). When taken in on top of the natural oestrogen produced by both men and women, plus the added oestrogen taken in by women on HRT, these chemicals can 'over-oestrogenise' a person. Too much oestrogen stimulates the excessive proliferation of hormone-sensitive tissue, thus increasing the risk of hormone-related cancers. The effect of these chemicals is not, however, quite so direct. Essentially, they confuse the hormonal messages the body sends out, changing our sexual and reproductive development. They are best thought of as hormone-disrupters, interfering with the body's ability to adapt and respond appropriately to its environment.

Such worldwide increased exposure to these hormone disrupters is even more worrying in the light of the finding that a very small change in hormone exposure during foetal development can lead to infertility and increased cancer risk in adulthood. 'We have unwittingly entered the ultimate Faustian bargain ... In return for all the benefits of our modern society, and all the amazing products of modern life, we have more testicular cancer and more breast cancer. We may also affect the ability of the species to reproduce,' says Devra Lee Davis, former deputy health policy advisor to the US government.

As we have seen in Chapter 2, girls appear to be reaching puberty earlier. The first signs of sexual maturity are now frequently appearing in younger children. According to Professor Richard Sharpe of the Medical Research Council, 'If you expose animals to low levels of extra oestrogen neonatally, they will have advanced puberty.'[9]

The lack of definitive proof on whether hormone-disrupting chemicals have the potential to harm human health leads to polarised opinions dominating this contentious field of enquiry. It is clearly not easy to identify cause and effect, particularly when health effects may not manifest until many years after initial exposure.

The accumulation of hormone-disrupting chemicals

It would appear that the increased incidence of breast cancer and testicular dysgenesis syndrome (low sperm counts, testicular cancer, undescended testes and the genetic condition in males, hypospadias) has driven the debate on how hormone-disrupting chemicals disrupt our own hormones and contribute to ill health.

It has been known for a long time that some hormone-disrupting chemicals, including many organochlorines, are oestrogenic and can also accumulate in breast fat. Although an initial study linked organochlorine exposure to a higher risk of breast cancer, most other research following this have not confirmed the link, including studies from different countries and those that took account of exposure to organochlorines for several years before breast cancer developed.

Two key researchers in the field, Sharpe and Irvine, reviewed the strength of the evidence between environmental chemicals and adverse effects on human reproductive health, and published their findings in the British Medical Journal.[10] They looked at which chemicals were being measured, over what time period, and what the effects of a mixture of these chemicals might be. They suggest that it may be more pertinent to focus our attention on the huge number of non-pesticide chemicals in the environment. Phthalates, for example, can leach out of plastics, carpets and fabrics into air, rainwater and food. They are also found in many creams, soaps and perfumes and emanate from exhaust, cigarette and combustion fumes.

The subtle effects

Our exposure to these synthetic chemicals is high, but just how high was appreciated only in about 2002. The effect of these chemicals now appears to be much more subtle than was previously thought. Rather than having a direct oestrogenic effect by occupying oestrogen receptors in the body, they appear to influence how much of the body's own oestrogen is made available to oestrogen-sensitive tissue, such as bone, the breasts, brain, ovaries, prostate and the womb. The discovery that phthalates could influence sexual differentiation in male foetuses was only discovered around the turn of the 21st century. Phthalates have been shown, for example, to reduce the ability of the testes to make testosterone during development in the womb and in this way interferes with sexual differentiation.

Another common hormone disrupter is BPA (bisphenol) found in many canned foods[11] – even those labelled as organic. BPA is used in the manufacture of polycarbonate and other plastics and has been linked to disrupted reproductive development in animals. The chemical is often found in drinking bottles, baby bottles and sipper cups as well as in the lining of aluminium food and beverage cans. Many experts believe that these should be banned for use in any baby bottles or baby food containers at the least.

Other related chemicals are PCBs (polychlorinated biphenyls), primarily found in insulating and cooling fluids, and PAHs (polyaromatic hydrocarbons), the products of burned or charred foodstuffs, both of which can prolong the action of oestrogen in the body by suppressing the action of an enzyme that enables oestrogen to be added to sulphur. In this 'sulphated' form, oestrogen is inactive and unable to influence oestrogen-sensitive tissues. This type of mechanism is a relevant consideration in the context of breast cancer.

It would appear that we have been chasing a bit of a red herring by looking for chemicals that have direct oestrogenic activity.

The anti-adaptogens

The chemicals listed above, and the broad spectrum of ill effects they appear to be generating, can be seen as anti-adaptogens, which interfere with our innate ability to adapt to our environment. They are a spanner in the works of our endocrine and immune systems whose job is to ensure that we adapt our body systems to maintain good health. Coupled with a poor intake of adaptogens – vitamins, minerals, essential fats and phytonutrients – which help to balance our hormones and increase our ability to adapt, these chemicals are leading us towards disaster in terms of ever-decreasing hormonal health.

Such substances are thought to disrupt the body's biochemistry because of their ability to lock on to hormone receptor sites. This alters the ability of genes to communicate with the body's cells (gene expression), which is vital for the orchestration of health. In some cases these chemicals block a hormone receptor, in other cases they act as if they were the hormone, and some simply disrupt the hormone message. If you think of this hormone → hormone receptor → gene expression → biochemical response sequence as 'communication', what such chemicals do is turn the 'sound' up or down and scramble the message. This is because they do not fit the receptor site perfectly. Our body's chemistry hasn't been exposed to them before and hasn't managed to adapt its response accordingly.

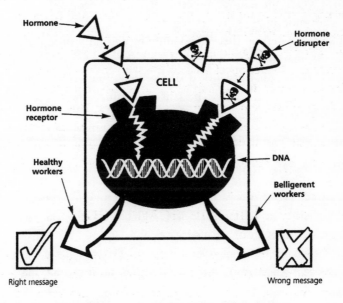

How hormones and chemicals affect genes

The trouble with synthetic hormones

The same is true of synthetic hormones. Take progesterone, for example, which is a hormone that is naturally produced by the body. It has a precise chemical structure: only this exact molecule can trigger a precise set of instructions which maintain pregnancy, bone density, normal menstruation and other functions of the hormonal dance that occurs in every woman. It has, even at levels considerably higher than those produced by the human body, remarkably little toxicity.

Yet, almost without exception, every contraceptive pill or HRT prescription – pill, patch or depot (a deposition of hormones under the skin which release over time) – contains synthetic progestins (altered molecules that are similar to, but different from, genuine progesterone). They are like keys that open the lock, but don't fit exactly; consequently they generate a wobble in the biochemistry of the body. Not surprisingly, toxicity increases – so much so that the side effects include increased risk of diseases such as breast cancer, against which the natural molecule actually protects us.

The same applies to oestrogen, or more correctly, oestrogens. Unlike progesterone there is a family of naturally produced oestrogens; the main three are oestradiol, oestrone and oestriol (see the box below). Many pharmaceutical drugs, including contraceptive pills and HRT, use synthetic oestrogens that mimic the effects of these naturally occurring molecules.

The inside story: oestrogens

Oestradiol is the strongest, most often used oestrogen in conventional HRT preparations and most associated with side effects, including the increased risk of breast and uterine cancer.

There is one HRT preparation, Hormonin, which contains all three oestrogens – oestradiol, oestrone and oestriol. Physiologically this

cont ▶

is more balanced, as it provides what the body produces. For post-menopausal women with low oestrogen and progesterone levels this, taken together with progesterone cream in equivalent amounts to those a woman produces, is a more logical way to restore hormone balance.

Oestriol is the major oestrogen in pregnancy and is considered more protective. It is produced in significantly larger quantities during pregnancy than at other times, when oestrone and oestradiol predominate.

Oestrone and oestradiol are potent forms of oestrogen and readily stimulate oestrogen-sensitive tissue. These two forms of oestrogen convert to other oestrogen compounds, known as oestrogen metabolites (see below), which, even in small quantities, can be highly toxic to oestrogen-sensitive tissue unless the body is able to produce specific compounds that help to keep them 'safe'. Making these compounds relies on a combination of good nutrition and our genes. (This topic will be further discussed in Chapter 25 – Testing for Hormone Imbalances.)

Oestriol only is available as a cream and in tablets as Ovestin. The cream is excellent for vaginal dryness, while the tablets often help women with hot flushes, with a fraction of the associated risk of oestradiol. It is best given together with natural progesterone cream (see Chapter 25).

Phytoestrogens are plant-based oestrogens that are very weak in comparison and appear to protect against oestrogen overload by occupying the same hormone receptor sites as oestrogen. These are found in beans, lentils, nuts and seeds and, especially, soya.

Xenoestrogens are environmental chemicals that mimic oestrogen and often attach to the same hormone receptor sites as oestrogen, triggering a growth message and potentially promoting cancer. These include the industrial pollutants, pesticides and herbicides listed on page 19. One of the best ways to limit your exposure to them is to eat organic food.

Danger from the first synthetic oestrogen

There could be no more dramatic example of the danger of altering our exposure to these powerful hormone disrupters than DES, the first synthetic oestrogen, created in 1938. Within 20 years, DES was being given to women and to animals in the UK and the US. For the latter it improved growth rates, while for women it apparently promised a trouble-free pregnancy and healthier offspring. Eventually, up to six million mothers and babies were exposed to DES. It wasn't until 1970 that the flaws surfaced. Girls whose mothers had been on DES during pregnancy started to show abnormal genital development and a substantial increase in cancer rates, especially vaginal cancer of a kind never seen before.[12] It was then discovered that boys whose mothers had taken DES also had defects in the development of their sexual organs.[13] Many DES children died and many more were infertile.

DES is no longer prescribed, but synthetic oestrogens and progestins are, and both are associated with increased cancer risk (see Part 4). The danger of synthetic hormones doesn't just lie in the subtle differences of their chemical structure and effect, but also the amounts given and their relative balance with other hormones. The level of hormones in a contraceptive pill or HRT treatment may be many times higher than the body would naturally produce. Oestrogen produced by the body in health is balanced with progesterone but, if this balance is lost (and oestrogen is no longer opposed by progesterone), health problems arise.

Unopposed oestrogen is linked to cancer

Excessive exposure to oestrogen, oestrogen metabolites and oestrogen mimickers may be a major factor in hormone-related cancers. Oestrogens make things grow. And too many oestrogens can promote hormone-sensitive cancers. The late Dr John Lee, a medical expert in female hormones, health campaigner and author of many books on the subject (see Recommended Reading), said this in the 1990s:

The major cause of breast cancer is unopposed oestrogen and there are many factors that would lead to this. Stress, for example, raises cortisol and competes with progesterone for receptor sites. Xenoestrogens from the environment have the ability to damage tissue and lead to an increased risk of cancer later in life. There are also clearly nutritional and genetic factors to consider. What is most concerning is that doctors continue to prescribe unopposed oestrogen to women.[14]

He was, of course, referring to the widespread prescribing of synthetic hormones in contraceptive pills and HRT, which we have seen have been mirrored by the rise in hormone-related cancers; for example, if breast epithelial cells are exposed to oestrogen, their rate of abnormal proliferation doubles. A study by Dr L. Bergkvist and colleagues involving 23,000 Scandinavian women showed that if a woman takes HRT for longer than five years she doubles her risk of breast cancer.[15] They also found that if the HRT included progestins that risk was even higher.

This was confirmed in a large-scale study, published in the *New England Journal of Medicine*, which showed that post-menopausal women in their sixties who had been on HRT for five or more years have a 71 per cent increased risk of breast cancer.[16] The longer a woman was on HRT, the greater the risk. Overall, there was a 32 per cent increased risk among women using oestrogen HRT, and a 41 per cent risk of those using oestrogen combined with synthetic progestin, compared to women who had never used hormones.

Oestrogen is usually kept in check by progesterone, which has an anti-proliferation effect. One study showed that when oestrogen levels were increased in pre-menopausal women with breast lumps, the proliferation rate of breast epithelial cells (those lining the breast) increased by over 200 per cent – more than twice the normal rate. According to the lead researcher, Dr Chang from the National Taiwan University Hospital in Taipei, if natural progesterone is given and the level in breast tissue is raised to normal physiological levels, cell multiplication rate falls to 15 per cent of that in women who have not been treated. So oestrogen promotes the proliferation of breast cancers, while progesterone is protective.[17]

HRT's effects on the womb

Breast cancer isn't the only concern. Early trials of HRT, which contained only oestrogen, showed a vastly increased risk of endometrial or womb cancer because one of the jobs of oestrogen is to stimulate cell growth there, preparing the womb for a potential pregnancy. The increase ranged from 200 to 1,500 per cent, depending on how long it had been taken, and the risk would still be significantly raised several years after it had been stopped.[18] So progestin, a synthetic hormone, was added to the mix, starting in the 1960s. The idea was that, by counteracting unopposed oestrogen, the womb lining would be protected from excess cell growth. Adding progestins to HRT did reduce the risk of endometrial cancer, although it didn't stop it.[19] Another study, carried out by the Emory University School for Public Health, followed 240,000 women for eight years; results showed that the risk of ovarian cancer was 72 per cent higher in women given oestrogen.[20]

The real clincher, however, was the Million Women Study in 2003. This study, published in the *Lancet*, followed a million women aged 50–64, half of whom had used HRT.[21] It was found that those who had used oestrogen and progestin HRT doubled their risk of breast cancer. The conclusion of Professor Valerie Beral from the UK Cancer Research Epidemiology Unit at Oxford, who was in charge of this study, was: 'Use of HRT by women aged 50 to 64 years in the UK over the past decade has resulted in an estimated 20,000 extra breast cancers, 15,000 associated with oestrogen–progestagen; the extra deaths cannot yet be reliably estimated.'

Fortunately, the practice of prescribing oestrogen-only HRT is now much rarer, as most doctors now recognise the risk, and research confirms that for those who stopped taking HRT their risk of breast cancer has been reduced. According to one UK expert, a 50 per cent drop in HRT use in recent years has probably stopped up to 1,000 breast cancer cases a year.[22]

However, as you'll see in Part 4, there is a big difference between natural, or bio-identical, hormones and synthetic forms.

Oestrogens and men

Although men are not exposed to oestrogen compounds from taking the Pill and HRT, their oestrogen load may come from xenoestrogens, oestrogens in food and the small amount of oestradiol produced in a man's body. These oestrogenic chemicals interfere with the male hormone testosterone, preventing it from being active. Also, older men do produce relatively more 'female' hormones later in life. The net effect is to 'oestrogenise' men, increasing the associated risks of getting prostate cancer and other hormone-related cancers.

Other sources of oestrogen

Oestrogen also comes from the food we eat.

Dietary oestrogens

We take in oestrogens from natural foods. Dairy produce, for example, contains significant amounts of oestrogen, as does meat. However, the high levels in these foods may indicate that they aren't perhaps as 'natural' as we would like to think. Much of the meat once eaten in the UK came from animals whose feed had hormones added to it. Wisely, this practice has been banned in the EU since 2006, although it still continues in the US; however, it is not uncommon for residues to be found in meat sold in the UK, either because the product may contain meat originating from the US or because some farmers are not complying with the regulations. Oestrogens, combined with a high-protein diet, artificially increase the growth of the animal, and this means more profit for the farmer. High levels of oestrogens can also be found in milk products. This can be attributed to modern-day farming practices which make it possible to milk cows continuously, even while they are pregnant, but during pregnancy oestrogen concentrations in milk go up substantially.

Meat and dairy products are also a storage site for non-degradable toxins which contaminate sources of water and then accumulate along the food chain. Millions of tons of chemicals, like non-biodegradable PCBs and DDT, have been released into the environment. Traces of these non-degradable chemicals are found in meat, fish and fowl. These creatures have fed on other animals, which in turn have fed on pastures or food in water that is contaminated with these non-degradable chemicals. The chemicals accumulate in the animals' fat and, when we eat animal fat, they accumulate in us.

Insulin and insulin-like growth factor

The hormone insulin helps control blood sugar levels by taking the excess out of the blood and delivering it to cells to make energy, or to the liver to turn into fat and put into storage. The body also makes insulin-like growth factor (IGF), which is also present in both breast milk and cow's milk. The most active form, called IGF-1, is a potent stimulator of growth, encouraging hormone-sensitive cells to grow. It also switches off the cell's normal 'suicide signal', called apoptosis, which is how overgrowing, misbehaving rogue cancer cells are normally destroyed. During pregnancy, and in early infancy, the body makes more IGF-1 to encourage rapid growth. Normally, IGF-1 levels are high during childhood, peaking during puberty to stimulate sexual maturation, and then falling off rapidly. But they continue to be high during adulthood if the diet includes foods containing them; that is, non-organic dairy products and meat from dairy cows.

The typical Western diet, high in refined carbohydrates and sugars (known as high-glycemic foods), and an inactive lifestyle, leads to ever-increasing insensitivity to insulin, called 'insulin resistance'. In response, the body produces more and more insulin. A typical breakfast of cereal, milk and coffee, for example, is going to raise levels of all three critical hormones – insulin, insulin-like growth factor (IGF) and oestrogens. If you think about it, drinking milk as an adult isn't natural – no other animal species does it.

The combination of high insulin levels, insulin resistance and high IGF-1 levels is strongly linked to weight gain, particularly around the middle, diabetes, high blood pressure, heart disease, dementia, cancer, increased risk of allergy, auto-immune diseases and acne.[23]

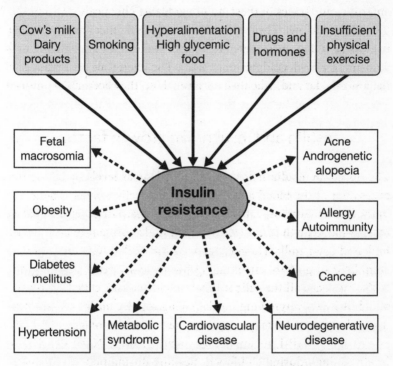

Risk factors of insulin resistance and associated diseases

(Reproduced with the kind permission of B. Melnik – see 'Permanent impairment of insulin resistance from pregnancy to adulthood: The primary basic risk factor of chronic Western diseases', *Medical Hypotheses* 73(5);(2009):670–681)

The effects on your body's metabolism

The shift to high insulin and IGF-1 levels parallels a shift in the body's metabolism towards 'metabolic syndrome' which also means higher cholesterol levels, more inflammation and hence pain, and poor blood sugar control – which is turn increases PMS symptoms and the risk of polycystic ovaries, endometriosis, breast lumps and cancer. All of this is rather like global warming in the body, as the inner ecology becomes more and more out of balance.

Metabolic syndrome also doubles your risk of depression[24] and memory problems[25] as well as increasing pain, accelerating ageing,[26] infertility and cancer, especially of the breast.[27]

The main risk factors that lead to this 'internal global warming' are eating a diet with too much sugar and refined carbohydrates – known as a high-GL (glycemic load) diet – regular consumption of milk products, smoking, the contraceptive pill, and a lack of physical exercise. (I explain about the glycemic load and its effects on the body in Chapter 7.)

What's wrong with milk?

It's not a good idea to drink lots of milk or to eat dairy products during pregnancy, as it increases insulin resistance and may be one of the reasons 'pregnancy diabetes' is on the increase. If you were bottle-fed as a baby on cow's milk formula you will have significantly higher levels of IGF-1 than babies who are breast-fed.[28] At any point in life the more dairy products you consume, including yoghurt, the higher your IGF-1 levels will be.[29]

Although milk is touted as not raising your blood sugar level significantly, it actually raises insulin a lot, as much as if you had eaten a refined carbohydrate or sugary food. Despite having a very low score on the glycemic index (a measure of the way that foods affect the body's blood sugar level), milk products produce three to six times more insulin than a non-dairy equivalent of an equally low-scoring food.[30]

The combination of dairy products and a carbohydrate snack is particularly bad.[31] Even worse is the addition of caffeine.[32] These combinations can triple blood sugar levels and insulin release, and therefore halve insulin sensitivity. So, starting your day with a refined cereal, such as cornflakes, with milk, or toast or a croissant with a latte is a recipe for disaster as far as your insulin sensitivity is concerned.

'Industrialised' milk production by pregnant cows contributes to insulin resistance as well as increasing your oestrogen overload, because these animals are kept permanently pregnant for up to five years to increase milk output.[33] The amount of extra hormones a high milk consumer receives is almost equivalent to what you'd get from taking oral contraceptives.

A cocktail of effects

Fat cells also make more oestrogen, adding to your burden. If you also take, or have taken, oral contraceptives for several years, and use oestrogen hormone therapy, smoke and are overweight, your body's hormone levels are going to be well out of balance.

If you are a body builder, stay away from milk protein drinks and growth hormone. Whey, the main protein in milk, promotes high insulin levels, while casein, the other protein, increases IGF-1 levels.[34] Body builders and those who are trying not to age often take growth hormone which can encourage muscle growth, but it does so at a cost. It directly raises IGF-1 levels and, in my opinion, is best avoided.

Furthermore, all of the above is a recipe for acne (both in adolescence and adulthood), weight gain and various overgrowth conditions, from polycystic ovaries to breast cancer.

What can you do to avoid this?

The good news is that simple changes to your diet, eating certain foods and taking particular herbs and supplements can help to reverse insulin resistance, lessen your oestrogen load, and balance your blood sugar and IGF levels, bringing your hormones back into balance. This will put an end to 'overgrowth' signals and will reduce

33

your risk of many common women's diseases. In Parts 3, 4 and 5 I am
going to tell you how.

Plant oestrogens may be protective

One simple way to protect your hormone balance is to eat more plant
food. Plants also contain natural, oestrogen-like compounds, known
as phytoestrogens. These are found in a wide variety of foods, including soya, legumes (beans, chickpeas and lentils), seeds, garlic, grains
such as oats and rice, and certain fruits and vegetables. The richest
source is soya and soya products, such as tofu or soya milk.

However, unlike oestrogenic chemicals such as PCBs, these
phytoestrogens are associated with a reduced risk of cancer. A high
dietary intake of isoflavones, the active ingredient in soya, is associated with a halving of breast cancer risk in pre-menopausal women,[35]
a halving of breast cancer in animals, and a substantial reduction in
deaths from prostate cancer in men.[36] Even more encouraging are
animal studies, which show that eating a small amount of isoflavones
in early infancy results in a 60 per cent reduced risk of breast cancer
later in life.[37] One theory is that these naturally occurring phytoestrogens may act as adaptogens; that is, they help the body to stabilise
hormone levels. The likely explanation for their protective effect is
that they may block the action of other more toxic environmental
oestrogens, perhaps by occupying the oestrogen receptor sites on
cells. Since they are about a hundred times weaker in their oestrogen
effect than xenoestrogens or the body's oestrogen, the net effect of
eating foods rich in phytoestrogens seems to be to lower the body's
oestrogen load and protect it against harmful hormone-disrupting
chemicals.

However, it is important to note that not all soya has equal benefits, and this depends on the treatment during processing. Some
processing methods involve the addition of harmful levels of aluminium and nitrates. For this reason, I recommend only buying soya
products that say they are made from the whole soya bean. Traditional
fermented sources of soya, such as tempeh, miso, natto, soy sauce

and tamari, are wise choices and are considered to provide more health benefits because fermentation helps to break down factors in soya that inhibit its proper digestion.

The potential negative effects of phytoestrogens

Although the effects of consuming phytoestrogens seem to be all positive, some researchers recommend caution, as many isoflavones tested in the laboratory, including genistein in soya, have the potential to prolong the action of a woman's own oestrogen; however, isoflavones have also been shown to increase the activity of the primary route for oestrogen detoxification (which happens in the liver) called glucoronidation and may well outweigh the negative potential.[38]

There is also some cause for concern over taking in very large amounts of phytoestrogens during the critical early years of development, which is exactly what would occur if an infant were bottle-fed using a soya-based formula. No one really knows if this is potentially beneficial or detrimental for hormonal health later in life. What can be said is that it is no more natural for an infant to be fed soya milk than it is to be fed cow's milk. There is no substitute for good quality human breast milk for infants. My recommendation is to eat phytoestrogen-rich foods in moderation, much like our ancestors have done for millennia.

Stress is another factor that affects the balance of your hormones, and in the next chapter I explore the effects that permanent stress has on the female body.

CHAPTER 4

The Problem with Stress

Although small bursts of stress are an inevitable, and necessary, part of everyday life, your hormone balance can be upset if you are permanently stressed. As I explain in Chapter 7, our bodies were designed to react quickly to stressful situations, by fleeing from the threat or fighting back, but our modern lives can feed us with underlying stresses on a daily basis, which inevitably means that the hormones whose job it is to cope with that stress become overused and unbalanced.

We produce many different hormones that keep our bodies in balance. These include insulin and glucagon to keep our blood sugar level even, adrenalin and cortisol to help us react to stress, thyroxine which controls our rate of metabolism, the female hormones (discussed in Chapter 1), and a whole host of hormones produced by the pituitary gland in the centre of the head that effectively conduct the hormonal orchestra of our bodies.

Whenever you take in a stimulant such as coffee or a cigarette, or if you react stressfully to an event, your body produces the adrenal hormone cortisol. Hormones are excreted into the bloodstream, and to exert their effect on cells they have to 'dock' onto a hormone receptor. Cortisol competes with progesterone for the same receptor but, effectively, cortisol wins because the receptor more readily takes up cortisol than progesterone. So the net effect of being permanently in a stressed or stimulated state is that your body has less active progesterone. What is more, when cortisol is locked into a receptor – therefore bound and unavailable – it sends a message to the brain to produce more. Too much cortisol leads to the breakdown of bone, contributing to osteoporosis and muscle loss. Maintenance of muscle mass as we age is a key determinant of overall health. It is believed that progesterone helps the body to burn fat and has also been shown to stimulate bone-building cells.

Since cortisol also increases the production of oestrogen, prolonged stress can contribute to oestrogen dominance. Normally the liver can easily deal with slight excesses of oestrogen, but if your diet isn't great, or if you have hidden allergies or you smoke or drink too much, your liver's ability to detoxify and eliminate oestrogen can be impaired.

Stress also upsets the balance of the 'male' hormone, testosterone, which is also present in the female body, as some is made by the adrenal glands, which are affected by stress. A disturbance in the balance of male and female hormones in women can lead to a lack of ovulation, a decreased desire for sex and the development of excessive facial hair and other male characteristics.

Stress and blood sugar control

The net result of stress, or a diet too high in sugar and refined carbohydrates, is an inability to keep blood sugar levels stable, known as dysglycemia. When you eat sweet foods your blood sugar level shoots up. The body then has to produce more insulin to get the sugar out of the blood and into body cells. When the blood sugar level is too low this stimulates the adrenal glands to make more cortisol. This scenario of disturbed hormone balance has many undesirable knock-on effects on your health, including a greater risk of PMS, polycystic ovaries and an underactive thyroid gland (leading to weight gain, fatigue and sluggishness). The vast majority of women with polycystic ovarian syndrome show this kind of hormone imbalance. No doubt it also contributes to many other female health problems.

This pattern of dysglycemia, with raised insulin and cortisol levels, is called metabolic syndrome, and it is associated with a greater risk of depression, memory loss, heart disease, high cholesterol, high blood pressure, cancer and diabetes.

Stress and weight gain

Metabolic syndrome may also be the reason why some women experience weight gain despite no apparent increase in calories consumed. Dr Kate Steinbeck and colleagues at the Royal Prince Albert Hospital in Sydney found that children who have metabolic syndrome have, in later life, a greater propensity to turn food into fat, as well as having a greater risk of diabetes and heart disease.

Hormone imbalances brought on by the wrong kind of diet, a stressful lifestyle and exposure to hormone-disrupting chemicals, can also lead to either an androgen (masculinising hormones) dominance or oestrogen dominance. Excessive androgen levels are now being linked to upper body and waist weight gain, while high oestrogen (feminising hormone) levels are associated with lower body weight gain. For this reason 'apple-shaped' people may be more likely to be androgen dominant, a factor associated with blood sugar problems and metabolic syndrome, while 'pear-shaped' people may be more likely to be oestrogen dominant. You can, of course, have both.

Without a doubt, we all need to control the levels of stress in our lives, and you may well also need to balance your blood sugar level and reduce your insulin load to reverse metabolic syndrome. In Chapter 7 I explain how do to this and how to lose weight effortlessly.

In the following chapter I explain how to protect your health by avoiding the hormone disrupters.

CHAPTER 5

How to Avoid Hormone Disrupters

A s you can see from the previous chapters, your diet, environment and lifestyle are all factors that can rock the boat of your hormonal health. If the load gets too great, the boat tips over and hormone-related problems may ensue. Once this happens, ignorance is not bliss, but armed with a good understanding of how to tip the odds in your favour, there is a lot you can do to protect, maintain and improve your health. The first step is to avoid hormone disrupters.

Recognising and avoiding hormone disrupters

Why, you may ask, don't we just ban all these hormone-disrupting chemicals? As Professor Louis Guillette, from the University of Florida says, 'Should we change policy? Should we be upset? I think we should be fundamentally upset. I think we should be screaming in the streets.' Since the first edition of this book many hormone-disrupting chemicals have been banned or restricted in their use. Yet, the reality is that – until large-scale government action is taken –

it isn't easy to eliminate all these substances because they are all around us: in our food, water, air and household products. There are, however, steps you can take to substantially reduce your own and your family's exposure.

First of all, you can buy organic produce wherever possible and avoid using pesticides or herbicides in your own garden or home. This immediately cuts down your exposure. It's a good idea to cut right back on meat and dairy produce or, at least, choose organic meat when you do eat it. Think carefully before going on the Pill or taking HRT (these are discussed fully in Part 4). Avoid excess sugar (explored in Chapter 7), stimulants and stress, as explained in the previous chapter.

The plastics in daily life

Plastic is impossible to avoid. It is, however, worth reducing your exposure to food in contact with plastic, particularly if the food is hot, liquid or acidic. Soft plastics used to contain plasticisers (substances which are added to plastics to increase their flexibility, transparency, durability and longevity), such as nonylphenol or bisphenol-A. These can pass into the foods and, as we have seen, disrupt hormones. Examples of this are packaged TV dinners, destined for the microwave, and some cans of food or juice cartons that are lined with plastic. Only this year, bisphenol-A was banned in the manufacture of baby bottles in Europe but it remains in the inner linings of many cans and lids. You can also reduce your risk by choosing drinks in glass bottles or unlined cans whenever possible or checking those products you do use. TetraPak, one of the main carton producers, have assured me that these harmful plasticisers were not used in any of their products. You might also want to use cling film sparingly, if at all, opting for non-PVC cling film. Put your sandwiches in a paper bag rather than cling film. Also, check household and cosmetic products you buy for the following chemicals: bisphenol-A, octoxynol, nonoxynol, noylphenol, octylphenol and ethoxylate.

Watch out for phthalates

Limit your exposure to potent phthalates. Although phthalates are being phased out of many products in the US and the EU because of health concerns, it is worth being aware and checking labels, as they can be found in many products, including adhesives and glues, building materials, personal-care products, detergents and surfactants, packaging, children's toys, pharmaceuticals, food products and textiles. It's best to use chemical-free, environmentally friendly household chemicals, toiletries and cosmetics (see Resources).

Chemicals shown to have oestrogenic effects

- Alkylphenol: synthetic surfactants used in some detergents and cleaning products
- Atrazine: weedkiller
- 4-Methylbenzylidene camphor (4-MBC): sunscreen lotions
- Brominated flame retardants (BFRs): widely used in furniture
- Butylated hydroxyanisole (BHA): food preservative
- Bisphenol-A: monomer for polycarbonate plastic and epoxy resin; antioxidant in plasticisers used in container liners
- DDT: insecticide
- Dichlorodiphenyldichloroethylene and dichlorodiphenyldichloroethylene dieldrin: breakdown products of DDT
- Endosulfan: insecticide
- Erythrosine (E127): food colouring banned in Norway and the US
- Ethinylestradiol (combined oral contraceptive pill): released into the environment as an xenoestrogen
- Heptachlor: insecticide
- Lindane/hexachlorocyclohexane: insecticide
- Metalloestrogens: a class of inorganic xenoestrogens
- Methoxychlor: insecticide

cont ▶

- Nonylphenol and derivatives: industrial surfactants, emulsifiers for emulsion polymerisation, laboratory detergents, pesticides
- Polychlorinated biphenyls (PCBs): in electrical oils, lubricants, adhesives, paints
- Parabens: lotions
- Phenosulfothiazine: a red dye
- Phthalates (plasticisers), DEHP: plasticiser for PVC
- Propyl gallate: food additive

At a glance advice

Some general guidelines are summarised below, while specific advice for particular health problems is discussed in Parts 2 and 3.

- **Eat organic** This instantly minimises your exposure to pesticides and herbicides. When you are eating non-organic produce wash it in an acidic medium, made by adding 1 tablespoon of vinegar to a bowl of water. This will reduce some, but not all, pesticides.

- **Filter your drinking water** I recommend getting a water filter that you install under the sink, made from stainless steel, not plastic or aluminium, or employing some kind of carbon-filtration system. The need to filter water in this way does depend to an extent on where you live; however, it is a good precaution. The alternative is mineral water, bottled in glass.

- **Increase your intake of plant-based phytoestrogens** Found in nuts, seeds and beans, these help protect against oestrogen over-load. Make these foods a regular part of your diet.

- **Reduce your intake of meat, milk and fatty foods** Meat, and milk particularly, leads to high levels of IGF-1, stimulating abnormal cell growth. Non-biodegradable chemicals accumulate up the food chain in animal fat. Minimising your intake of animal fat (meat and dairy produce), therefore, lessens your exposure. Opt for organic meat and dairy but, even so, have this infrequently. There is no need to limit essential fats in nuts and seeds.

- **Don't heat food in plastic*** This means saying goodbye to micro-waved TV dinners. If you have to have them, transfer the food into a glass container before heating.

- **Minimise fatty foods in plastic*** Some chemicals that keep plastics flexible easily pass out of the plastic into fatty food, including crisps, cheese, butter, chocolate and pies.

- **Minimise liquid foods in plastic*** This not only includes fruit juices in cardboard packs, which have a plastic inner lining, but also some canned fruits and vegetables, which may also have a plastic inner lining.

- **Minimise exposure of food to plastic*** This means using paper bags to put your vegetables in, as opposed to buying everything in plastic trays, covered with cling film.

- **Switch to natural detergents** Use only ecological detergent products, for washing up, washing clothes and body washing, from companies who declare all their ingredients. Also, rinse well after washing up.

- **Don't use pesticides in your garden** Some pesticides are hormone disrupters. Unless you're sure yours isn't, it is better not to spray. Research is suggesting a link between higher rates of childhood cancer and homes whose gardens are sprayed with pesticides.

- **Don't use the contraceptive pill or HRT** There are many safer ways to avoid conception and restore hormonal health.

* Until the plastics industry either stops using all suspect chemicals, or discloses which chemicals are contained in their products, you have no way of knowing if hormone-disrupting chemicals are present or not.

In Part 2, I explain the role your digestive system has in keeping you well and your hormones balanced, and the importance of keeping your blood sugar level. I then discuss the common hormone problems that many women are suffering on a regular basis and the natural ways that you can alleviate them.

PART 2

○◡

STAYING HORMONALLY HEALTHY

There are many critical factors that determine your hormonal health, starting with the food you eat. As you will see in this part, eating the right food, digesting it well, avoiding dysbiosis (imbalance of bacteria) and eliminating hidden food allergies all have a role to play in hormonal health. Your ability to keep your blood sugar level even is also essential, as this is linked to stress which, as we have seen, leads to hormonal imbalances, which in turn contributes to the development of many diseases experienced by women. Also, the symptoms of digestive and blood sugar problems often overlap with the symptoms of hormonal imbalance so it's best to sort these out first before assuming that you have a hormonal imbalance. This part tells you how. It then explains what you can do to solve common hormonal health issues that many women experience at some point during their life – from PMS and painful periods to a loss of energy and sex drive, and menopausal symptoms.

CHAPTER 6

The Gut–Hormone Connection

Many of the symptoms attributed to imbalances in the female hormones, such as irritability, anxiety, depression, lack of energy, joint pains, water retention, weight gain and bloating can have their origins in digestive problems. Therefore, having a healthy digestive tract is essential to achieve hormonal balance and optimum health.

Hormones are made by your body from the foods you eat. Therefore, eating the right food is essential for both making and keeping your hormones balanced. The gut is the body's largest endocrine gland, producing many hormones that affect your ability to digest and absorb the essential nutrients required to make other hormones and keep them balanced.

If you supply your body with second-rate fuel, over time your body is likely to give you second-rate performance. This chapter explains about the importance of eating foods that will *aid* and not strain the digestive system and your body's ability to cleanse itself of toxins. It also emphasises how a healthy digestive system will help your body to make the hormones it needs.

Throughout this book you will find that I refer again and again to vital vitamins such as B_6 and folic acid, and minerals such as zinc and magnesium, to name a few which, along with essential fats and amino acids from protein, help to control hormonal balance. Achieving 'optimum nutrition' by taking in the correct levels of essential nutrients is the first step to keeping your body hormonally healthy, and this begins with how your digestive system deals with the food you eat.

You are what you eat

It's not just what you eat that determines your health but also how well you digest, absorb and use the food. A healthy digestive tract, therefore, is essential if you are to enjoy good health. If it was laid out flat, your digestive tract would have a surface area about the size of a tennis court, and it is a quarter the thickness of a sheet of paper. This is the barrier between you – that is, the cells that make up your body – and the food you eat.

Each morsel of ingested food passes through three processes: the breakdown of food into simple units (digestion); the transport of nutrients across the gut membrane into the blood (absorption); and the selective ejection of waste (elimination). For this process to work efficiently your digestion needs good food. Giving your digestive tract 'low-grade fuel' puts undue strain on the system, because the extra effort required to deal with inappropriate foods is wasted energy and it draws on your body's reserves of nutrients in an attempt to cope. These valuable nutrients would be better spent balancing your energy, mood and hormones.

According to the late nutrition expert Dr Abram Hoffer, 'Modern diets are designed to appeal to the senses. Modern food bears little relationship to our physiological needs. Modern high tech-food processing has robbed us of the use of our senses in determining whether a food is or is not good for us.'

It is only recently that it has become necessary to educate ourselves about the composition of food. Our ancestors learned very effectively which foods were safe to eat using trial and error. Foods that were bland, salty or sweet were preferred and, as a rule, are not poisonous. These were balanced whole foods needed to maintain health. Today, our food supplies have been manipulated in such a way that we no longer recognise what is and what is not a healthy food.

The process of detoxifying

The body has to expend a lot of energy detoxifying – in other words cleansing from the body – every man-made chemical, pollutant or inappropriate food that goes into it. Yet every process in the body, especially detoxification, depends on nutrients such as amino acids, vitamins and minerals, which come from the foods we eat. The problem with man-made chemicals, pollutants and inappropriate foods is that they either do not supply any nutrients or may require even more to detoxify them than they provided in the first place. Combined with poor quality food choices, this leads to ever-increasing nutritional depletion and impaired detoxification potential.

This is particularly concerning because used-up hormones and derivatives of hormones also have to be detoxified, as do the hormone-like substances we inadvertently take in from pesticides, plastics, industrial pollutants and detergent residues. If they are not adequately detoxified, imbalances such as oestrogen dominance are created. Furthermore, we now know that even small amounts of oes-trogen derivatives (also called oestrogen metabolites) can be quite toxic if they accumulate because of poor detoxification. (However, is now possible to test for these, and a nutritional therapist might recommend such a test depending on your symptoms.)

Problems with digestion

Eating the wrong foods and living in a state of stress, which inhibits digestion, can play havoc with your digestive system. In order to deal with food, whether good or bad, the digestive processes need to be in good working order. The first major obstacle happens when food reaches the stomach. Here the body starts to digest the complex proteins found mainly in animal produce, nuts, seeds, pulses and grains. Conditions in the stomach need to be very acidic in order to break down the complex proteins. Zinc is a key nutrient to help make the conditions in the stomach sufficiently acid. (In fact, the body has a high demand for zinc, which is involved in over 200 reactions: it is required at every step of the reproductive process and is used in vast amounts when we are stressed.) When the acid in the stomach starts to work on the proteins, the minerals are freed up ready for absorption. A lack of stomach acid impairs mineral absorption.

The symptoms of low stomach acid are similar to having too much acid: mainly indigestion and heartburn. Many women over 50 do not produce enough stomach acid and are commonly prescribed antacids or proton pump inhibitor (PPI) drugs, which further deplete production. Rarely are they given any dietary advice, but taking antacids and continuing to eat a high-protein diet is only likely to compound the problem.

The body produces about 10 litres (17½ pints) of digestive juices containing digestive enzymes to break down food. Poor digestion leads to larger particles of food entering the small intestine than would be expected. The larger particles of food can act as local irritants on the gut membrane, contributing to increased permeability, which is commonly called 'leaky gut syndrome'. When larger particles of food enter the large intestine (the colon), which is the home of the body's microflora, the bacteria residing there feed off the unexpected feast and create flatulence and bloating, and general dysbiosis (an imbalance of the flora residing in the colon).

You can support your digestion by supplementing digestive enzymes with major meals.

Leaky gut syndrome

In health, the gut has a specific permeability that allows for the transfer of nutrients: digested proteins, fats and carbohydrates, and vitamins, minerals, phytonutrients and water. Anything that damages the gut – including painkillers, alcohol and antibiotics, as well as excessive bloating, food allergies and inflammatory conditions such as colitis – can make the inner membrane more permeable or 'leaky'. Three main problems may then arise:

1 Increased risk of food allergy If larger particles of food enter the small intestine and irritate the gut membrane making it more leaky, then they are able to cross over into the bloodstream. The immune system sees these incompletely digested food particles as foreign and can trigger an allergic reaction. Prolonged stress can also suppress proper immune-system function in the digestive tract.

2 Decreased mineral absorption Contrary to what may seem logical, if the gut becomes more permeable, its ability to absorb minerals is reduced. This is because minerals are normally picked up actively by a protein carrier and taken across the gut membrane into the blood. When the gut membrane is damaged, the carrier proteins are also damaged. This, combined with a low level of stomach acid and high exposure to pollutants and alcohol, is especially bad news for nutrient absorption. Alcohol can also destroy B vitamins in the gut. On top of this, if your diet is too high in wheat and soya – two major sources of phytates in food – the problem is further compounded, as phytates are capable of binding with minerals such as calcium, iron and zinc, preventing them from being properly absorbed. Too much caffeine from coffee, and tannin from tea, rob the body of the same minerals.

3 Increased risk of absorbing toxins If the gut is of a normal permeability then most toxins don't get through. Nature did not design the digestive tract to be permeable to toxins, but when the gut membrane becomes more leaky than it should, they can be absorbed into the blood more readily. Man-made hormone-disrupting chemicals, such as pesticides, may also find their way across a normal gut membrane, as can toxic metals such as lead and cadmium, particularly if your intake of essential minerals like calcium, magnesium and zinc is low or you drink alcohol on a regular basis.

The common causes, besides incompletely digested food particles, of the gut membrane becoming too leaky are:

- Prolonged stress

- Excessive growth of the yeast organism *Candida albicans*

- Certain drugs, including synthetic hormones, chemotherapeutic agents, antibiotics and, especially, non-steroidal anti-inflammatory drugs (NSAIDs) such as aspirin or ibuprofen, which irritate the digestive tract

- Surgery and radiotherapy

- Infection, especially gut infections

- Regular ingestion of alcohol

- Nutritional deficiencies leading to a weakened gut membrane

- Inflammatory bowel disorders such as IBS or colitis

- Poor immune function

A simple urine test can help to identify whether your gut membrane is of normal permeability or not. Nutritional therapists can provide you with this test.

Do you have hidden food allergies?

The classic definition of an allergy is 'any idiosyncratic reaction where the immune system is clearly involved'. Classical allergies – such as those to shellfish and peanuts – are more easily identified. They often present as asthma, eczema, hay fever and hives, and may even be life-threatening by causing immediate reactions such as swelling in the throat. These allergies are recognised in the blood by a marker which is a type of antibody called IgE (immunoglobulin E).

However, the emerging view now is that most food allergies are not IgE-based but involve another marker known as immunoglobulin

G (IgG). These antibodies work in a different way, the consequence being that you don't always get an immediate reaction. According to allergy expert Dr James Braly, co-author of *Hidden Food Allergies*:

> Food allergy is not rare, nor are the effects limited to the air passages, the skin and digestive tract. Most food allergies are delayed reactions, taking anywhere from an hour to three days to show themselves, and are therefore much harder to detect. Delayed food allergy appears to be simply the inability of your digestive tract to prevent large quantities of partially digested and undigested food from entering the bloodstream.

Many food allergies are likely to occur when the lining of the gut membrane is more leaky than it should be. Foods can act as a local irritant to the gut membrane and make it more porous. If larger particles of food escape into the bloodstream through the gut membrane, the immune system sees them as 'foreign' and sets up an inflammatory reaction. Headaches, joint pains, flatulence, bloating, mood swings, water retention and food cravings may result. Food allergens may also give the body a stress signal, setting up an inappropriate response in the body.

Because many, if not the majority, of food intolerances do not produce immediate symptoms, this makes them hard to detect by observation. Because they do not present in a classical way, as asthma or hives, for example, many people do not realise that the unpleasant symptoms they are experiencing could be associated with a food that they are eating regularly. IgG reactions are associated with the overuse of particular foods in the diet.

If you score high on the questionnaire overleaf, there's a good chance that you have hidden food allergies. The symptoms overleaf are the most common signs of increased likelihood of allergy.

Questionnaire: do you have allergies?

	Yes	No
1. Are you chronically tired?	☐	☐
2. Can you gain weight in hours?	☐	☐
3. Do you get bloated after eating?	☐	☐
4. Do you suffer from diarrhoea or constipation?	☐	☐
5. Do you suffer from abdominal pain?	☐	☐
6. Do you sometimes get really sleepy after eating?	☐	☐
7. Do you suffer from hay fever?	☐	☐
8. Do you suffer from rashes, itches, asthma or shortness of breath?	☐	☐
9. Do you have recurrent colds or sinus problems?	☐	☐
10. Do you suffer from water retention?	☐	☐
11. Do you suffer from headaches or migraines?	☐	☐
12. Do you suffer from other aches or pains, from time to time, possibly after certain foods?	☐	☐
13. Do you suffer from 'brain fog' or patches of inexplicable depression?	☐	☐
14. Do you get better on holidays abroad, when your diet is completely different?	☐	☐

Score 1 for each 'yes' answer   Total score: ☐

Score

Any 'yes' answer to these questions means there's a real possibility that you have an allergy.

5 or more
It's pretty much guaranteed that you have an allergy.

Wheat and dairy products

The two most common allergens in Britain are wheat and dairy produce. Wheat is the cheapest and easiest grain to grow, and its flour is not only used to bake bread, cakes, biscuits, and so on, but also as a filler in many processed foods. The gluten in wheat allows it to rise when fermented with yeast. The lighter the loaf the less raw ingredients the producer needs to use, which means more profit. This has led to the development of high-gluten strains of wheat. The quantity of wheat in the average person's diet is much higher than it was 50 years ago, particularly as so many of us are partial to a piece of toast as a snack or a quick pasta or pizza dish in front of the TV after a hard day's work.

It is quite common now, not only because of convenience foods but also as a part of an increasing emphasis on healthy eating (even for vegetarians), to be very dependent on wheat and dairy produce; for example, it is not untypical to have bran flakes and skimmed milk for breakfast, a wholemeal low-fat cheese sandwich for lunch, and a wholemeal pizza or pasta dish for supper, interspersed with fruits and vegetables. Effectively, the main food components are wheat and dairy for breakfast, lunch and supper, just assembled in different forms.

Strangely, it is quite usual for people to crave a food that they are intolerant of. If it is a slice of bread or a biscuit that you crave, then consider that you may be reacting to wheat. Similarly, if it is a glass of milk or a lump of cheese that gets you raiding the fridge, consider a dairy allergy. This is thought to be because wheat and milk protein can be converted into opioid-like chemicals that make you crave. Common symptoms are mood swings, irritability, foggy brain, flatulence, bloating, water retention and joint pains.

Coeliac disease is a particularly severe type of wheat allergy, suffered by about one in 40 people with digestive problems, but it is rarely diagnosed. It was originally believed that it was caused by a reaction to gluten, but there's growing evidence that the offending protein in wheat is something called gliadin. Gliadin is not present in oats and the vast majority of coeliac sufferers do not react to them.[1] If you want to test yourself for coeliac disease there's a simple, relatively inexpensive pinprick test called the Biotech BioCard Celiac Test, which gives you an instant result (see Resources).

Testing for hidden food allergies

Because the body sometimes delays its allergic reaction to a food, it is difficult to identify the food simply by avoiding certain foods and then reintroducing them. This is because you may not suspect the food culprit and so not test for it. Or you may suspect only one food, yet be allergic to a range of them, so you'll continue to have a background of allergic reactions.

The best and truly accurate way to find out what you are allergic to is to have what's called a quantitative IgG ELISA test. This is the gold standard of allergy testing. 'Quantitative' means the test shows not only whether you are allergic but also how strong your allergic reaction is. Many of us live quite healthily with minor allergies, but stronger allergies can create all sorts of problems, including weight gain. 'ELISA' is the technology used and I believe it to be the most accurate system. If it's done properly, it is at least 93 per cent reproducible. It's chosen by the best allergy laboratories in the world because it actually measures your body's antibody reactions against food. Three out of four people who have had this test and then acted upon its results report a considerable health improvement.[2]

All that's needed for testing is a pinprick of blood, which is absorbed into a tiny tube and sent to a laboratory. The lab then sends back an accurate readout of exactly what you are allergic to. Your body doesn't lie. You either show IgG 'bouncers' that react to wheat (for example) or you don't. Your diluted blood is introduced to a panel of liquid food 'testers' and, if you've got IgG for that food, a reaction takes place.

There are a number of laboratories who carry out IgG testing, and one that offers a handy test kit you can use at home. YorkTest have devised a clever procedure that involves a painless pinprick device and an absorbent material that you place against the pinprick. This material is then sent to the laboratory for testing (see Resources). They also do a useful 'first step' test that is relatively inexpensive so that if you don't have any reactions you don't need to pay for testing hundreds of foods.

The good news about IgG-based allergies is that if you avoid the offending food strictly for three to four months, the body is likely to forget that it is allergic to it. The reason is that there will no longer be any IgG antibodies in your system to that food. So, provided you've removed the underlying cause of the allergy, such as intestinal permeability, and don't over-eat that food every day, there's a good chance that you won't react to it any more. This doesn't hold true for IgE-based reactions, however. They last for life.

To give you an example, I have an IgE allergy to milk – that's the kind that causes rapid reactions. I react within 15 minutes by my nose becoming blocked up, often followed by a headache. Even if I avoid dairy products for a year, I still react if I consume some. I used to have an IgG allergy to wheat. I avoided it for three months and now I no longer react. In my case, I used to have migraines every other week from the ages of 6 to 20, until I discovered that wheat and milk were triggering them.

For more information about why allergies develop and how to prevent or reverse them, read my book *Hidden Food Allergies*.

Is it hormones or allergies?

Food allergies, overgrowth in the gut of the yeast organism *Candida albicans* (responsible for causing thrush – see Chapter 16), other gut infections and dysbiosis can all give rise to symptoms often associated with hormonal imbalances. Unless you already know that you have a female hormone imbalance I recommend that you pay special attention to the advice in this chapter and the next before you assume that an imbalance in your hormones is the cause of your symptoms. In so many cases, when women address these issues, their health problems clear up. Even those women with diagnosed female hormone imbalances often do very much better when they take these factors into account.

I cannot emphasise enough how important the digestive tract is in achieving hormonal balance and optimum health. Here are some ways you can improve your digestive health right now:

- Eat the right food (see Diet for the Good Life, Chapter 26) and minimise sources of hormone disrupters, including non-organic food.

- Find out what you are allergic to and avoid it.

- Reduce or avoid wheat and dairy products for a trial period of a fortnight.

- Take a daily multivitamin and mineral supplement that provides vitamin B_6, zinc and magnesium – all vital for healthy digestion.

- Supplement probiotics, digestive enzymes and glutamine for a month. Some supplements contain all three (see Resources).

- Minimise gut irritants, including painkillers, alcohol and caffeinated drinks.

CHAPTER 7

Cut Sugar and Control your Weight

I explained in Chapter 4 how stress affects the activity of progesterone in women, resulting in oestrogen dominance, which can lead to putting on fat. In this chapter I will explain how this and eating too much sugar affects your body's ability to control glucose in the blood, resulting in the sugar being converted to fat as excess weight, but also creating the environment for a number of female diseases. Controlling stress and your sugar balance are therefore essential for good hormonal health.

Our increasing sweet tooth

Most of us like sweet foods – in nature they are usually safe – and modern food processing has cashed in on our sugary inclination. From early infancy, when sugar is added to baby drinks and cereals we become 'hooked' on the desire for something sweet, and the more you have the more you want.

In the 1820s the average daily intake of sugar amounted to two teaspoons, which is the amount of glucose (sugar) that we have in our blood at any one time. By the 1980s the average intake of sugar had risen to an amazing 38 teaspoons a day! When you consider that the average confectionery bar contains 10–15 teaspoons of sugar, and a cola drink around 7 teaspoons, and then consider what is added to tea, coffee, cereals, biscuits and cakes, it soon adds up.

However, eating sugar is not the only way to increase the level of glucose in your body. Stress, and stress-inducing stimulants such as coffee and cigarettes, do this very efficiently, without us ever having to put a teaspoonful of sugar into our mouths. A difficult day at work or at home with the children, having a cup of coffee and a cigarette, eating too much red meat or salt, or just watching a horror movie, all effectively raise sugar levels. It's part of the 'fight or flight' response that is triggered by adrenalin, and it gets your body ready to escape from danger by running like hell!

The stress connection

In modern times, it is difficult not to be stressed. Many of us live 'shoulder to shoulder' in towns and cities, or have moved further out but still need to commute to work every day. Our busy lives are stressful, but we all experience stress differently: some of us enjoy it; others perform badly under it; and there are some people who feel stressed because there isn't enough stress in their lives.

How does the body react to stress?

Whatever the stressor, the body will respond to it in the same way: by releasing a variety of chemicals to deal with the situation. The adrenal glands release the hormone adrenalin, which releases the stores of sugar into the blood, and the hormone cortisol (which is needed to help regulate glucose and energy balance as well as to moderate any inflammatory reactions). The released sugar is taken from the blood to the cells by the hormone insulin, to be burned for energy to deal with a perceived emergency or put into storage as fat if not needed. The essential mineral chromium helps insulin to work. Without it you become insensitive to the effects of insulin, and this is known as being insulin resistant.

As part of this reaction, calcium is released from its store in the bones in preparation for an immediate 'fight' by increasing the heart rate and the ability of the muscles to contract. Calcium is also involved in blood clotting, which would be necessary in the event of any injury in the 'fight'.

When the 'fight' doesn't happen

The problem is that we are not in a real 'fight'. More often than not, we are just dealing with another work or family pressure or another cup of coffee. If we were dealing with a true emergency, like stopping a young child from running across the road at the wrong time, then the chemicals released to deal with the situation would be appropriate and the body would use them up. After the emergency was over, your body's chemistry would settle down and regain balance. However, modern-day stressors are continually present in our lives. Almost every hour of every day, we are likely to be stressing our bodies for one reason or another. So, regaining chemical balance is difficult because our bodies do not receive a clear message that the emergency is over. It is important to consider the body as inherently wise, but its wisdom is moment-by-moment, not long term. It acts according to the immediate priorities. So how do our bodies react to these 'fake emergencies'?

- If the sugar that is released is not used for energy, it is converted to fat, which may end up in your artery walls, be converted to cholesterol and stored as body fat.

- If the calcium that is released does not receive the body's natural signals to return to the bones after the perceived emergency, then it, too, may end up on artery walls (contributing to hardening of the arteries), or be deposited into joint tissue (contributing to arthritis) instead of the bones and increase your risk of osteoporosis.

The body has to respond in this way. It has no other option, because excess sugar in the blood is life threatening, and the level of calcium circulating in the blood has to be kept within strict limits to maintain life. The body is effectively 'dumping' dangerous material from circulation into places where it can do no immediate harm. The fact that coronary artery disease, obesity, arthritis or osteoporosis may develop years hence, is not relevant at the time.

Stress hormone testing

It is possible, through a saliva test taken at specific times over 24 hours, to measure the impact that stress might be having on your health. The test tracks the normal flow of adrenal hormones over 24 hours. If the tests show that you might have reached adrenal fatigue they can help a nutritional therapist to target a diet and lifestyle programme that is best for you (see Chapter 25).

Recognising problems with glucose balance

The problems are not all long-term ones. Many people experience unpleasant symptoms on a daily basis for years as a result of adrenal stress. When the body responds to an adrenal stimulant with a surge of sugar entering the bloodstream it makes us feel good. But what usually happens 30 minutes or so later is that we experience the downside. Too much insulin is released, bringing the blood sugar level down too low. When we are not physically active, the majority of sugar in the body feeds the brain, so mental well-being is affected first when your blood sugar levels drop. Having relied on artificial stimulation throughout the day, it is not uncommon to find it difficult to sleep at night. The body may be tired, but the mind is still racing. Equally, it can be difficult to get going in the morning until we have had our first 'fix' like tea, coffee or a cigarette.

Symptoms of glucose imbalance (dysglycemia)

Irritability, anxiety, insomnia, depression, dizziness, mood swings, poor concentration, food cravings, irritability after six hours without food, excessive thirst, sugar cravings, cold hands, need for excessive sleep or drowsiness during the day, lack of energy, needing more than eight hours sleep at night, barely awake within 20 minutes of rising, needing something to get going in the morning like tea, coffee or a cigarette, excessive sweating, avoidance of exercise due to tiredness.

As most of us do not like feeling this way, the tendency is to turn to another cup of coffee or tea, a chocolate bar or a cigarette to pick us up again. This vicious cycle can keep us addicted all our lives unless we know better or choose to do something about it. This chapter will help you break this cycle.

On page 323 you will find a Hormonal Health Questionnaire. The higher your 'G' score when you take this check, the more likely you are to have dysglycemia.

How sugar and stress unbalance your hormones

Adrenal stress and glucose imbalance is inextricably tied up with female hormone imbalance. As described in Chapter 4, the stress hormone cortisol competes with the same binder as progesterone, so the net effect of being permanently stressed is less active progesterone. Since cortisol can also increase the production of oestrogen, prolonged stress can contribute to oestrogen dominance. Oestrogen also encourages the body to lay down fat, particularly around the hips and thighs, while high blood sugar levels, too much cortisol, together with insulin resistance, all lead to dumping sugar as fat, especially around your middle. In addition, high cortisol levels can also reduce the production of a helpful immune substance that protects the membranes of the gut, the airways and the urinary tract, called secretory IgA, and increase the risk of having a 'leaky' gut as described on page 50, as well as conditions such as cystitis. Polycystic ovaries are also strongly linked to this chain of events. Premenstrually, any tendency to glucose imbalance is exacerbated. That's why the symptoms of PMS look like the symptoms of poor blood sugar control (dysglycemia).

So, you can see just how stress and dysglycemia can wreak havoc in the body and can be a significant contributory factor in the development of many diseases experienced by women (which I explain in detail in Part 3). Given that most of our lives are stressful to varying degrees, it is essential that this factor is addressed as part of any programme to manage imbalances in the female hormones.

Why being overweight increases your risk of disease

You read a lot about how being obese or significantly overweight increases your risk of many diseases. In fact, the World Health Organization believes that being overweight has become a bigger threat to global health than being underweight! In America being obese has overtaken smoking as the single biggest preventable contributor to premature death. Being overweight, having insulin resistance and metabolic syndrome also increase your risk of hormonal health problems, ranging from polycystic ovaries to breast cancer. Indeed, you double your chances of developing cancer if you've gained weight with every decade of your life since your teens.[3] Being obese is considered a major risk factor for diabetes, heart disease and high cholesterol, arthritis, polycystic ovaries, cancer and many other diseases. But I believe that being overweight is just another symptom of an underlying change in your body's chemistry, often called metabolic syndrome (see page 38). The hallmark of metabolic syndrome is losing your blood sugar control.

Losing weight the healthy way

Excess weight around the middle, as I have explained, indicates blood sugar problems, and if you gain weight on your hips and thighs particularly, this often indicates oestrogen dominance. Another less common cause of weight gain is eating foods you are allergic to (see Chapter 6). Fat cells are also a storage site for oestrogen and many chemicals, including toxic metals like mercury, and pesticides, because when the body's ability to detoxify toxins is overloaded they are dumped into storage.

Each time weight loss occurs, many toxins can be liberated from fat cells and enter the circulation, so implementing a 'safe' weight-loss programme is essential. It involves ensuring that your diet includes a good base of protein, as many of the amino acids in protein are used to detoxify toxins. The critical process of detoxifying is called methylation and it relies on amino acids and other nutrients, such as B vitamins, to work efficiently. Levels of one of the amino acids found in the blood, homocysteine, can tell us how well our body is detoxifying and also gives us an indicator of our state of health, as the box below explains.

What is methylation and homocysteine?

Methylation is the orchestral conductor of your body's chemistry. Every second there are over a billion adjustments made in your body to keep you healthy and alive. Biochemicals in your body pass 'methyl groups' (made of one carbon and three hydrogen atoms) from one partner to another to help your body make the substances it needs or to break down those that it doesn't.

Homocysteine is an amino acid found naturally in the blood. Our levels of it – or our 'H score' – tell us how well our bodies are performing the process of methylation, which is why your H score is probably your most vital health statistic. In fact, it is more accurate than a cholesterol

cont ▶

reading in terms of predicting your risk of a heart attack or stroke, and a better measure than genes of your risk of having many other conditions, including Alzheimer's and osteoporosis (see Chapter 21).

Measuring your homocysteine
Your homocysteine level is easy to measure at home (see Resources). Your doctor can also test you, although few do. Homocysteine is measured in mmol/l. At one time experts thought that a 'high' level was above 15 units (mmol/l). This is what increases your risk of a heart attack and doubles your Alzheimer's risk. Up to 30 per cent of people with a history of heart disease have a homocysteine level above 14 units. The average level in Britain is 10.5; however, most experts now believe that a level below 6 or 7 units is ideal.

If you find your level is higher than 6, read my book, *The H Factor*, co-authored with Dr James Braly. This explains fully how to lower it to a safe level by making simple dietary changes and supplementing the correct vitamins, including folic acid, B_2, B_6, B_{12} and zinc.

Weight loss and toxins

During weight loss, an increased number of free radicals are formed. These are the dangerous by-products of normal bodily functions, such as breathing and eating, and they can destroy cells and damage body tissue. The body protects itself from free radicals with antioxidant nutrients (which we obtain from specific fresh foods). There is therefore an increased need for antioxidants during weight loss. Many extreme weight-loss and detoxification diets are low in calories and therefore low in protein and antioxidants, as well as important B vitamins and nutrients, and have a higher potential for toxic compounds liberated into circulation to cause harm.

Toxins can also slow down how quickly you convert what you eat into energy by reducing the activity of many of the enzymes that convert one substance into another, thus interrupting the flow of energy production. This can make it very hard for some women to lose weight. Based on the accepted theory of 'calorie input must be less than calorie output' in order to lose weight, some women are struggling on a combination of relatively low-calorie diets and high-energy output, and yet still find weight loss difficult.

Maintaining muscle mass with age is a good predictor of overall health. Combining a good protein-to-carbohydrate balanced diet with exercise and stress management are vital components of becoming a master of your weight and maintaining your muscle mass, which then burns more calories than fat.

A low-GL diet is the most effective for health and weight loss

The healthiest, and most effective way to lose weight is by eating a low-GL diet, which means limiting foods that cause your blood sugar level to rise sharply.

The measure of what a food does to your blood sugar is known as the glycemic load (GL). Neither protein nor fat (for example, meat, fish, cheese or eggs) have any substantial effect on your blood sugar balance, but sugary and carbohydrate-rich foods cause your blood glucose levels to soar. This is because the sugars and starches in foods with a high GL (refined carbohydrates, such as white bread, sweets and biscuits) are broken down and absorbed quickly into the bloodstream. When this happens you are likely to experience an increase in energy followed by an energy crash when your blood sugar drops, and you will probably reach for something sweet in order to relieve the symptoms of low blood sugar. The sugars and starches in foods with a low GL (the complex carbohydrates such as whole grains, vegetables, beans or lentils, or simpler carbohydrates such as fruit), however, take longer to digest than refined carbohydrates. As a result, the glucose released from these foods trickles slowly into the bloodstream. This means that it's used for energy rather than being stored, leaving blood glucose levels on an even keel, and preventing dramatic changes in your mood, behaviour and energy.

Eating a low-GL diet means that you eat healthily and keep your blood sugar even by choosing foods with a low GL score over those with a high one. You will find a chart showing the GL values of foods on page 328 and I'll be explaining the principles of this healthy diet later in the chapter.

The low-GL diet provides all the nutrients you need for healthy detoxification and it stops insulin resistance from occurring: when the body tries to cope with a diet high in fast-releasing carbohydrates by releasing lots of insulin to bring blood sugar levels down. This is another hallmark of metabolic syndrome. When your blood sugar is too high the excess sugar damages your blood and arteries.

Testing for blood sugar control

Damage to your blood and arteries caused by excess sugar is called glycosylation. By measuring your level of glycosylated haemoglobin (red blood cells) (also called HbA1c) you get one of the best measures as to whether you are losing your ability to control blood sugar. There's a simple pinprick home test, called the GL Check (see Resources) that measures this. Ideally you want a score below 5.5. If your score is 7 or more you are heading for diabetes and need to follow the advice in this book immediately.

Fast-release and slow-release foods

So what makes your blood sugar level unbalanced? Obviously, eating too much sugar and too many sweet foods; however, the kinds of food that have the greatest effect are not always the ones you might expect.

Alcohol, a chemical cousin of sugar, also upsets blood sugar levels. So do stimulants, such as tea, coffee, cola drinks and cigarettes. The combination of too much sugar, stimulants and prolonged stress taxes the body and results in an inability to control blood sugar levels, which, if severe enough, can develop into diabetes.

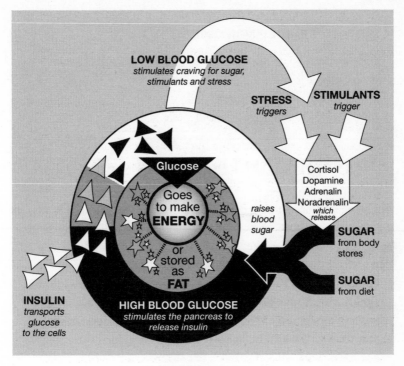

The sugar cycle

Eating sugar increases blood glucose levels. The body releases insulin into the blood to help escort glucose out and into body cells, to make energy or convert into fat. The result is low blood glucose. Either stress, causing more adrenalin, or induced stress, caused by consuming a stimulant such as caffeine, which raises adrenal hormones, causes breakdown of stores of sugar in the liver and muscles, called glycogen, which raises blood sugar levels. Low blood glucose causes stress or cravings for either something sweet or a stimulant.

The only way out of this vicious circle is to reduce or avoid all forms of concentrated sweetness, tea, coffee, alcohol and cigarettes, and start eating foods that help to keep your blood sugar level even. The best foods are all kinds of beans, peas and lentils, oats and whole grains. These foods are high in complex carbohydrates and contain special factors that help release their sugar content gradually. They are also high in fibre, which helps to normalise blood sugar levels.

How to balance your blood sugar

There are three golden rules to mastering your blood sugar balance:

1 Eat low-GL foods.
2 Eat protein with carbohydrate.
3 Graze, don't gorge – eat little and often.

The carbs that keep blood sugar even

Although you need to eat carbohydrate with every meal, it is important to choose those carbs that are healthy and will not cause your blood sugar level to rocket and then to dip. In Appendix 2 you will find a chart that gives the GL score of an average serving of a range of common foods. Foods with a GL of less than 10 (shown in bold) are good and should be the staple foods of your diet. A GL of 11–14 (shown in regular type) can be eaten in moderation. Foods with a GL higher than 15 (shown in italics) are to be avoided.

Healthy snack options

It's good for you to have a snack both in the morning and the afternoon to keep your blood sugar even, but don't go for the usual ones. Try these alternatives instead:

- **Instead of crisps** have oatcakes, pumpkin seeds, roasted snack mix or plain popcorn.
- **Instead of biscuits** have sweet oatcake biscuits (such as Nairn's) or fruit or nut bars (such as Fruitus bar by Lyme Regis Foods).
- **Instead of sweets and chocolate** have fresh fruit (apple, pear, peach, plum, berries), dried fruits such as apricots (these are a concentrated source of natural sugars, so eat in moderation).
- **Instead of sugar** (in drinks and home baking) have xylitol – it tastes just like sugar but doesn't upset blood sugar balance or cause tooth decay. cont ▶

* **Instead of sweetened drinks** drink water, fruity/herbal teas, diluted fruit juice (gradually increase the amount of water to let your taste buds adjust), diluted apple and blackcurrant concentrate, such as Meridian, or cherry concentrate such as CherryActive.

Eat protein with carbohydrate

The more fibre and protein you include with any meal or snack, the slower the release of the carbohydrates, which is good for blood–glucose balance. So, combining protein-rich foods with high-fibre carbohydrates is an excellent rule of thumb. Here's how you do it:

- Eat unsalted seeds or nuts with a whole fruit snack.
- Add seeds or nuts to carbohydrate-based breakfast cereals.
- Top wholemeal toast with eggs, baked beans or nut butter.
- Serve salmon or chicken with brown basmati rice.
- Add kidney beans to pasta sauce served over wholemeal pasta.
- Put cottage cheese on oatcakes, or hummus on pumpernickel-style whole-grain rye bread.
- Make sandwiches with sugar-free peanut butter and wholemeal bread.

What about high-protein diets?

Very high-protein diets have proved effective in managing blood sugar (as well as providing you with an abundance of amino acids), but they are not great for your health in the long term. This is because too much protein, especially from meat and dairy products, can have negative effects on the kidneys and bones, as well as being associated with a higher incidence of breast, prostate and colorectal cancer.

You can get the best of both worlds – that is, good health as well as a plentiful supply of amino acids – by eating protein-rich foods together with low-GL carbohydrates.

Protein and carbs with every meal

Remember: you need some protein with every meal because protein provides essential amino acids, and you need low-GL carbs to give you energy.

For breakfast, you can achieve the correct balance and amount of protein and low-GL carbohydrate by, for example, eating some seeds, yoghurt or either skimmed milk or soya milk, with your cereal and fruit. If you have an egg on toast, or kippers and oatcakes, you've done it already.

The fibre factor

Most people think of fibre as roughage – the indigestible part of plant foods, which helps to clean out our insides. What fibre actually does is absorb water in the digestive tract, thereby bulking out faecal matter, which then passes more easily through the body. This means that our exposure to carcinogen-containing foods is shorter. It also minimises the formation of carcinogens, which can happen if the food passes through slowly and, in effect, rots inside us.

There is little doubt that the modern diet – high in alcohol, sugar and fat, and low in fibre – wreaks havoc on the digestive tract. Such a diet disrupts the sensitive balance of beneficial bacteria, inflames the digestive tract wall and disturbs the gut-associated immune system, causing dysbiosis. Beta-glucuronidase is a carcinogen made within a digestive tract in a state of dysbiosis and it interferes with the liver's ability to break down oestrogen, which results in its continued circulation, thereby contributing to oestrogen dominance. Dysbiosis can easily be tested by stool analyses, which measures the presence of beta-glucuronidase as well as butyric acid – a kind of fat that actually feeds and nourishes the digestive tract. A certain proportion of fibre is fermented into butyric acid. Without this source of fuel, the digestive tract is more likely to become inflamed.[4]

The best way to increase your fibre intake is to eat whole foods, such as whole grains, lentils, beans, nuts, seeds and vegetables, all of which contain fibre. Some of the fibre in vegetables is destroyed by cooking so you should also eat something raw every day.

The balanced food plate

The simplest way to visualise your meals, as far as lunch and dinner are concerned, is to divide your plate into quarters. Visualise a protein-rich food portion (roughly the size of the palm of your hand), filling one-quarter on the left side of your dinner plate, and an equivalent-sized serving of any carbohydrate-rich food filling the other quarter on the left, then a large salad or two servings of vegetables filling the rest of the plate. So, half of what's on your plate is vegetables, one-quarter is a protein-rich food and one-quarter is a carbohydrate-rich food.

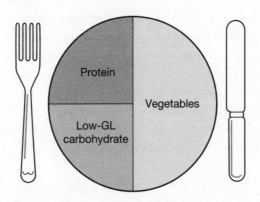

The perfectly balanced dinner plate

You need to quit stimulants

As I mentioned on page 68, you need to address stimulants like caffeine and nicotine. The research data is conflicting on whether tea and coffee per se are beneficial, or contribute negatively towards health. Coffee certainly raises homocysteine, which increases the risk of many diseases, including osteoporosis (see Chapter 21). Tea, particularly green and white tea, and coffee also contain many compounds that confer antioxidant protection.

The stimulating effects of caffeine, however, are real and some people rely on tea and coffee to bump up their low energy. Many people recognise the need for a cup of tea or coffee to get going in the morning or drink excess coffee to keep awake in order to complete a job or to study for an examination. Others notice withdrawal effects – like headaches and mood swings – when trying to quit caffeine, which makes them give up and continue with the habit.

Other culprits are cola and energy drinks, chocolate bars and chocolate drinks. Instead of these, have herbal teas or rooibos (redbush) tea, or green tea in moderation (a maximum of three cups a day). You can also have decaf tea or coffee, but these still contain some stimulants. A stimulant-free alternative, such as a grain or dandelion coffee substitute, is better. My favourite coffee substitutes are Teeccino and Caro Extra. These are available in health-food stores. Stabilising your blood sugar is an important part of decreasing the severity of any symptoms you may suffer while giving up caffeine.

The most effective way to give up caffeine, in my experience, is to choose a day and just stop, but if you do this expect to experience withdrawal symptoms for a few days. Occasionally, withdrawal symptoms can go on for much longer, so it's also wise to prepare for caffeine withdrawal; you might want to choose a time when you have a few days off work to cope with the side effects, which will be fewer if you eat a low-GL diet and take supplements, as detailed in Chapter 28.

It is also likely that you will be able to enjoy tea and coffee again in moderation once you are no longer reliant on them; however, some people notice that after a period of withdrawal they notice the 'buzz' effect of caffeine and no longer like the feeling.

Cigarettes

Nicotine is a highly addictive compound and may need to be tackled differently. Tobacco has many potentially hazardous compounds. Supporting yourself with a good diet and other lifestyle strategies should in principle help to limit the damaging health effects of smoking and help towards being able to withdraw from nicotine in due course. For more information on dealing with addictions, read my book, co-authored with David Miller and Dr James Braly, *How To Quit without Feeling S**t*.

Nutritional supplements can be helpful

I recommend that supplements are taken from day one of starting a programme to address either weight or sugar cravings. I have found that clients do much better when supported with extra nutrients that are known to assist in blood sugar control.

Vitamins B_1, B_2, B_3, B_5 and C, CoQ_{10} and the minerals magnesium, manganese, iron and copper are needed to turn glucose (sugar) into energy. Vitamin B_6 and the mineral zinc are required for the production of adrenalin. Chromium helps the action of insulin. Vitamins B_5 and C are needed to support the adrenal glands. A balance of calcium and magnesium is required so that each can be used effectively.

Supplementing a high-strength multivitamin and mineral that gives you at least 20mg of the B vitamins would be a good place to start. Pick a multi that also provides at least 150mg of magnesium, 200mg of calcium and 10mg of zinc. You may also wish to add 1g of vitamin C a day and 200mcg of chromium, if you suffer from sugar cravings. For those with diabetes I often recommend more chromium, up to 600mcg a day. The three most effective supplements for weight loss are chromium, HCA (which is an extract from tamarind) and 5-HTP, a type of tryptophan that is also a natural mood booster (see page 80).

Summary

To help control your weight, put an end to sugar cravings and become a master of your blood sugar control, and therefore help to keep your hormones in balance:

- Eat low-GL foods.
- Eat protein with carbohydrate to help balance blood sugar.
- Eat little and often.
- Eat wholefoods, such as whole grains, lentils, beans, nuts, seeds and vegetables every day – all of which contain fibre.
- Balance your meals by filling half your plate with vegetables, one quarter with a protein-rich food and one quarter with a carbohydrate-rich food.
- Avoid alcohol and cut right back on caffeine, sugar and fat.
- Take the right supplements.
- Maintain a healthy weight and engage in regular physical exercise to help reduce insulin levels.

You can read more about the low-GL diet in my book *The Low-GL Diet Bible*. (If you find it hard to stick to any diet, check out my Zest4Life 10-week programmes at www.zest4life.eu, which are run by experienced nutritional therapists and weight-loss coaches.)

CHAPTER 8

Beating PMS with Diet

Many women suffer the monthly problems of premenstrual syndrome (PMS), which is believed to be hormone related. PMS hit the health agenda in the 1970s and it is only since then that it has been recognised as a genuine health problem. Before it became a 'syndrome', it was called premenstrual tension (PMT) and referred to the variation of physical and mood symptoms that begin during the last one or two weeks prior to a period and usually end an hour to a few days after menstruation starts.

The specific combination of symptoms is very individual, but common ones include acne, anxiety, fatigue, irritability, fluid retention, forgetfulness, mood swings, bloating, breast tenderness, sweet cravings and weight gain.

Eight in ten women experience some kind of PMS, with an estimated one in ten having severe symptoms. About 3–5 per cent of women have symptoms so severe that it affects their work, education, relationships and/or daily activities. This is equivalent to 500,000 women in the UK alone.

The average age of onset of PMS is 26 and it generally gets worse with age, with the most severe form affecting more women in their forties. As women get older they spend more time in the premenstrual phase as the cycle gets shorter and shorter towards menopause, giving rise to more frequent symptoms.

Premenstrual dysphoric disorder (PMDD) is a diagnosis used by psychiatrists and other mental health workers to describe a specific set of particularly pronounced mood symptoms, appearing the week before, and going away a few days after, a period starts.

Sometimes it is difficult to differentiate between a true depression and PMS. A telling difference is when your symptoms are only partially relieved when the period starts. In which case, it is worth exploring the possibility of an underlying mental or physical health problem with your doctor or health-care professional, as many conditions may give rise to similar symptoms.

However, the good news is that once you have ruled out any other underlying condition, and you know that PMS is your problem, you can put an end to these unwanted symptoms after just a few months of following my optimum nutrition principles.

Case Study: Elaine

Elaine had suffered from PMS for as long as she could remember. Her moods were so bad in the week before her periods that her children would flee and her husband would cower. Here's what she told me:

'My PMS starts a week before a period. For the first two days I can handle it, my stomach starts churning, I get worse and worse, won't listen to anyone, I go nuts, get breast tenderness, and have heavy, painful periods.'

Two months later here's what she said:

'I haven't had any PMT – should be really bad right now. None of my outbursts. I've stuck to the diet completely. My energy has gone through the roof. I just feel like a completely different person. I can't believe it's happened so quickly. My husband can't believe the change. No breast tenderness. My middle daughter said, "What have you been doing to your skin? You look so much younger!" I'm really enjoying the diet. I'm trying new foods and the taste is great.'

What causes PMS?

PMS does not occur before the onset of the first period, during pregnancy or after natural or surgical menopause. Although the precise cause remains elusive, ovulation appears to be an important factor, with evidence suggesting that the symptoms are generally a result of changes in brain chemistry triggered by fluctuations in ovarian hormones.

Both oestrogen and progesterone levels generally fall sharply before a period, and this sudden change is thought to trigger PMS. Two major brain chemicals (neurotransmitters) seem to be affected by this change – serotonin and gamma-aminobutyric acid (GABA).

Serotonin – sometimes called the 'happy hormone' – has been shown to help control appetite and carbohydrate cravings. Oestrogen helps to improve mood by keeping up the levels of serotonin. Antidepressants, such as Prozac and Seroxat, are thought to work by helping to maintain levels of serotonin, although there are more natural ways to achieve the same thing (see below).

Similarly a derivative of progesterone enhances the production of GABA, which is a calming neurotransmitter that switches off adrenalin, helping to reduce anxiety and irritability. So, falling levels of oestrogen and progesterone before a period could plausibly trigger PMS symptoms. Peri-menopausal and postnatal depression seem to bear this theory out, as in both cases there is a major decrease in both hormones.

Dopamine is another neurotransmitter involved, as you will see later.

Having a well-balanced diet (see Chapter 26) is the best way to provide the nutrients needed for all three of these neurotransmitters to work effectively.

Supporting serotonin levels naturally

Choosing the right foods will help to boost your serotonin levels. There are also supplements that you can take.

The importance of protein

The protein that you eat is made up of amino acids, which are vital for many processes in your body, including making hormones, enzymes and neurotransmitters. There are 22 altogether, 8 of which are 'essential', which means they cannot be made in the body and therefore must come from the diet.

Tryptophan is one of these essential amino acids and is the raw material from which your body makes serotonin; however, it is the least abundant essential amino acid in food. Meat, beef, game, poultry, eggs and almonds are among the best sources. Dairy products, grains and chocolate also provide good amounts. Although chocolate is a stimulant and the sugar it provides makes it doubly attractive if you are having a blood sugar dip, it would be best not to rely on chocolate for your source of tryptophan. Tryptophan is also carried into the brain by insulin so it is possible that carbohydrate cravings serve the purpose of increasing serotonin production when needed. Therefore, it is possible that low levels of serotonin explain sugar, carbohydrate and chocolate cravings before a period, so make sure your diet contains good sources.

Vital vitamins and minerals

Many vitamins and minerals are needed to convert tryptophan to serotonin. Vitamin B_6 in its active form – pyridoxal-5-phosphate (P5P) – is perhaps the most well known vitamin required for this conversion; however, the B vitamins niacin (B_3), biotin and folate, plus vitamin C, as well as the minerals zinc and iron, are also needed.

Interestingly, women taking the contraceptive pill are often deficient in B_6. This vitamin plays a vital role in controlling mood and depression and was first prescribed in the 1970s to treat women on the Pill suffering from depression. It is also needed for clearing oestrogens from the liver. If oestrogens are not cleared efficiently, symptoms relating to oestrogen excess will be observed. According to the late Dr John Lee, 'A surplus of oestrogen or a deficiency of progesterone during the two weeks before a period allows an abnormal month-long exposure to oestrogen dominance, setting the stage for the symptoms of oestrogens side effects', which include an increased risk of breast cancer, endometrial growths, polycystic ovaries, PMS, an underactive thyroid, as well as accelerated ageing, breast tenderness, depression and fatigue. (See Dr Lee's book *What Your Doctor May Not Tell You About the Menopause*.) Too much oestrogen also increases copper levels; high copper can deplete the body of zinc, and both high copper and low zinc are associated with depression.

A low thyroid function may also simulate the symptoms of PMS, and since oestrogen competes with the thyroid hormone thyroxine at hormone receptor sites, oestrogen overload can lead to symptoms of an underactive thyroid. Your doctor or nutritional therapist can recommend and interpret a thyroid function test for you (see Chapter 14).

Vitamin B_3 (niacin) is also essential for balancing hormones and helping to prevent PMS. It is needed for energy production and sugar balance in the body. If your blood sugar levels are unstable, you are more likely to be tired, irritable, depressed and have hot flushes.

Only a small amount of dietary tryptophan is converted to serotonin, as the majority of tryptophan is used to make vitamin B_3. Vitamin B_3 is considered an essential nutrient; that is, it must be eaten in the diet. If your diet is deficient in vitamin B_3, your body has to make it from tryptophan. Vitamin B_6 needs zinc to convert into P5P, which is vital for converting tryptophan to B_3.

Metabolites of oestrogen have been shown to impair the activity of enzymes converting tryptophan to vitamin B_3. Mild deficiency of B_3 is quite common. Abnormal use of tryptophan converting to B_3 has been reported in women using the Pill. The Pill has been shown to deplete many nutrients including vitamin B_6, folate and magnesium.

Insomnia, anxiety and impulsive behaviour are associated with low serotonin levels and all three symptoms are associated with PMS. The body uses serotonin with the aid of magnesium to make a major hormone called melatonin, which helps to regulate sleep (and is also a very powerful antioxidant). Magnesium, known as 'nature's tranquilliser', is a valuable mineral for treating PMS, and magnesium levels are linked to poor appetite, nausea, tiredness, mood swings and muscle cramps. If you suffer from PMS it is likely that you will have lower levels of magnesium than women without symptoms.[5] As magnesium works together with vitamin B_6, I suggest taking magnesium and a B-vitamin complex containing both niacin and the P5P form of vitamin B_6.

The essential fats

Essential fats, which also improve serotonin status, may also play a role. The most beneficial fat for PMS is called GLA, found in evening primrose oil and borage oil.

Since we need both omega-3 and omega-6 fats, and more people are omega-3 than 6 deficient, a good starting point is to supplement, on a daily basis, an omega-3 and 6 supplement, ideally containing ten times more omega-3, from fish oil, than omega-6, from borage oil; for example, if you took two capsules providing 750mg of fish oil (giving you about 650mg of active omega-3) plus 250mg of borage oil (giving you about 50mg of GLA) this is a good insurance policy.

However, most studies show best effect from supplementing the equivalent of up to 300mg of GLA a day.[6] That's the equivalent of six 500mg evening primrose oil capsules; however, you can get concentrated GLA capsules using borage oil, containing 150mg or 300mg in one capsule. If a basic change in diet, plus a daily omega-3 and 6 combination supplement doesn't sort out your PMS try taking 150mg or 300mg of GLA in the week before your period.

PMS supplements at a glance

You can get relief from PMS by supplementing:

- High-dose B vitamin complexes containing B_3 (50mg), B_6 (50mg), B_{12} (10mcg), folic acid (200mcg) and biotin (50mcg)
- Extra vitamin C (1–2g a day)
- Magnesium (300mg a day)
- Omega-3 and especially omega-6 essential fats (up to 300mg of GLA)

Supplementation with 5-HTP

Tryptophan is converted to the amino acid 5-hydroxytryptophan (5-HTP – the precursor of serotonin) and then into serotonin. Many women find that supplementing 5-HTP relieves symptoms. Vitamin B_6, biotin and the mineral zinc are still required to convert 5-HTP to serotonin. Supplementing 5-HTP is thought to spare dietary tryptophan for converting to vitamin B_3, as described above. It's best to choose a 5-HTP supplement that also contains these B vitamins, starting with 100mg, up to 300mg a day. 5-HTP is much better absorbed away from a protein-rich meal, ideally with a carbohydrate snack, such as a piece of fruit or an oatcake. 5-HTP is not recommended if you are on an antidepressant drug, because many of these block the breakdown of serotonin, whereas 5-HTP helps you to make more. The combination could theoretically result in serotonin overload.

Ensuring adequate dietary tryptophan, and the vitamins and minerals needed for it to function in the body, is very important. Supplementation with 5-HTP does not displace the importance of a balanced diet but could help in the short term as an aid while you tune up your diet. In the long term you should be able to be PMS-free without relying on 5-HTP.

Interestingly, animal studies have shown that artificially reducing serotonin levels leads to weight gain and an insatiable appetite.[7] Dieting and stress lower the level of tryptophan in the blood and when the level of tryptophan falls in the blood it makes you hungry, especially for carbohydrates.[8] Weight gain and carbohydrate cravings are common symptoms of PMS.

Supporting levels of GABA naturally

GABA is the major relaxing neurotransmitter that works throughout our central nervous system, helping to keep it calm. Benzodiazepine drugs, like Valium, activate GABA neurons and receptor sites in the brain helping to induce a sedative, sleep-promoting, anti-anxiety effect in the body. A new class of 'non-benzodiazepine' drug also acts on GABA. They can be addictive and are therefore only recommended for short-term use.

As with serotonin, good-quality protein is necessary in the diet to make GABA. The amino acids glutamine and glutamic acid both help make GABA and also work interdependently with GABA and have been described as the Three Musketeers – 'one for all and all for one'. Vitamin B_6 is important for regulating the production of GABA in the brain. The non-essential amino acid taurine is similar to GABA and also acts as a powerful calming neurotransmitter. Animal produce is the major source of taurine, so vegetarian and vegan diets can be short of this amino acid.

Two forms of GABA also act as calming neurotransmitters, and alcohol has been shown to increase their levels, which may help explain why some people use alcohol as an antidote to stress. One of these two compounds, gamma-hydroxybutyric acid (GHBA), helps to promote sleep. The function of GABA is also enhanced by a derivative of progesterone called allopregnenelone, which acts like a sedative, decreasing anxiety and irritability. In the US you can buy GABA supplements over the counter. A dosage of 500–1,000mg has a relaxing effect. In Europe, look for formulas that contain glutamine, taurine, magnesium and the relaxing herbs passion flower and hops, for a natural relaxant effect.

Dietary principles

A fundamental principle for managing PMS for most women is to eat meals and snacks that provide both protein and carbohydrate, as described in Chapters 7 and 26. Also follow the advice below:

Don't be afraid of carbs One of the most important dietary factors for balancing hormones is to keep your blood sugar level even. Eat plenty of complex, unrefined carbohydrates such as whole grains (oats, brown rice, whole-grain bread and pasta, millet), beans (lentils, soya beans, kidney beans, and so on) and plenty of vegetables.

However, do cut out all refined carbohydrates such as white bread, white pasta and rice, cakes, biscuits and sweets, and any foods containing added sugar (check labels as there will be more foods than you think – even bread, for example, often has sugar added to it).

Get the right five a day Although eating plenty of fruit and vegetables has many benefits, vegetables such as broccoli and cauliflower are especially beneficial for PMS sufferers, as they contain a substance called diindolymethane (DIM). DIM has been shown to mop up excess oestrogen and therefore relieve the associated problems such as weight gain, PMS, acne and menopausal symptoms.

Out with the bad, in with the good Cut back on 'bad' saturated and hydrogenated fats (found in meat, dairy products and processed foods, such as cakes, biscuits and junk food), as these have no nutritional value. Replace these fats with the essential fats found in oily fish, nuts, seeds and vegetable oils. These good fats are especially important for menstruating women as they help to prevent inflammation and reduce abnormal blood clotting. Cutting out saturated fats should also help to reduce headaches, menstrual cramps and endometriosis discomfort. In fact, it has been shown that diets high in saturated fats increase oestrogen production and prevent the absorption of the beneficial essential fats.[9]

Bulk up Not only does fibre help with digestion and reduce cholesterol levels, but it also plays a key role in balancing female hormones. Fibre found in vegetables, fruit and whole grains can absorb excess oestrogen in the gut and prevent it from re-entering the blood. Oat fibre from whole oats or rough oatcakes is particularly good.

Cut the caffeine Caffeine not only removes vital minerals and vitamins from your body due to its diuretic effect but it's also linked to PMS, in particular breast pain and tenderness. Caffeine in tea, coffee, chocolate, soft drinks and headache tablets is also a stimulant, as we have seen, affecting blood sugar levels. See page 74 for my recommendations for substitutes.

... and the alcohol Although it has been all-too-easily accepted that red wine is 'good for the heart', research has actually shown that these effects are only evident in women post-menopause. The liver is one of the key organs for controlling and balancing hormones, as this is where excess hormones can be removed. If the liver is over-taxed by a poor diet and alcohol, this elimination will not occur.

Fight symptoms with phytoestrogens As explained in Chapter 3, phytoestrogens are oestrogen-like, plant-derived substances which are found in high amounts in soya products and various vegetables such as peas and beans; however, despite being similar to oestrogens, they can actually reduce the problem of oestrogen dominance. This is because they lock onto, and block, the body's oestrogen receptors, so protecting against the negative effects of too much oestrogen. Research has found that soya supplementation can help with many premenstrual symptoms, including headache, breast tenderness and cramps.[10] Asian women, who typically eat a lot of soya products, have fewer symptoms of the menopause, suggesting a beneficial effect on hormones. Remember to bear in mind, however, that the majority of soya eaten by Asian women is the fermented kind, which is safer and has greater health benefits, as explained on page 34. The herb red clover also contains several phytoestrogens which may help balance oestrogen dominance.

Herbal and supplemental help

As well as following a well-balanced diet with the addition of some valuable vitamins and minerals, there are a number of herbs that I recommend to help with hormonal imbalances.

- **Black cohosh**, originally used by the native North American Indians, may help to counteract excess oestrogen. It may also act on serotonin receptors and raise levels of the 'happy' neurotransmitter, serotonin. This makes it a useful supplement for treating PMS-related depression.

- **Agnus castus/chasteberry** is a herb that has been shown to increase progesterone while decreasing excess oestrogen levels. In women suffering with PMS, taking agnus castus (20mg daily) can reduce symptoms by 42.5 per cent.[11]

- **Dong quai** Another herb I often recommend is dong quai (*Angelica sinensis*), which is one of the most commonly prescribed herbs in Chinese medicine for female problems. It promotes normal hormonal balance and helps sufferers of menstrual cramps, as it has muscle-relaxing qualities.

- **Dandelion** If you suffer from water retention, I recommend the natural diuretic dandelion, as it not only helps with the removal of fluid, but also supports the liver and can help in the removal of excess hormones.

In terms of supplements, the most important are vitamins B_3, B_6, zinc, magnesium and a combination of fish oil omega-3 fats with borage oil for omega-6 fats. If these don't work, try adding 100mg of 5-HTP. (See page 317 for guidance on doses.)

Summary

I cannot stress enough the importance of following the Diet for the Good Life in Chapter 26 as the basis for addressing PMS and other hormone-related problems. Follow a varied, well-balanced diet that includes plenty of whole foods, fruits and vegetables (in particular cruciferous vegetables); swap saturated fats for essential fats; and cut out all stimulants such as caffeine, alcohol and sugar. If you are suffering from menstrual cramps, take a magnesium supplement and a B-vitamin complex plus the herb agnus castus or dong quai. For bloating, dandelion can help, either in a tea or in capsule form.

If all this doesn't help, a nutritional therapist can help you to address PMS symptoms more specifically than a trial-and-error approach. It is very difficult to determine an individual's exact hormonal imbalance

cont ▶

without a simple saliva test, which I recommend you take (see Chapter 25). If you are found to be oestrogen dominant, follow all the recommendations in this book for reducing oestrogen levels, including increasing your intake of fibre, ensuring a good intake of phytoestrogens and B vitamins, eating organically grown produce, limiting your exposure to xenoestrogens and reducing your consumption of high-fat meat and dairy produce. Most women obtain freedom from PMS within a few cycles.

CHAPTER 9

Natural Solutions for Heavy and Painful Periods

Painful or heavy periods are not uncommon, particularly in young women before they have had a baby. Many women gain relief from painful and heavy periods by following a general optimum nutrition programme and dealing with allergies and/or candidiasis (see Chapters 6 and 16). Fibroids, however, cause painful and heavy periods and these arise because of oestrogen dominance, as I will explain in this chapter.

Painful periods

The muscles of the womb, like other muscles in the body, can become unbalanced in their ability to contract and relax. During a period these muscles are working extra hard to shed the womb's inner lining. Calcium and magnesium are the two major nutrients needed to control this process. Calcium helps the muscle to contract and magnesium helps the muscle to relax. Eating healthy foods rich in calcium and magnesium, and taking supplements, helps many women. However, many diets that rely heavily on dairy produce are rich in calcium but relatively poor in magnesium. Including nuts, seeds and dark green, leafy vegetables in your diet often helps, as these foods are rich in both calcium and magnesium.

Essential polyunsaturated fats, vitamin E and the mineral zinc may also help. It is worth taking a multivitamin and mineral supplement to boost your intake of these nutrients. Essential polyunsaturated fats are particularly likely to help if the pain is associated with a heavy blood loss that has a tendency to clot. These oils make a type of prostaglandin that controls blood thickness. It is best to take an essential fat supplement that provides both omega-6 (GLA) and omega-3 (EPA, DPA and DHA) fats. Vitamin E can also help reduce cramps. Cutting down on red meat and dairy produce should help too, as these high-fat foods can promote inflammatory prostaglandins.

The contraceptive pill is often recommended for period pains; however, I don't recommend this approach, as the Pill interferes with the working of many essential nutrients. Many women recover from painful periods naturally, with help from the same nutrients that are depleted by the Pill.

Heavy periods

Follow the Diet for the Good Life (Chapter 26) and test for any food intolerances (see Chapter 6). Some women find that their periods get heavier in the first few months of an anti-*Candida* diet (see Chapter 16), but it usually settles down.

A lack of vitamin A is associated with heavy periods. Levels do appear to fluctuate over the month, indicating a correlation with the fluctuating female hormones. Another study clearly indicated that women with heavy periods had less than half the normal levels of vitamin A in their bloodstream. Researchers found that, when treating heavy periods with high levels of vitamin A daily for 35 days, over half of the participants' heavy periods were completely cured, and 14 more women showed a marked improvement. In all, 93 per cent improved.[12]

Sometimes, it may not be that vitamin A is actually deficient, just a lack of another nutrient prevents it from being used properly in the body; for example, zinc is required for the enzyme that releases vitamin A from storage in the liver, and is also needed to produce a protein that transports vitamin A through the circulation to the tissues. So, lack of zinc could lead to an apparent vitamin A deficiency, and sometimes correcting zinc status is all that is required for the proper use of vitamin A.

The Pill can create a high level of vitamin A in the blood[13] and, while taking the Pill, a woman's artificial periods are usually fine. The Pill creates this high level of vitamin A in the blood by moving it from its store in the liver; however, when a woman stops taking the Pill, the level of vitamin A in the blood can fall dramatically, consequently depleting stores in the liver. It is therefore common for some women to experience heavy periods after stopping the Pill.

Vitamin C and bioflavonoids have been shown to help control heavy periods. Bioflavonoids are found mainly just beneath the surface skin of fruit. It is unclear whether low iron levels are an effect, as well as a cause, of heavy periods, but correcting iron status is an essential part of any programme. Taking vitamin C with iron-rich foods increases the absorption of iron from non-animal sources.

If you are iron-depleted after a heavy period, which is likely, supplement 20–30mg a day for at least a week. A decent multivitamin and mineral supplement should give you 10mg. So you'll need an extra iron supplement providing 10–20mg a day. Iron chelated with glycine, called ferrous bisglycinate, is the best-absorbed and gentlest on digestion.

Irregular periods

Depending on the cause, irregular periods can be perfectly normal. Towards the menopause it is expected that periods will become irregular, and they stop altogether during pregnancy. If your periods are either absent or irregular, and you do not come into either of these categories, it is worth checking out the cause. Absent or irregular periods are associated with low weight, strenuous exercise, anorexia nervosa, taking the Pill, or extreme stress. Extreme stress can lead to either missed periods or more frequent periods. Also read Chapter 18 to ascertain if polycystic ovaries (PCOS) might be an issue.

Fibroids

Fibroids are the most common growths in the female reproductive system. They are benign, firm, round lumps (usually more than one) that attach themselves to the muscular wall of the womb. They often grow to the size of a grapefruit and routinely disappear after the menopause. They are, however, one of the most common reasons why pre-menopausal women have their womb removed. Symptoms are irregular, heavy and painful periods, while the weight of the fibroids can weaken the pelvic floor muscles, leading to stress incontinence. The usual treatment is to remove them surgically.

Fibroids are mostly a result of oestrogen dominance, so when levels fall at the menopause the fibroids shrink. According to the late Dr John Lee, when the oestrogen dominance is addressed by using natural progesterone, fibroid tumours usually decrease in size and can usually be kept to a minimum until the menopause is over, when they will naturally shrivel up. Oestrogen dominance can be easily detected by a simple saliva test to measure oestrogen and progesterone levels (see Chapter 25). Use natural progesterone only with the guidance of a medical doctor familiar with its use.

Iron is the most common mineral deficiency in women during their reproductive years –mostly a result of very heavy periods. Iron is vital for energy, stamina, brain function and immunity. The declining intake of red meat compounds the problem, as it is a readily absorbable source of iron whereas vegetable sources of iron are not so easily absorbed, although taking vitamin C will assist absorption. Ask your doctor or nutritional therapist to run a haemoglobin and ferritin blood test, if you think you might be short on iron. This is an easily correctible nutritional deficiency.

CHAPTER 10

Promoting a Healthy Sex Life

You may be surprised to learn that the sex drives of both men and women are on the wane. We're told that men apparently think about sex every five minutes, but the continuing sales of Viagra are proof enough that many men are having difficulties, and although sexual impotence is more physically obvious in men, women are experiencing it too. So what's going on? In this chapter I'll be explaining the role that hormones play in women's sex lives and how to maintain a healthy sex drive.

Sex drive is a complex issue. Desire is not only generated by the excitement and feelings you get when you're attracted to someone but it is also a question of physiological processes that are essential for that desire to be translated into actually wanting to have sex.

Sexual difficulties are extremely common

Sure, sex is a less taboo subject than it used to be, so we are more likely to state our demands and complain if our partner is unable to meet them or if we are having difficulties. But the fractured taboo does not explain the increased outspokenness about the decline in sex drive. Surveys are showing that nearly a third of women never reach orgasm and a fifth don't enjoy their sex life.[14] According to Catherine Kalamis, author of *Women Without Sex*, 'Research from

America, Britain and now other countries including China suggests that women have more sexual problems than men – probably around 43 per cent of women compared to 31 per cent of men are experiencing sexual difficulties at any one time,' she explains. Catherine's view is supported by Dr Kevan Wylie, Consultant in Sexual Medicine at the Royal Hallamshire Hospital in Sheffield. 'One thing seems fairly consistent in the epidemiological studies to date – around 40% of women are describing some degree of sexual dissatisfaction or actual dysfunction,' he says. Researchers compared data from the 52 published studies on sexual dysfunction that have been generated in the past ten years,[15] and found the following problems reported by women:

- Orgasm: 4–24 per cent

- Arousal: 8–19 per cent

- Low libido: 5–46 per cent

- Painful sex: 9–21 per cent

A GP-based UK survey[16] found that 41 per cent of female respondents reported an ongoing sexual problem, with 68 per cent saying they experienced a sexual problem at some time in their lives. The most common complaints were vaginal dryness and difficulty achieving orgasm.

Although many men suffer from erectile dysfunction (not being able to have or sustain an erection), many more are finding their libido is low in the first place.

One clear finding from the wealth of research is that sex drive is complicated. It is not simply a matter of taking a potion. There are insidious things happening in our lifestyles and environment that are undermining our desire to have and enjoy sex.

Of course, past experiences, lack of communication, insecurity and other emotional triggers can interfere with the ability to want sex and become aroused. But those aside, after the initial flush of excitement with a new partner, you may be wise to take some steps to keep your sex drive strong.

The feminisation of nature

Apart from being attracted to someone, our sex drive is largely dictated by our hormones. Over the last 50 years, there's been an undeniable escalation in hormone-related problems such as infertility, breast and prostate cancers and an array of hormonal imbalances, particularly in women. These problems are associated with overexposure to hormone-disrupting chemicals, excess oestrogens and insulin.

When men are exposed to high amounts of such xenoestrogens, they can develop female characteristics such as breast growth. At the same time, these hormone disrupters affect sex drive and other particularly male characteristics such as muscular strength and development. In other words xenoestrogens can interfere with the role of the male hormone, testosterone, in the body.

Women produce testosterone too, although in smaller amounts, in the adrenal glands and ovaries. Studies have shown that giving women testosterone implants raises their sex drive – with significant improvements in sexual desire, fantasy and response and a decrease in painful sex caused by lack of excitement and insufficient natural lubrication.

Stress – the libido killer

Xenoestrogens are not the only factor in decreasing testosterone and sex drive. Rather than looking at adding testosterone (which may be more useful in women who have had hysterectomies or after menopause), it's useful to look at why testosterone levels – in both men and women – may be down. Stress appears to be a major contributing factor to the widespread decline in libido.

If your stress reserves are low, not only will a tough day at the office or a family crisis take its toll but so will a hard night's partying or a strenuous session at the gym. Although the body needs its stress response to deal with everyday life, if stress is prolonged or extreme, the response can have negative effects on many aspects of health, including your hormone balance, as I explained in Chapter 7. Prolonged stress is often a factor in developing an underactive thyroid (a common symptom of which is low sex drive), as I will explain in Chapter 14. Thyroxine is also needed for nitric oxide regulation, a key factor in sexual stimulation (see below).

Testosterone is a steroid hormone, derived from cholesterol. Another important steroid hormone is cortisol, which is secreted as part of the body's response to stress. Both testosterone and cortisol are derived from progesterone. So, you can see that if your body is stressed, and is therefore making cortisol from progesterone rather than testosterone, there can be a testosterone deficit. Although in more serious cases, testosterone medication (on prescription only) may help, it is still necessary to deal with some of the potential root causes of deficiency.

So, rather than just adding testosterone, or even taking so-called aphrodisiacs, it makes sense to help control the body's stress response. This must primarily take the form of reducing the stress in your life and your attitude towards life's events, but it can also be given a hand by modifying your diet and taking certain supplements.

Avoiding stimulants, such as coffee, tea, alcohol, cigarettes and sugary foods and drinks can go a long way to stabilising your body's response to stress by helping to balance your blood sugar levels. (Caffeine, nicotine and alcohol also impede blood flow, which interferes with the proper function of the male and female sex organs during sex.) It's also helpful to eat regularly, have some protein at each meal and eat fresh, unprocessed, fibre-rich foods. Essential fats from fish, nut and seed oils are also important for hormone production and effective hormonal messaging. Include oily fish, nuts and seeds (such as walnuts, pecan nuts, pumpkin and chia seeds) in your diet at least three times a week.

Nutrients for combating stress

The body's main stress response comes from the adrenal glands, which rely on a good supply of several nutrients to work efficiently.

An important one is vitamin C (take 1g a day), others are B_5, also called pantothenic acid (best taken as part of a high-strength multivitamin–mineral supplement or B complex), as well as the minerals magnesium and chromium (which is particularly important for helping to balance blood sugar levels; take 200mcg daily). Vitamin B_5 helps to convert choline, found richly in eggs and fish, into the important neurotransmitter acetylcholine, which plays a role in sex drive and vaginal lubrication. It is best to take all of these nutrients if you consider yourself under considerable stress.

Natural aphrodisiacs

There are several nutrients and herbs that may help to give your libido a direct boost. These include B vitamins, zinc and antioxidants. Oysters are the richest known food source of zinc, so no wonder they have a reputation for being a powerful aphrodisiac. Antioxidants include nutrients such as vitamins A, C, E, the minerals zinc and selenium and plant nutrients such as bioflavonoids, which protect the body's cells from damage by oxidants.

Dong quai A widely used Chinese herb, dong quai (which I've discussed on page 87), tones the female reproductive organs and may therefore help increase the desire for sex. The dose of powdered herb is between 2 and 4g per day. The herbs muira pauma, maca and damiana all have reputed libido-boosting effects (see pages 100–1).

Zestra is a feminine arousal oil that's become the best-selling female lubricant in the US. Unlike other lubricants on the market, many of which are made from chemicals that irritate that vulva area to create a temporary warming effect, Zestra is made entirely from natural ingredients (evening primrose and borage seed oils with extracts of angelica and coleus).

What's particularly interesting is that it's also the only product I've seen that's clinically proven to enhance sensation and sexual satisfaction. A study published in the *Journal of Sex and Marital Therapy* tested the effects of Zestra on a group of 20 women, half of whom suffered with 'female sexual arousal disorder'.[17] Despite the small sample group, the study was designed as a randomised, placebo-controlled, double-blind crossover trial – which is the most scientifically robust. After examining evidence from participant questionnaires, diary entries and interviews with sex therapists, the researchers concluded that Zestra 'improved level of desire, satisfaction, arousal, genital sensation, sexual pleasure, ability to have orgasms and enhancement of sexual experiences'. The study also found that Zestra eliminated 'the undesirable sexual side effects of SSRI antidepressants in women'.

Zestra is irritant-free as well as chemical- and parabens-free. It comes in single-use sachets that can be applied to the vulva area during foreplay. It takes effect within 5 minutes and generally lasts for 45 minutes. Zestra is not available to buy in shops or pharmacies, but you can buy it online.

Arginine The amino acid arginine is often claimed to be a natural alternative to Viagra. The reason why Viagra works in men is that a substance called nitric oxide (NO), produced by the body, is vital for improving blood flow and smooth muscle contraction required both for a man to get an erection and also for stimulating a woman's genitalia. NO is made from arginine, the natural form of which is called l-arginine. Arginine is a non-essential amino acid, which means it can be made from other amino acids in food. Some say that our levels decline with age and there may be advantage in supplementing extra; however, although the Internet is full of claims of people, especially men, enjoying improved sex lives by supplementing 1–3g of arginine (usually one or two hours before sex), the evidence for it working, especially in women, is a bit thin on the ground. In combination with other herbs, arginine has been shown to help improve sexual arousal[18] in two studies. With so much interest in arginine it won't be too long before better studies are published; however, there is unlikely to be any harm from trying it. (There's also the added benefit that it helps the body make muscle rather than fat.)

Supplements for better sex

Here are the nutrients and herbs I recommend increasing to support a healthy sex life, together with the diet and lifestyle factors recommended in Part 5.

Antioxidants

How they work Antioxidants minimise oxidant damage to sex organs and optimise blood flow to sex organs.

Cautions None at the recommended dosage.

How much? Take a good antioxidant formula that contains the vitamins A, C and E plus zinc, selenium and perhaps lipoic acid and CoQ_{10}. Make sure your daily multivitamin contains many of these antioxidants.

Arginine

How it works Promotes nitric oxide production, necessary for improving blood flow and muscle relaxation during sex.

Cautions None in sensible doses.

How much? 1–3g a day, ideally within two hours of sex. Best taken on an empty stomach.

B vitamins

How they work B vitamins are needed for testosterone production, adrenal support, energy production and healthy nerves. Vitamin B_1 is needed for healthy thyroid function; B_3 is a vasodilator, enhancing blood flow to the sex organs and essential for pituitary function, which controls hormone balance.

99

Cautions None in sensible doses. Excess B_3 and B_6 can have adverse effects (in doses above 1,000mg a day). Vitamin B_3, as niacin, acts as a vasodilator, improving circulation and causing blushing at doses above 50mg. This may improve sensitivity.

How much? Niacinamide (B_3) 50mg, niacin (B_3) 50mg, pyridoxine (B_6) 50mg, cyanocobalamine (B_{12}) 50mcg, folic acid 500mcg a day.

Damiana

How it works The central American shrub damiana is said to stimulate the production of testosterone and increase the sensitivity of both the clitoris and penis. Preliminary trials suggest it helps recover sexually exhausted men[19] and helps improve sexual satisfaction in women[20] in combination with other nutrients.

Cautions No toxicity known.

How much? 400–800mg × 3 daily.

Ginseng

How it works The herb ginseng is widely regarded as a 'sexual rejuvenator', and animal studies have shown it increases testosterone levels, helps the body adapt to stress and boosts energy.

Cautions None at recommended doses. Make sure you get a brand whose dose is standardised to contain particular amounts of active ingredients.

How much? Panax ginseng 200mg (standardised to 10 per cent ginsenosides) × 3 daily, Siberian ginseng 200mg (standardised to 1 per cent eleutherosides) × 3 daily.

Maca (*Lepidium meyenii*)

How it works A native to Peru's central highlands, maca has been used in traditional Andean culture to awaken healthy passion for over 2,000 years. Inca warriors are said to have eaten it before battle for extra power. And during the conquest of the South American continent, the Spaniards fed maca to their horses to combat weakness and infertility in the high altitude.

For women, maca was not only used for its libido benefits but was also used to help promote normal menstrual cycles, minimise menopausal symptoms and to help alleviate vaginal dryness.

Experiments on mice showed increased sexual performance and improved erectile function even in testes-removed rats! It's also been shown to help men with erectile dysfunction,[21] post-menopausal women[22] and those on antidepressants with reduced libido.[23] Exactly how it works remains a mystery.

Cautions None known.

How much? 3–5g of ground maca.

Muira pauma

How it works Muira pauma is a native to the Brazilian Amazon. Its mechanism of action remains unknown, but it appears to boost the libido and enhance sexual experience in both sexes. (In a study in France, 62 per cent of the men claimed it had changed their lives.) It is traditionally used to alleviate menstrual cramps and the discomforts of menopause; it also tonifies the female sex organs.

Cautions None known.

How much? 1g a day.

Zinc

How it works Zinc is needed to convert testosterone to its active form, dihydroxytestosterone. It is needed to help sustain lubrication of the vaginal wall, as well as for pituitary function.

Cautions Smoking, alcohol, coffee and some drugs deplete zinc. It is only toxic at excessive levels – that is, above 150mg per day.

How much? 15mg daily (best taken as part of a multivitamin–mineral).

CHAPTER 11

Fertility Rights and Wrongs

Infertility has been recorded since ancient times and was historically seen as the woman's problem – and often that she was somehow responsible for her own condition. It is only relatively recently that we have discovered that up to 40 per cent of infertility problems relate to the man and around 80 per cent of birth defects are the result of damaged sperm. Around one in four couples have fertility problems. Even for those who don't, it is not uncommon for successful conception to take between 6 and 18 months.

The causes of infertility

The most common cause of infertility in women is blocked fallopian tubes, most frequently arising after abdominal surgery because of scarring and adhesions. Gynaecological problems, such as pelvic inflammatory disease, endometriosis and infections, can also contribute to blocked fallopian tubes and infertility. Excess acidity of the cervical mucus is also associated with the problem, as it creates an environment that is hostile to sperm from the moment they enter the vagina.

Improving your diet, with particular emphasis on increasing your intake of alkaline-forming foods (see Chapter 26), will help to normalise excess acidity in the body.

Being underweight is also associated with difficulties becoming pregnant, because when a woman's weight is too low there will be an absence of periods, or anovulatory cycles, and these are a major cause of infertility. In earlier centuries, when women were producing offspring in times of fluctuating food supplies, it was important for her to carry on her body all the energy required – stored as fat – to complete the growth of the developing baby even if food supplies ran short. Therefore, for your body to maintain regular periods and fertility, it would seem that you need to have about 22 per cent body fat. Women with anorexia nervosa often have no periods. Loss of periods is also not uncommon in young women athletes who have a hard training schedule and therefore very little fat. If you are concentrating on physical training and trying to conceive it would be sensible to change to a less demanding regime.

In contrast, women who do not regularly ovulate and who are also significantly overweight are at as much risk, if not more, of infertility as underweight women. Maintaining an ideal body weight increases your chances of becoming pregnant.

Infertility programmes

In the 21st century, we have discovered ingenious ways of helping infertile couples have babies. The technique of in vitro fertilisation (IVF), whereby an ovum is fertilised by a sperm outside the body and then replaced in the womb, has already transformed the lives of many childless couples.

IVF pregnancies, however, are usually supported by heavy doses of synthetic hormones. So, if you are having trouble conceiving, it is important to give your body the best chance to conceive naturally, particularly when you have no known, specific condition that is affecting your fertility, before you embark on complicated and potentially toxic, hormonal programmes to increase your fertility. Even if you do have such a condition, good nutrition will help to support the success of an IVF-induced pregnancy.

Nutrition for fertility

If you are being advised to go on a hormonal programme because your partner's sperm count is low, encourage him to see a nutritional therapist to identify any deficiencies and to embark on an optimum nutrition programme. Ideally, a preconceptual-care programme would be for a minimum of three months, and preferably six, for both of you. A nutritional therapist can work with you to optimise your diet and help to identify, through testing, any nutritional imbalances or other factors that may be affecting your ability to conceive. Several nutritional therapists specialise in preconceptual care and can be contacted through Foresight, an organisation committed to helping couples increase their chances of conception and having a healthy baby (see Resources).

Fertility wrongs

As part of an overall programme to maximise your chances of conception there are also several factors to avoid – many are described in detail in the next chapter. It's also important to reduce your homocysteine level to below 7, if it is above this (see page 65). Obvious substances to avoid when trying to conceive are alcohol, cigarettes, caffeine and drugs – both recreational and some prescription drugs. Antidepressants, for example, are associated with an increased risk of pregnancy problems.[24] It is also wise to avoid supplementing more than 2,250mcg (7,500iu) of vitamin A daily in the form of retinol; this is the animal form of vitamin A (whereas beta-carotene, the vegetable form, is not known to be toxic). Retinol in very high doses is associated with foetal abnormalities, but these are well above the safe level given here.

Synthetic hormones

Many women have spent years on the Pill, a method of contraception that works by preventing ovulation. Although one in every 200 women's periods will cease after stopping the Pill, fertility will return in most cases within two years.

As part of an infertility programme, many women are treated with drugs to stimulate ovulation, even when they are shown to be ovulating spontaneously. These are often the same women who have previously taken the Pill. What is often not considered as part of most infertility treatments is that natural hormone production and hormone receptor sites within the cells need a good supply of zinc and magnesium to work effectively, but these vital minerals are both somewhat depleted by the Pill and are commonly deficient in women having problems conceiving.

The use of synthetic hormones before and during pregnancy exposes a developing baby at its most critical stages of development. This is the time when sex, intelligence and future health are being determined. It is known that hormones taken by the mother in early pregnancy can increase the risk of cancer and genital abnormalities in her children.[25] The results of a study involving 5,700 pregnancies showed a remarkably low incidence of congenital abnormalities in children born to women who had never taken the Pill, compared to women who had regularly taken it.[26]

Depo-Provera and Noristerat are injectable progestogens (synthetic forms of progesterone). Provera carries the warning that its use in early pregnancy may increase the risk of early abortion or congenital deformities of the foetus. In order to give the body a chance to restore its natural hormone balance, women are generally advised to wait at least three months before attempting to conceive once they have stopped using the contraceptive pill. I recommend that you wait at least six months to allow the synthetic hormones to be eliminated from your body.

Natural family planning

Pregnancy will occur only if a viable sperm meets an egg. The egg survives for only up to 24 hours after release, whereas the sperm can survive for three to six days. It is therefore important to capture this period of time to maximise your chances of conception. Given that many cycles do not fit into the classic 28 days, it can be difficult to know when you have ovulated. There is a simple method available that can help you identify this. A good book to read on this subject is Marilyn Glenville's *Getting Pregnant Faster* (see Recommended Reading). Essentially, the method involves three steps:

1 **Checking cervical mucus** With increasing oestrogen levels, the cervical mucus changes at ovulation from being cloudy, thick and sticky to a more watery, clear and slippery fluid. It also becomes alkaline, which sperm like.

2 **Checking the cervix** Changes occur in the cervix in synchrony with the changes in the cervical mucus. When the egg is about to be fertilised, the mouth of the cervix opens, to enable the sperm to meet the egg. Otherwise the mouth of the cervix remains closed. The cervical mucus changes and becomes clear, slippery and stretchy, just like raw egg whites.

3 **Checking your temperature** The rise of progesterone just after ovulation increases body temperature by at least 0.2°C. This is a simple test that many women use to identify whether they have ovulated. In an average four-week cycle, ovulation usually takes place on day 14. By taking your temperature each day and recording it on a graph, you can easily tell when you have ovulated because your temperature will rise by at least 0.2°C. For those with longer, shorter or irregular cycles, the graph is a useful means of identifying when ovulation has occurred.

The success of the natural method depends on how motivated the woman wishing to become pregnant is and how well she has been taught. Some women do find it difficult to identify the different states of the cervical mucus, although one researcher found that 97 per cent of women could do so,[27] and others find the process of self-examination unpleasant.

Ovulation predictor kits, which are also useful, are now widely available in large chemists. Both the natural method and predictor kits can be used to avoid pregnancy, as well as enhancing the chances of becoming pregnant.

To find out more about making healthy babies, once you do conceive, and how to avoid problems during and after pregnancy, including how to wean your child, read my books *Optimum Nutrition Before, During and After Pregnancy* and the *Perfect Pregnancy Plan*, co-authored with Susannah Lawson and Fiona McDonald Joyce.

CHAPTER 12

Balancing Your Hormones During Pregnancy

There is no time when hormone balance is more important than during pregnancy. When conception takes place it triggers the increased production of both progesterone and oestrogen, as well as other hormones, which are essential to maintain a healthy pregnancy; inadequate levels of hormones are an extremely common cause of miscarriage. Some women sail through pregnancy whereas others experience awful sickness, especially during the first three months – this, again, is due to hormone imbalance. Also many women, despite looking forward to motherhood, find themselves suffering from the 'Baby Blues' after giving birth. For most women this is short-lived, lasting for a few days to a week or so, but for about one in ten, postnatal depression becomes more serious and long lasting.

In this chapter I want to address those problems associated with hormonal imbalances in pregnancy, and am grateful for the input of Dr Tony Coope who has worked with many women who have suffered from postnatal depression.

Minimising miscarriage risk

The first problem that can occur if a woman has a hormonal deficiency is a greater risk of miscarriage. As we saw in Chapter 1, the hormone progesterone is aptly named because it does everything to maintain a healthy pregnancy. When a woman becomes pregnant the corpus luteum keeps growing and producing progesterone. Too little, and the pregnancy cannot be maintained. In the case of many women who fail to become pregnant, or who experience early miscarriage, this is often the result of progesterone deficiency.

Although good nutrition is vital – by applying all the principles in Part 5 – it is also well worth getting your hormone levels checked. If you are deficient, I recommend taking a natural or bio-identical progesterone, delivered through the skin using a transdermal skin cream, at a level consistent with that which your body should be producing. Since progesterone rises from the time of ovulation this is normally started at the mid-point of the cycle, continued until menstruation, then stopped. If you become pregnant the transdermal progesterone should be continued for up to three months, after which the placenta is sufficiently developed and produces its own. How to use bio-identical hormones, and how to find a practitioner to prescribe them, is explained in Part 4.

Morning (noon and night) sickness

Another hormonal health problem, experienced by many women, is known as morning sickness, even though for some it lasts throughout the day.

During the first three months of pregnancy, all of the baby's organs are completely formed. It is during this period – and, of course, before conception – that optimum nutrition is most important. Yet many women experience continual sickness and don't feel like eating healthily. The most common signs and symptoms are nausea, which is usually worse on an empty stomach, and is often triggered by the smells of certain foods or perfumes; vomiting after eating; aversions to some foods and cravings for others; a metallic taste in the mouth; a feeling of hunger even when feeling nauseous; and relief from nausea by eating.

Pregnancy sickness is one example of a condition that usually only manifests in women whose nutritional status is less than optimum. It is probably caused by an increase in a hormone called human chorionic gonadotrophin (HCG), and women with poor diets are particularly at risk.[28] HCG is produced by the developing placenta from the moment of conception and it usually reaches its peak around nine to ten weeks after the last period, before declining by weeks 14–16. In very undernourished mothers, HCG may not be produced in sufficient quantities at all, which may explain why women who miscarry early are less likely to have experienced any pregnancy sickness. Conversely, very well nourished women appear to ride the storm of these hormonal changes with little or no symptoms of nausea at all.

Other possible explanations for nausea or sickness are connected to the body trying to eliminate toxins, or may involve difficulty maintaining blood sugar balance. Chapter 7 explains the importance of balancing your blood sugar level for hormonal health, and how to become a master of your blood sugar control. The diet I advocate also serves as a natural detox. The other important point is to make sure you are getting enough nutrients, especially B vitamins, since these can mitigate feelings of nausea. That is why it is very important to take the supplements recommended in Chapter 28. Far from being cautious about taking nutritional supplements during pregnancy, this is the time you really need to make sure you do. After all, you are building a baby as well as maintaining your own health.

If you still suffer, however, try the following:

- Always eat breakfast, preferably containing some protein foods such as yoghurt or eggs.

- Eat small meals and frequent snacks of fruit and seeds.

- Avoid refined and sugary foods – eat a low-GL diet instead.

- Avoid high-fat junk food containing long lists of additives and preservatives.

- Decrease your intake of dried fruit or undiluted fruit juice, both of which provide concentrated sugar.

- Drink plenty of water between meals.

- Avoid or decrease your intake of coffee and tea.

- Take a multivitamin containing a good level of all the B vitamins and zinc.

- If sickness persists, take 50mg of vitamin B_6 twice a day and 200–500mg of magnesium once a day until the sickness subsides.

- Ginger may also help to relieve the sickness and settle your stomach – take either in capsules or as tea.

Gestational diabetes

Gestational diabetes is an extreme form of poor blood glucose control (see Chapter 7), where the body is unable to maintain a constant energy level. It usually occurs during the second half of pregnancy and disappears after birth, but it can be an early warning sign of developing diabetes later in life. Your baby may be bigger, increasing the chances of Caesarean delivery, and baby also has a greater risk of developing diabetes. This condition affects up to three in every 100 women and manifests as a whole host of symptoms including fatigue, poor concentration, irritability, nervousness, depression, excessive thirst, sweating, headaches and digestive problems. If you are diagnosed with gestational diabetes, the diet outlined in this book will help you to control it. Specifically:

- Eat complex carbohydrates that release their energy slowly (such as rye bread, oats, brown rice and vegetables) and avoid refined carbohydrates (such as white bread, biscuits and cakes) and any foods with added sugar.

- Balance your meals and snacks with protein. So, eat some seeds and yoghurt with your breakfast cereal or have a boiled egg;

make sure main meals include some lean meat, fish, pulses or dairy products; and balance snacks – for example, have an apple with ten almonds, or hummus and carrot or celery sticks, or nut butter on oatcakes.

- Make sure you include lots of fibre in your diet, as this slows down the release of glucose into your blood. Eating plenty of whole grains will help, as will lots of vegetables and fruit (but balance your fruit with protein, as above).

- Take a multivitamin and mineral to boost nutrient levels, but supplement extra chromium, ideally in combination with a cinnamon extract called cinnulin, to specifically help your body manage glucose. Chromium – an essential mineral – is required for the insulin receptors to work in making insulin (the hormone that balances your blood sugar) more responsive. An extract in cinnamon, called MCHP, also helps. You can usually buy these combined. See Resources for suppliers.

Depression during pregnancy

About 10 per cent of pregnant women – 13 per cent to 15 per cent among new mothers – develop depression severe enough to interfere with their functioning. That's the equivalent of about 70,000 women a year suffering in the UK!

Many mothers experience the Baby Blues after the birth of the baby, which usually start around the time when the milk comes in (roughly the third day) and last just a few hours or days. Other women, however, suffer with depression after the birth. The symptoms are not surprising, given the intense and mixed emotions that a mother may suddenly feel on the birth of her baby, especially a firstborn; feelings of overwhelming love and protectiveness; and/ or terrifying responsibility and fears for the future. If the mother is particularly exhausted after a difficult or lengthy birth, she may experience feelings of guilt or inadequacy. If there is no past history of depression or other mental illness, then a positive and supportive cast of family and friends is all that is needed.

You can do a lot to reduce your risk of experiencing depression either before the birth or after by being optimally nourished while you are pregnant. Three main players in pregnancy-related depression are zinc, essential fats and hormonal deficiency.

In a study of 11,721 British women, researchers found that those who consumed greater amounts of seafood (a rich source of both essential fats and zinc) during the last three months of their pregnancy were less likely to show signs of major depression before and for up to eight months after the birth. Women with the highest intakes of omega-3, who consumed fish two or three times a week, were half as likely to suffer from depression as women with the lowest intakes.[29]

Before a woman gives birth, she transfers a large supply of zinc to her baby. Without a good supply herself, the chances are she will become deficient, especially if she goes on to have a long and difficult labour. Depression is a common side effect of zinc deficiency, as are white marks on more than two fingernails, a poor appetite, stretchmarks and a poor immune system. So if you have any of these additional symptoms, increase your supplementary zinc intake to 15mg twice a day until your mood improves. As zinc works with the B vitamin family, particularly B_6, also taking a multivitamin that provides at least 10mg of zinc, plus 20mg of B_6, is essential. The late Dr Carl Pfeiffer, one of the world's leading authorities on treating mental-health problems with nutrition, said, 'We have never seen postnatal depression or psychosis in any of our patients treated with zinc and B_6.' By following my hormonal health plan in Part 5, your intake of zinc and essential fats will be optimal.

If all this good nutrition doesn't work, the most likely reason for depression after the birth is a precipitous drop in the mother's progesterone level after the separation of the placenta from the womb, because the placenta is responsible for raising progesterone levels by as much as 50 times during the pregnancy itself. There is some disagreement about this in different quarters of the medical profession, as oestrogen shows a similar (but less dramatic) fall, and there are also other factors to consider, which I address on page 233.

Dr Tony Coope adds:

This fall can be the trigger for a more serious, and longer-lasting depression called PND or postnatal depression. Apart from the misery experienced by these mothers, and the knock-on stress and unhappiness to partners and families, this also creates a serious potential disruption in the bonding process between mother and baby. If she is not fully present mentally or emotionally in the first 9–12 months of the baby's life, this can lead to problems of self-esteem and the ability to relate to others, which in turn has an effect on the child's future chances of achieving fulfilment in work and love.

In more extreme cases, self-destructive 'borderline' and narcissistic personality disorders can develop in such children, with painful consequences for them, their family and all that come into contact with them. This is well covered by Dr James F. Masterson in his book *The Search for the Real Self*. In a way, all the fundamental problems of life start here, with the cycles of difficulties being passed on from one generation to the next.

In addition, symptoms of the mother's depression may be hidden from family and friends by her apparently 'bright' exterior until, in the most severe cases, the devastating reality of suicide comes like a bolt out of the blue. In the past I have spoken in depth to several women who fortunately failed in their attempt, recovered fully, and were aghast at what they so nearly had done.

On each occasion of this very severe form of PND, the pattern was the same: they had become overwhelmed and confused, and depression was robbing them of motivation until they seemed to improve and the family were beginning to relax. Behind the lighter façade, however, there came a point where it became extremely clear to the mother that she believed her life was of no value, and that her husband and even their children really would be better off without her. With this belief she felt great peace, becoming even more able to hide her very clear intentions. If taken to the final conclusion, these events are tragic in the fullest sense of the word.

The third degree of postpartum illness is known as puerperal psychosis (from the Latin *puerpera* meaning 'woman in childbirth').

This is much rarer than PND, occurring in only one or two mothers per thousand, so an individual GP may see only two or three cases in a working lifetime, out of an official incidence of 700–1,400 in the UK a year. Although a tiny proportion of the number of births (0.1–0.2 per cent), it contributes disproportionately to the sum of human pain.

This depression is usually sudden and acute, sometimes immediately after the birth. Persisting anxiety, insomnia and agitation are early signs, followed by suspicion, confusion, bizarre thoughts and sometimes rejection of the baby. In more extreme cases mania or schizophrenia-like symptoms may appear, with paranoia, delusions, hallucinations and an irrational disconnection of thought and feeling. Thus the mother may struggle to resist horrifying thoughts of murder, but never confide these to anyone for fear her child may be taken away.

Puerperal psychosis is a much more dangerous condition than PND. It is much more difficult for carers and family to deal with. There is always the possibility of violence to self, baby or others, and for these reasons urgent hospital admission is usually the best option. Especially because it is often impossible to be sure of what is going on in the mother's mind.

Treating PND

Given the importance of these illnesses in the postnatal period, what are the best forms of prevention and treatment? Set against all the above is the compelling work of two doctors – Katharina Dalton in the UK and John Lee in the US – who both extensively studied the roles of bio-identical progesterone, the former in post-partum illness and PMS, the latter more in the menopause and peri-menopause. Dr Dalton's excellent work seems to have been forgotten by the medical mainstream, possibly because of her 'larger than life' personality and lack of 'rigorous' research methods. Her book *Depression After Childbirth* is, however, a classic.

If we also take into account the personal experience in the use of progesterone of the relatively small number of doctors in the UK, a broader perspective emerges. So how can we make coherent sense of this? The answer lies in the precipitous drop in progesterone, and to a lesser extent oestrogen, after birth. This has a destabilising effect on the emotional resilience and resistance to stress of the majority of mothers (70–80 per cent). If they are psychologically and emotionally stable, however, the effects are short lived – hence the Baby Blues.

If the mother is more vulnerable, such as having a previous history of depression or PMS, then depression is the result. If she is more severely vulnerable, with a more defined previous mental/emotional instability, then psychosis is the result.

Thus the abrupt hormonal change is the 'trigger', acting on the stability or otherwise of the mother and altering the threshold at which these symptoms appear. With regard to the differing views of doctors and researchers, each discipline – whether psychiatrists, gynaecologists or family doctors – all see the problem through the filters of their own training, conditioning and experience. Each leans towards the interpretation with which he or she is most comfortable. Neither should we forget that there are different groups of patients who will be subtly drawn to the doctors that are in alignment with their own beliefs and symptoms.

That said, my own experience is mainly of women who are relatively 'oestrogen dominant' in relation to progesterone and whose symptoms worsen if prescribed oestrogen. I believe this problem is likely to become increasingly prevalent with the passage of time.

Regarding prevention and treatment, Tony Coope and I believe the best option in postnatal illness to be a combination of the appropriate therapy for the depression or psychosis (which I explain in my book *The Feel Good Factor*) and bio-identical progesterone in cream or pessary form to reduce the likelihood of the postpartum fall in hormones triggering symptoms (see Chapter 24).

There's a lot you need to know to maximise your chances of a trouble-free pregnancy, and a healthy baby as a result, but that is not the purpose of this chapter. My book *Optimum Nutrition Before, During and After Pregnancy*, explains all this. The book is co-authored with nutritional therapist Susannah Lawson, a Foresight practitioner who specialises in preconceptual care.

Summary

If you are suffering from pregnancy sickness or postnatal blues it's really important to:

- Get your nutrition up to scratch by eating a healthy low-GL diet.
- Supplement a high-potency multivitamin, possibly with extra B_6, folic acid, zinc and magnesium as well as omega-3 and 6 essential fats.
- Have your hormones checked, especially if you are experiencing chronic Baby Blues – you may need natural progesterone (see Chapter 24).

CHAPTER 13

The Secrets of a Trouble-free Menopause

Usually, when a woman is in her forties she enters what is known as the peri-menopausal phase, during which she has more menstrual cycles when ovulation doesn't occur even though menstruation appears normal. These cycles are followed by more irregular menstrual periods and some symptoms associated with the menopause. Finally, when she is in her fifties, her periods will stop completely. The menopause should occur gradually, allowing the body to adapt to the changes with ease – this is controlled by the female hormones.

With the menopause is the increased risk of osteoporosis, breast cancer or heart disease but, for many women, it is not the fear of those illnesses that most concerns them but how to cope with the debilitating symptoms that affect their daily lives: the hot flushes, vaginal dryness, joint pains, fatigue, headaches, irritability, insomnia, depression and decreased sex drive. The degree to which a woman experiences any or all of these symptoms is highly dependent on how good her nutrition is. Indeed, you don't have to suffer at all.

Case Study: *Karen S*

Here's what Karen told me in relation to her plethora of health issues that accumulated around the menopausal years:

> 'My weight had ballooned up to 15 stone [95.25kg/210lb], partly due to stress. A blood test confirmed I was going through the menopause and a scan had confirmed that my bone density in my lower spine was getting thinner. I felt I needed to sort my life out. In December 2004, I started your low-GL diet. I did the homocysteine test and the food intolerance test. My homocysteine result came back high so I have added supplements to help reduce it. Bread was out, as was milk, replaced by soya products. I also reduced chocolate and tea considerably. I added more vegetables, fruit and supplements. I do Psychocalisthenics [an exercise system I recommend, see Appendix 6] four or five times per week and also use my rebounder. I aimed to lose a pound [450g] a week. I have lost weight and inches, I feel much calmer and in control of my life. Psychocalisthenics and then 20 minutes on the rebounder makes me feel so much better, there is a definite calm, but a good feeling afterwards. Mood swings are less evident now. Overall I feel good.'

What is it that makes the menopause so potentially dramatic in effect? It happens when a woman's production of oestrogen and progesterone begin to decline because they are no longer needed to prepare the womb lining for pregnancy. As oestrogen levels fall, the menstrual flow becomes lighter and often irregular, until eventually it stops altogether. Even before the menopause, often when a woman is in her forties, many cycles occur in which an egg is not released. These are known as anovulatory cycles. Whenever this happens, levels of progesterone, produced from the sac that's left once the egg has been released, decline rapidly.

Progesterone is oestrogen's alter ego and the two need to be kept in the right balance. Too much oestrogen relative to progesterone – so-called 'oestrogen dominance' – results in too many growth signals to cells of the breast and womb, raising the risk of cancer.

Consequently, many women in their forties, although low in oestrogen, are in a state of oestrogen dominance because their progesterone levels are even lower.

Symptoms of oestrogen dominance can include water retention, breast tenderness, mood swings, weight gain around the hips and thighs, depression, loss of libido and cravings for sweets. The symptoms of progesterone deficiency overlap these, and also include insomnia, irregular periods, lower body temperature and menstrual cramps.

Many of these symptoms can show up during the menopause along with the more common hot flushes, vaginal dryness, and other symptoms described above. So, if your hormones are in real disarray, you experience a distressing burden of symptoms. There is much you can do about this, however, but women are rarely told by their doctors how they can help themselves to cope with the menopause naturally. The usual remedy that doctors used to prescribe with some success was HRT; however, since the risk of HRT increasing breast cancer is now well known, many doctors – and women – are unwilling to go down this route. To read about the chequered history of HRT, see Chapter 23. The intelligent use of bio-identical hormones, which I explain in Part 4, is a valid alternative; but before considering even bio-identical hormones there's a lot that you can do for yourself. The best way to start is to complete the questionnaire on pages 324–7 – if you haven't done so already – to find out how well balanced your hormones are at the moment. Then read on and follow the advice that relates to you.

Hot flushes – how to turn the heat down

Three-quarters of all British menopausal women, particularly those who are thin, experience some hot flushes. These are not directly a sign of oestrogen deficiency, but a result of increased activity of the hypothalamus gland in the brain, which makes two hormones – follicle stimulating hormone (FSH) and luteinising hormone (LH). Extra-high levels of these two hormones occur as the menopause approaches, in an attempt by the brain to stimulate any remaining eggs to develop. Meanwhile, oestrogen levels fall, ovulation becomes infrequent and progesterone levels decline rapidly. Using 'natural' or bio-identical progesterone cream has been shown to help. (This is discussed in detail in Chapter 24.) Although wild yam extract, which can be processed in a lab to produce progesterone but doesn't actually contain any progesterone, doesn't appear to work.[30]

Supplementation with phytoestrogens, which are structurally and functionally similar to the body's own oestrogen, has been shown to reduce the frequency and severity of hot flushes. Four studies show that the oestrogen-like, plant-derived substances known as isoflavones, found in high concentrations in soya and red clover, approximately halve the incidence and severity of hot flushes.[31] While some studies have not found this effect (at least at a level of statistical significance), they have shown that the higher the isoflavone levels in the urine of the women studied, the lower the incidence of hot flushes.[32] This suggests that a high intake of isoflavones from diet or supplements is likely to help reduce hot flushes in some women, but not all. This is certainly consistent with the low incidence of hot flushes in Chinese women with a daily intake of soya. I recommend fermented sources of soya where possible, including miso, tempeh, natto and tamari. Tofu, soya milk and soya yoghurt contain less phytoestrogens than fermented sources and also have other disadvantages, as explained in Chapter 27. Highly processed forms of soya like burgers often have very little. Opt for organic, not genetically modified, sources of soya.

If you have dysglycemia (see Chapter 7) – which means your blood sugar level goes up and down like a yo-yo – you are much more likely to experience fatigue, irritability, depression and hot flushes. Specifically, research has found that when you have a blood sugar low this can trigger a hot flush.[33] By keeping your blood sugar level even through 'grazing' rather than gorging, and by choosing low-GL foods, you can considerably reduce the number of hot flushes you have. The advice here is no different from that for preventing diabetes: eat a low-GL diet and consider supplementing chromium. For more details see Chapter 7.

Other nutrients that may help during the menopause are vitamins C,[34] E and essential fats (both omega-3 and omega-6). Choose a vitamin C supplement that contains berry extracts rich in bioflavonoids, as there's some evidence that these help too. When vitamin E levels are low, there is a tendency for FSH and LH to increase. Vitamin E also helps to stabilise hormone levels and has been reported to help alleviate vaginal dryness.

Helpful herbs

The most promising of the herbs used to treat the symptoms of menopause is black cohosh, which can help reduce hot flushes, sweating, insomnia and anxiety. This is one of most commonly used herbs by women in China. Three double-blind trials have been published.[35] One showed no effect, the other was beneficial and the third showed reduced sweating but no reduction in the number of hot flushes. Also encouraging is new research that seems to indicate that black cohosh neither increases cancer risk nor is anti-oestrogenic.[36] It also helps relieve depression by raising serotonin levels. Even so, I'd recommend that you take black cohosh three months on, one month off, and avoid it if you are taking liver-toxic drugs or have a damaged liver. Take 50mg twice a day.

The other 'hot' herb for hot flushes is dong quai, whose scientific name is *Angelica sinensis*. In one placebo-controlled study from 2003, 55 post-menopausal women who were given dong quai and chamomile instead of HRT had an 80 per cent reduction in hot flushes. These results became apparent after one month.[37] An earlier study didn't find this effect, however.[38] If you want to try dong quai, which doesn't appear to have oestrogenic or cancer-promoting properties, I recommend 600mg a day for relief from hot flushes.

Another popular herb, Vitex agnus castus (also called chasteberry), can also help with hot flushes, although it is most well known for being helpful for menstrual irregularities, PMS (see Chapter 8), and especially for the symptoms of breast tenderness. Agnus castus's therapeutic powers, proven in a series of double-blind trials in 2005, are attributed to its indirect effects on decreasing oestrogen levels while increasing progesterone and prolactin.[39] Raised prolactin is known to lower oestrogen levels. In most trials, 4mg a day of a standardised extract (containing 6 per cent agnusides – one of the active ingredients) was used.

Side effects There are no known serious adverse effects from black cohosh or agnus castus (although it is always wise to be cautious about herbs during pregnancy and when breast-feeding). Dong quai may thin the blood and is therefore contraindicated for women on blood-thinning drugs such as warfarin.

Exercise and belly breathing

Both regular exercise and learning how to breathe deeply have proven benefits for menopausal symptoms (see box below). According to a 2003 study conducted at Lund University in Sweden, if you stay active you can reduce the impact of menopausal symptoms. Researchers interviewed nearly 4,500 women 58 to 68 years old about their sociodemographic, lifestyle and current health conditions. They found that women who did more vigorous physical exercise were less likely to suffer from hot flushes.[40]

Breathing from the belly

The basic principle of all breathing exercises is to use your diaphragm, rather than the top of your chest as we tend to do when we are anxious or stressed. If you're unsure where the diaphragm is, it's the dome-shaped muscle at the bottom of the lungs. Three trials have shown that this type of breathing can reduce the frequency of hot flushes by about 50 per cent.[41]

Breathing in this way works best at the start of a hot flush. Breathing from the diaphragm is part of many health systems such as yoga. (See

cont ▶

Appendix 6, page 340, for more precise instructions on this kind of breathing.) The exercise system Psychocalisthenics, which takes 15 minutes a day to do, combines this kind of breathing with exercises that keep you strong and supple. It is excellent for minimising menopausal symptoms and improving your vitality and mood. See www.patrickholford.com/psychocalisthenics.

Sexual problems

A lack of sex drive can result for a variety of reasons, not all nutritional. Chapter 10 discusses some of the other possible causes.

Vaginal dryness is another reason for declining interest in sex. The vagina is kept moist because it produces vaginal secretions, but declining oestrogen levels tend to dry up these secretions; however, the adrenal glands continue to produce oestrogens, as do fat cells, during and after the menopause. Supplementing vitamins A, C and E plus zinc, are also important for keeping vaginal membranes healthy and encouraging normal mucus production. These nutrients are available in good high-potency multivitamin and mineral supplements, which are worth taking on a daily basis. Vitamin E cream used locally has helped many women with vaginitis. There's also evidence that a phytoestrogen-rich soya-based gel can help.[42]

There are also natural hormone creams that help, especially if you are deficient in hormones; for example, progesterone. Natural oestrogen creams such as Ovestin, which provides the much gentler oestriol, have been successful in treating dryness and vaginitis and can also reduce the occurrence of urinary tract infections, restore normal vaginal mucous membranes, and provide the right environment in the vagina to inhibit the growth of unfriendly organisms. The late Dr Lee found that, when women used progesterone creams rubbed into the skin to treat their vaginitis, they experienced similar benefits to those using oestrogen cream. Progesterone cream is preferable for women who are advised against using oestrogen therapy because of a history of breast, ovarian or uterine cancer; however, hormonal creams should be given with the supervision of a medical doctor familiar with their use. These are discussed in Chapter 24.

Vaginitis

As a woman nears the menopause, mucus production in the vagina changes, alongside declining levels of oestrogen. Vaginal infections are more common at this time and women on the Pill appear more susceptible. The oral contraceptive pill suppresses natural hormone production and it may be as a result of this that mucus production is affected.

Natural progesterone can help post-menopausal women with recurring urinary and vaginal infections, helping to lessen symptoms and improve mucus production. Oestrogen replacement may be inappropriate for some women who might be at risk of breast or uterine cancer.

Insomnia

There are many factors that underpin our ability to stay well. These include eating a good diet, keeping hydrated, breathing properly, daily exercise, having a positive frame of mind and, importantly, getting good quality sleep; however, women the world over sleep less as they get older, which may be a protective mechanism so that the young are protected by their elders in the small hours. As long as the sleep you experience is refreshing, if you wake up early it's best to get up to do something productive and enjoy the peace, rather than worrying about not sleeping. For those of you who like to meditate, the early hours of the morning are reputed to be the best time and can compensate for sleep.

There are a number of ways to ensure you get all the sleep you need. Stimulants, such as caffeine in tea and coffee, and nicotine in cigarettes, can disrupt sleeping patterns and are best avoided, or at least limited after midday. Caffeine also acts as a diuretic, causing frequent visits to the bathroom during the night. Green tea (as previously discussed under PMS), chamomile or lime blossom tea have relaxing properties. So too does the mineral magnesium, which is found plentifully in green, leafy vegetables and in nuts and seeds.

Oats and a particular type of cherry, called Montmorency, are natural sources of the hormone melatonin, which is derived from serotonin. Melatonin is the hormone that aids sleep and is also a powerful antioxidant. A hot or cold glass of Montmorency cherry juice not only tastes good but should also help you to achieve quality sleep. You could also consider a bowl of oats in the evening rather than for breakfast. The meadow grass *Festuca arundina*, known as asphalia, is also a good natural source of melatonin. Both Montmorency cherries and *Festuca arundina* are available for supplementation in capsule form (see Resources).

Hundreds of people have also reported great results listening to a CD called *Silence of Peace*; this is piano music that is specifically designed to put you into the 'alpha' brain-wave state that is the prerequisite of sleep (see Resources).

My favourite strategy for sleep is caffeine avoidance; taking a combination supplement providing both 5-HTP, magnesium and calming herbs an hour before bed; and listening to *Silence of Peace* as you go to sleep. If this doesn't work, try melatonin, available on prescription or over the counter in most countries outside the EU. Start with 3mg.

Preventing headaches

Some headaches are caused by blood vessels in the head narrowing, possibly as a result of declining oestrogen levels, since oestrogen dilates blood vessels, improving blood flow. Coffee, alcohol and red wine frequently give rise to headaches, as can a food allergy, candidiasis, or glucose imbalance. This is covered in detail in Chapter 15.

Reducing menopausal joint pains

There are many reasons for joint pains, but following the Diet for the Good Life in Chapter 26 is the place to start for reducing any symptoms. Weight management, supported by a balanced diet and exercise, is key to preventing and managing joint pains; however, you may need to reconsider the type of exercise that is best for you at a later stage if you continue to have pain.

Vitamin B_6 supplementation has been shown to help painful nodules on finger joints if treated early. Vitamin B_6, like all B vitamins, is best taken as part of a B complex. Food intolerance may become more prevalent at the menopause and can be a cause or contributor to joint pains. Wheat and dairy produce are the most common offenders (see Chapter 6). The omega-3 fat EPA has potent anti-inflammatory properties and can help to reduce the inflammation that contributes to joint pain. Vitamin B_6, B_3, biotin and vitamin C, plus the minerals zinc, calcium and magnesium, all play an important role in helping essential fats create anti-inflammatory prostaglandins. Too much red meat and full-fat dairy produce, on the other hand, help to create too much of a type of prostaglandin that in excess increases inflammation in the body. Culinary herbs like turmeric and ginger, as well as red onions and olives, also contain natural anti-inflammatories. Progesterone has anti-inflammatory properties. My book *Say No to Arthritis* explains everything you can do to banish joint aches and pains, including the role of supplements containing glucosamine and potent natural anti-inflammatories (see Resources). Dr John Lee found with many of his patients that rubbing progesterone cream directly onto the joint or tissue that hurts was helpful. As previously mentioned, natural progesterone is best used under the direction of a medical doctor familiar with its use.

Preventing memory loss

If you are worried about losing your memory as you age I cannot stress enough how important it is to eat well now to prevent this happening; however, even this may not provide enough nutrients, especially vitamin B_{12}, which is increasingly poorly absorbed as you age. All the evidence suggests that both age-related memory loss and Alzheimer's is, in almost all cases, completely preventable if you follow the right diet, take the correct supplements and have a healthy and active lifestyle. (My book *The Alzheimer's Prevention Plan* explains exactly how to do this.) Increasing your intake of B vitamins, omega-3 fats and antioxidants all contribute to reducing your risk. B vitamins, especially B_{12}, folic acid and B_6, are most important because they lower your level of homocysteine, which I discussed on page 65.

Acetylcholine, another neurotransmitter, is important for memory, particularly the first stage of memory, called encoding. This first stage includes the initial making of the memory and, to an extent, the second stage of consolidating memory; that is, the creation of long-term memories.

Acetylcholine is made from choline, a vital nutrient found in fish, organ meats and, especially, eggs. It is also found richly in lecithin granules and capsules, derived from soya, for vegetarians. B vitamins are needed to help convert it into the memory-boosting acetylcholine.

Hormones and your mind

There's a strong link between hormones, your mind and mood. Serotonin, acetycholine and noradrenalin (made from dopamine) are thought to be the most important neurotransmitters involved in memory. Oestrogen stimulates receptors for serotonin and noradrenalin in the brain and also seems to slow the process of these neurotransmitters being broken down. Similarly oestrogen helps raise levels of acetylcholine.

Oestrogen appears to have a mild ability to dilate blood vessels, helping to improve blood flow and nutrient supply to the brain, and helping the brain to function more efficiently; however, studies using oestrogen hormone replacement therapy (ERT) have largely proved inconclusive. The risks and benefits also need to be considered in terms of the increased risk of breast and uterine cancer associated with ERT.

If you are concerned about your memory, or have a family history of early cognitive decline read *The Alzheimer's Prevention Plan* and consider getting your homocysteine level tested (see Resources) as this is one of the best predictors of risk. Homocysteine is lowered by increasing your intake of vitamins B_6, B_{12} and folic acid. A nutritional therapist can assess your risk and advise on how to reverse it.

Solving menopausal mood dips

The causes of depression are many, and some of them can be helped by nutrition. Causes can include neurotransmitter and hormonal imbalances, stress, blood sugar imbalances, nutrient deficiencies, secondary to chronic and life-threatening illness, chronic pain, loss and social deprivation. Our mood is very dependent on the foods we eat, so implementing the Diet for the Good Life (see Chapter 26) provides a sound basis for supporting your mood.

As discussed above, oestrogen appears to improve the function of serotonin and noradrenalin and, through this mechanism, improve mood; however, the risks and benefits of using HRT, as discussed above and in Part 4, need careful consideration. For natural ways to support serotonin, GABA and dopamine production, see Chapter 8, and also the discussion in Chapter 15 regarding an important enzyme called monoamine oxidase.

An elevated level of homocysteine is also increasingly linked to depression (see Chapter 7). Omega-3 fish oil and supplements of 5-HTP have proven particularly effective.

St John's wort, a herb renowned for its antidepressant effects, has been demonstrated to relieve other menopausal symptoms, including headaches, palpitations, lack of concentration and decreased libido. In fact, a German study found that 80 per cent of women felt their symptoms had gone or substantially improved at the end of 12 weeks.[43] The combination of black cohosh and St John's wort (300mg a day) can be particularly effective for women who are experiencing menopause-related depression, irritability and fatigue.[44]

St John's wort, at this dosage, has no reported serious adverse effects, but be aware that it is best to consult your doctor if you are on an antidepressant. Work with a nutritional therapist to help identify triggers that may be contributing to your depression or low mood. There are a number of nutritional and hormone-related tests that could help in the design of a programme more personalised to your needs. The Brain Bio Centre, my clinic in Richmond, London, specialises in a nutritional approach to depression and other mental health problems.

Preventing associated increased risk of heart disease and stroke

Deaths related to disorders of the circulatory system have shown a steady decline since the 1970s, and particularly over the last decade; however, circulatory disorders remain the leading cause of death in women after the menopause.

Although oestrogen is known to reduce coronary heart disease and stroke in post-menopausal women, studies demonstrate that long-term use of HRT, or oestrogen replacement, can increase the incidence of breast cancer, stroke and heart attacks, not reduce it, as was suggested back in the 1980s and 1990s.

Apart from eating more fruit and vegetables, upping your intake of omega-3s from fish, nuts and seeds, and increasing your intake of homocysteine-lowering B vitamins are essential for reducing risk. Stroke and heart attack risk is better predicted by homocysteine than by cholesterol, and better lowered with B vitamins than drugs. Exercise also helps reduce risk, as does increasing your intake of antioxidant nutrients. All these steps help to reduce oxidative stress, which is the process by which we age.

Oxidative stress, meaning an excess of oxidants to antioxidants, is also associated with accelerated brain degeneration. The brain consumes a lot of oxygen, has a relatively low antioxidant capacity, and has a high content of polyunsaturated fats, prone to oxidation, and minerals, like iron, which increase the likelihood of oxidative damage to the brain.

Even under the best of conditions, about 5 per cent of oxygen is converted to potentially damaging oxidants. Just through the process of breathing, fighting infections and converting fuels into energy we produce oxidants. Dietary antioxidants help to a large extent, but we all age and eventually die.

An excess of oxidants is implicated in most chronic illnesses, including ageing itself. Antioxidant nutrients and compounds shown to be of potential benefit include lipoic acid, acetyl-l-carnitine, CoQ_{10} and vitamin E. Other compounds that have been shown to have benefical effects include phosphatidylcholine, phosphatidyl serine, omega-3 fats, omega-6 fats and B vitamins, especially folic acid and B_{12}. Compounds showing memory-boosting potential include turmeric, green tea, blueberries and resveratrol, an antioxidant found in red grapes.

Combine good nutrition with exercise

The benefits of regular exercise throughout life cannot be overstated. Weight management, mood, concentration, sleep and memory may all be improved by good exercise, which helps to supply nutrients to the brain. Both improving your diet and increasing your exercise is the winning formula, as the following study illustrates.

The study followed 21 women using HRT and 27 non-HRT users over 24 weeks through supervised aerobic exercise three times a week. The women were at least two years post-menopause and between the ages of 50 and 75. The participants' diets were stabilised for six weeks on the American Heart Association Step 1 Diet, which was low in saturated fats, rich in fruits, vegetables, whole grains and fat-free or low-fat dairy products.

Oxidative stress, as previously discussed, results when there is too much free radical activity and inadequate antioxidant reserves. The generation of excess free radicals has long been implicated in heart disease and stroke, and post-menopausal women have been found to have higher levels of oxidative stress. Although high-intensity aerobic

cont ▶

exercise is associated with oxidative stress, what was shown is that moderate-intensity exercise appeared to reduce oxidative stress in these women by increasing the activity of antioxidants. Both HRT and non-HRT users had an 11–18 per cent drop in markers associated with oxidative stress. Exercise also has profound effects on keeping your bones strong and protecting you from osteoporosis (see below).

Get moving on the menopause

The two main forms of exercise that boost the health of your bones and increase bone mass are weight-bearing exercise and resistance exercise. Note that the recommendations here are for both younger people and women in the menopause, as prevention is vital.

A weight-bearing exercise is one where bones and muscles work against the force of gravity. This is any exercise in which your feet and legs carry your weight. Examples are walking, jogging, dancing and climbing stairs.

Resistance exercise involves moving your body weight or objects to create resistance. This type of exercise uses the body areas individually, which also strengthens the bone in that particular area.

For women before the menopause

You can either do all the following suggestions or a combination of them based on your level of fitness:

- Jumping or skipping on the spot (50 jumps daily).
- Jogging or walking for 30 minutes (five to seven days per week).
- Resistance weight training (two or three times per week).
- High-impact circuit or aerobic-style class (one or two times per week).

For post-menopausal women

You can either do all of the following suggestions or a combination of them based on your level of fitness:

- Weight training (one set of 8–12 repetitions using maximum effort. If 12 can be reached on a regular basis then the weight is slightly too light).

- Jogging/walking for 10–20 minutes (five to seven days per week).

- Stair climbing (10 flights of 10 steps per day).

- Exercise classes such as yoga or aqua aerobics (one or two per week).

(The above regime is also suitable for men over 50.)

With thanks to Joe Sharpe for compiling this information.

Although you can try any of these recommendations individually, a combination of all these herbs, nutrients, diet and lifestyle suggestions will yield the best results.

Summary

In summary, if you do your best to bring most of these pieces together into your diet and lifestyle, and take the right supplements, the chances are that any menopausal symptoms you experience will be minor and short-lived.

- Eat good sources of phytoestrogens every day, including beans, chickpeas or fermented soya products such as miso, tempeh, natto and tamari (not too much of this as it is high in salt). You probably need the equivalent of 30–40g a day for an effect, which is about one cupful.

cont ▶

- Up your intake of anti-ageing antioxidants by eating lots of brightly coloured fruits and vegetables.
- Balance your blood sugar by eating a low-GL diet (see Chapter 7) and possibly supplementing chromium, 200mcg in the morning.
- Take a high-strength multivitamin, with an additional vitamin C supplement (1–2g) that also contains berry extracts, and an essential-fat capsule containing both omega-3 and omega-6 oils.
- Check your homocysteine level. If it's high, supplement additional folic acid, B_6 and B_{12} (see Chapter 7) accordingly.
- Consider using natural, or bio-identical hormones, prescribable by your doctor (see Part 4).
- Try these herbs: black cohosh (50mg a day) or dong quai (600mg a day) with 300mg St John's wort a day if you're prone to depression, or Vitex agnus castus (4mg a day of a standardised extract).
- Get fit with frequent weight-bearing exercise to minimise your risk of osteoporosis.
- Learn 'belly breathing' and Psychocalisthenics (see Appendix 6) or join a yoga class.

PART 3

STAYING FREE FROM HORMONE-RELATED DISEASES

In this part I'll delve into the more chronic and serious health problems that often result from hormonal imbalances. These are the insidious health issues – from polycystic ovaries to endometriosis, breast disease and osteoporosis – that can only be solved by understanding the complex factors that contribute to their origin.

CHAPTER 14

Underactive Thyroid – A Common Cause of Chronic Fatigue

The thyroid hormone thyroxine is produced from a tiny gland that curves across the windpipe just below your Adam's apple; its job is to keep the body working at the right pace. Too much and everything goes too fast – you lose weight, you can't sleep and your heart races; too little and your system slows down, causing fatigue, low sex drive, low body temperature, weight gain, poor memory, dry skin and constipation. Regulating thyroid function helps prevent the development of many chronic diseases associated with ageing. Thyroid problems are not connected to the female hormones and affect men and women, although women are more likely to be affected with certain thyroid problems than men.

Many people who feel tired all the time unknowingly have underactive thyroid function – known as hypothyroidism. This is often the result of poor nutrition, too much sugar and refined carbohydrates, caffeine and prolonged stress or intake of certain drugs which can damage your thyroid. A less common cause of an underactive thyroid is an autoimmune disease, Hashimoto's disease, whereby your body makes antibodies that attack the thyroxine-producing cells. This is associated with food allergies (see Chapter 6). Some women may also develop hypothyroidism after pregnancy. Radiation treatments and congenital defects of the thyroid gland are other causes. Patient groups, such as Thyroid-UK – set up in 1999 to fight for better treatment for this condition – claim pollutants and even a lack of fruit and vegetables can also reduce your thyroid gland's output.

Testing your thyroid

The official medical line is that if the level of a marker for thyroid levels in your blood is within the 'normal' range, then you aren't hypothyroid and you shouldn't be given a hormone supplement; however, many practitioners report great results in people given low levels of thyroxine who have all the symptoms of an underactive thyroid, but only low–normal blood levels of thyroxine.

In fact, whether you are found to be inside or outside the normal range can depend on where the test is being done. In the UK, the healthy range for the most commonly used test – known as TSH (thyroid stimulating hormone) – is between 0.5 and 5, although many experts will refuse to treat a patient until the level reaches 10 (the job of TSH is to make the thyroid produce more thyroxine, so when it is high it means the thyroid is in trouble). Yet four years ago, the American Association of Clinical Endocrinologists recommended that: 'Doctors consider treatment for patients who test outside a TSH range of 0.3 to 3.' Thyroid expert Dr Leonard Wartofsky, from the Department of Medicine at Washington Hospital Center in the US, thinks an upper level of 3 may even be too high. 'According to the latest thinking, the upper level should be about 2.5,' he says. 'My UK colleagues say there's no evidence that treating below 10 is beneficial but I'd say it was mixed; studies showing benefit are coming in. We certainly see dramatic improvements in patients treated within UK reference levels here.'[1]

So there is certainly hot academic debate going on about just what counts as a healthy thyroid level. In fact, as Lynn Mynott of Thyroid-UK points out: 'The Department of Health guidelines say that "blood tests are useful but should not be used in isolation".' In other words, you need to take symptoms into account as well.

Testing for thyroid problems

So the first thing to do if you are worried about your thyroid levels and have had them tested by the doctor, is not to accept vague phrases about their being 'high' or 'low' but instead to ask for actual numbers and what the testing lab considers to be a normal range. If possible, get a copy of the actual report.

If the report shows that your TSH level is above 2.5 or 3 and you are told that this is normal, point out that the American Association of Clinical Endocrinologists (AACE) now recommends treating when TSH goes above 3.

A more detailed test is the Total Thyroid Screen which tests for TSH, anti-thyroid antibodies and the two kinds of thyroxine (your thyroid hormone) called T4 and T3. Thyroid hormones are made from the amino acid tyrosine, which is converted into T4 then T3, the active form of thyroxine. How this works is shown below. A nutritional therapist can arrange this test for you.

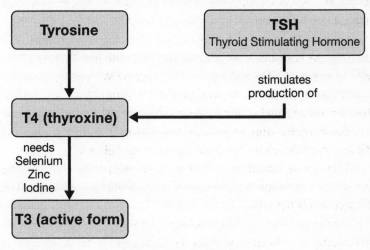

The thyroxine pathway

Sometimes you can have a normal T4 but a low T3, which means your ability to convert T4 into T3 is below par and you may feel tired as a result. If this is the case, follow the nutritional guidelines below.

If your TSH is high, but your thyroxine levels (T4 and T3) are normal, one possibility is that you have no problem making enough, but have excess circulating oestrogen, which competes with thyroxine at hormone receptor sites. In other words, the message isn't getting through. Eating a lot of dairy products can promote excess oestrogen, so reduce or exclude dairy, but do increase nuts or seeds to make sure you get enough calcium.

Having too much cortisol, the stress hormone, can also compete with thyroxine. So stress can play a part too. Cortisol is also stimulated by blood sugar imbalances.

With all the mainstream emphasis on blood tests, the issue of thyroid dysfunction diagnosis has become a highly controversial one. Much of this controversy has swirled around Dr Barry Peatfield, who has been treating thyroid patients holistically for a long time. He had his licence suspended by the General Medical Council in 2001 for this approach and has since resigned; he now runs a complementary therapy clinic – The Peatfield Clinic for Metabolic Health (see Resources). His book *The Great British Thyroid Scandal* is well worth a read if you have thyroid problems.

Dr Peatfield is one of a growing number of thyroid experts who don't rely on blood tests alone, but also diagnose low thyroid on the basis of symptoms as well as a detailed physical examination. He frequently asks patients to use the Barnes temperature test, which involves taking your temperature first thing before rising on five consecutive mornings (for women, in the first half of their cycle). If it falls below 36.6°C, it can be a sign of hypothyroidism.

Although some doctors dismiss it as unreliable, Dr Peatfield claims it is supported by good evidence and that it gives a more accurate picture of the state of your system than the snapshot provided by a blood test.

Anti-thyroid antibodies

A thorough investigation of thyroid function should always include measuring for the presence of 'anti-thyroid antibodies'. Some research groups find that more than half those with underactive thyroids have anti-thyroid antibodies[2] so this really is something that should be tested. If positive, this indicates that you have an autoimmune condition, where your body produces antibodies that attack the thyroid. If so, there's a good chance you may have an unidentified food allergy. What appears to happen, in some cases, is that your immune system reacts against a food protein (the most common being wheat, milk and soya) and cross-reacts against thyroid tissue. So the next step is to test yourself with an IgG food intolerance test (see Chapter 6).

Case Study: *Jill*

Jill was feeling tired all the time despite eating a healthy diet and practising yoga on a daily basis. When she had her thyroid tested she had both low thyroxine and anti-thyroid antibodies. She was then investigated for allergies and found to be allergic to wheat. When she eliminated wheat, her thyroid function returned to normal.

Synthetic thyroxine or Armour Thyroid?

If your doctor is prepared to treat you, you will almost certainly be offered levothyroxine, a synthetic version of T4, which the body then turns into the useable form T3. (If you are only tested for T4 it can be misleading, because if your problem is that T4 is not being properly converted into T3, it won't be spotted – you will have plenty of T4 and may still feel terrible.)

Some people don't respond well to doses of T4, so a few doctors are prepared to offer an older form of treatment known as Armour Thyroid. This is a dried extract of pig thyroid which was used regularly on the NHS until over 30 years ago. Mainstream doctors will say that T4 is more consistent in quality and lacks the risks associated with treating with animal extract. But its supporters claim that Armour Thyroid is more like the natural human hormone and that some patients do very well on it. It is no longer licensed in the UK but can be obtained from the US and doctors can issue a private prescription for it.

Just how many people could benefit from thyroid hormones, even though official guidelines say they should not get it, is unknown. Women are about ten times more likely to be affected than men. One lower UK estimate says that low thyroid could affect a million women – more than have diabetes.

Nutritional support for your thyroid

From a nutritional perspective, the two most common causes of an underactive thyroid are 'endocrine burnout', which we will come to in a minute, or an autoimmune condition where your body produces antibodies that attack the thyroid, in which case it's vital to investigate the possibility of unidentified food allergies (see Chapter 6).

As I highlighted in the diagram on page 141, thyroid hormones are made from the amino acid tyrosine, which is converted into thyroxine, then into T3. This is carried out by enzymes that depend on zinc, selenium and iodine. B vitamins are also important. So, make sure you are taking a high-strength multivitamin that contains iodine, zinc (at least 10mg) and selenium (at least 35mcg). You might want to try adding extra zinc (up to 20mg a day in total) or extra selenium (up to a maximum of 200mcg in total). Kelp is also a good source of iodine, as is seafood.

You need about 1,000mg of tyrosine (some people need twice this), taken on an empty stomach, or with a carbohydrate snack such as a piece of fruit or an oatcake. This improves absorption. Some supplements provide tyrosine together with adaptogenic herbs such as the ginsengs.

Most of all, put yourself on a strict low-GL diet (see Chapter 7), eating lots of fresh fruit, vegetables and whole foods, and minimise stress and stimulants (caffeine and nicotine). You may also want to supplement 200mcg of chromium, since this often helps to lift low energy and low mood, improving insulin sensitivity which helps to stabilise both your blood sugar levels and stress hormones, which compete with thyroxine.

All these steps can help to reverse endocrine burnout. But if none of this works, I recommend exploring the possibility that you have an underactive thyroid and may benefit from a low dose of thyroxine. With the right nutritional support, the chances are you won't need very much to feel a lot better.

If you'd like some help interpreting any of these home tests or getting your nutritional programme right, I recommend you see a nutritional therapist. The best place to find a list of sympathetic doctors is through one of these two patient support groups (see Resources):

- Thyroid Patient Advocacy-UK

- Thyroid UK

CHAPTER 15

Migraines, Headaches and Hormones

There are several nutrition-related causes of headaches and migraines, including blood sugar dips, dehydration, unidentified food allergies, caffeine sensitivity and a lack of B vitamins. There are also other factors, such as the cervical vertebrae in the neck being out of alignment. If you suffer from frequent headaches or migraines, all these are potential culprits. Many women complain of headaches and migraine in relation to the menstrual cycle. In this chapter I'd like to explore and explain why hormone imbalances can trigger these kinds of headaches.

The most common reason for hormonal headaches is an oestrogen imbalance – either oestrogen excess or premenstrual deficiency.

Excess oestrogen is more common in those eating larger amounts of meat and dairy products and those who are overweight, since fat cells make oestrogens. Too much oestrogen suppresses the activity of an enzyme called monoamine oxidase, which oxidises or breaks down 'amines' such as serotonin or adrenalin, which are made from one amino acid (hence 'mono-amine'). Amines are potent constrictors of blood vessels, and having too many in circulation promotes vasoconstriction, which is an underlying cause of migraines.

Amines are naturally present in many foods (see the box opposite for common sources). It is known that diets rich in these amines, such as cheese and chocolate, can increase blood pressure and cause migraine specifically in patients taking monoamine oxidase inhibitors (MAOIs), which are a type of antidepressant.[3] So, logic follows that, if this enzyme is inhibited by other means – such as high levels of oestrogen – this too may lead to migraine in susceptible people.

Oestrogen is usually at its highest mid-cycle and some women experience migraines at this time of the month. Lowering dietary amines a few days before and after the mid-point of the cycle often helps if you are prone to mid-cycle headaches.

Amine-rich foods to avoid[4]

Cheese, especially ripe cheeses (except cottage, ricotta, cream cheese and Quark)

Avocados

Aubergine

Tomatoes

Beers and wines, and other fermented drinks

Cultured dairy products (such as yoghurt)

Bananas, pineapples, raspberries, red plums and dried fruits

Broad beans, lima beans and lentils

Chocolate

Vanilla extract

Chicken liver

Picked herrings, salted or dry fish

Yeast extracts, soy sauce, MSG and all fermented foods, such as vinegar, miso and soya

Any overripe vegetables or fruit

Amines are also produced by fermentation and by gut bacteria – even more so if you have the wrong balance of bacteria with too many bad guys and not enough good. Vitamin B_6, zinc, magnesium and sulphur are important nutrients for the breakdown of amines. Magnesium also helps to relax blood vessels. A good daily supplement programme will provide all of these (see Chapter 28), except for sulphur, which is best supplemented as MSM 1,000mg a day. Vitamin B_3 (as niacin) helps to widen blood vessels and can be taken preventatively in a 100mg dose if you feel a headache coming. This form of vitamin B_3, which you can buy in a health-food store, can cause a temporary hot flushing sensation that lasts for about 20 minutes, because it widens the blood vessels. It's not harmful as such, but not everybody likes it. The good news is that it often ends a headache or migraine, especially if taken early enough.

Addressing the balance of gut flora is also a useful strategy to help lower amine levels as well as ensuring adequacy of B_6, zinc, magnesium and sulphur. In practical terms this means taking a probiotic supplement daily for a fortnight, and sticking to a good-quality twice-a-day multivitamin plus 1,000mg of MSM, the most absorbable form of sulphur. Make sure your multi gives you at least 150mg of magnesium, 10mg of zinc and 20mg of B_6.

However, some women can be oestrogen dominant throughout the month and may experience migraines on an ongoing basis so would not necessarily relate their migraines to oestrogen dominance. If this applies to you, and as long as you've ruled out other potential causes, I recommend you try a low-amine diet to see if it helps reduce the number and severity of your migraine attacks. Amines, as the box overleaf indicated, are in a wide range of foods, many of which would be considered healthy foods, such as fish and fruits like raspberries, tomatoes and bananas; however, amine intolerance is not an allergy and there is no need to avoid any one particular food – just be mindful of the total load and construct your meals around lower amine food choices.

There's some evidence that a particular sulphur-dependent enzyme called M-form sulphotransferase produced in the gut may become overwhelmed by a large dietary intake of amines; for example, serotonin in bananas, phenylethylamine in chocolate and tyramine in cheese. Also, migraine sufferers have been shown to have low levels of another form of sulphur enzyme, called P-form sulphotransferase, which reduces the body's ability to detoxify amines and other naturally occurring chemicals in many fruits called phenols.[5] Once again, supplementing MSM might help.

The homocysteine connection

High levels of oestrogen can also suppress the ability of the liver to make the non-essential amino acid taurine (non-essential means the body can make taurine from other amino acids). A low taurine status is linked to a high incidence of migraines, and so too are high homocysteine levels.

Taurine is a calming neurotransmitter and a potent antioxidant, supporting the immune system. It may also improve the action of insulin, which aids blood sugar balance. Taurine also helps cells to retain magnesium. The non-essential amino acid cysteine can be directly converted to taurine and this requires vitamin B_6.

Taurine is mainly found in animal produce, so vegetarian and vegan diets tend to be low in it. The essential amino acid methionine becomes vital when dietary taurine is low. Converting methionine all the way to taurine requires folate and B_{12} as well as B_6. It's the same biochemical pathway that lowers blood levels of homocysteine (see Chapter 7). Twice as many migraine sufferers compared to non-sufferers have a gene mutation that can lead to a high level of homocysteine, which suggests that lowering homocysteine might make a difference. A high level of homocysteine is increasingly linked to heart attacks and strokes as well as other chronic illnesses. It's worth testing your level with a home-test kit (see Resources) and supplementing homocysteine-regulating nutrients B_6, B_{12}, folate and magnesium, as well as TMG and zinc. These can be found in a homocysteine-lowering formula.

Premenstrual migraines

The vast majority of women suffering with menstrual migraines experience a headache a few days before, or a few days after, the start of their period. Here, it's not an excess of oestrogen that's thought to be the trigger, but the rapid drop in oestrogen that can happen just before a period. Oestrogen deficiency is also a likely trigger in menopausal migraines. Although the exact mechanism is not fully understood, sudden hormonal changes are thought to affect blood vessels and, where a person lacks the capacity to adapt, headaches can be the result; however, simply improving your nutrition often helps your body to cope better with all the hormonal changes that occur throughout the month and adapt more quickly without suffering any side effects.

Migraine sufferers appear to have low levels of serotonin and, for these people, supplementing 100–200mg of 5-HTP a day helps. (5-HTP is the amino acid that serotonin is made from.) One of the more popular class of drugs for migraine, called triptans (such as zolmitriptan), also works by promoting serotonin. Magnesium supplementation can also reduce the intensity and duration of migraine headaches at this time of the cycle. To test the effect of magnesium you need to take in 300mg a day. A good multivitamin may provide 100mg. So you'll need to supplement a further 200mg.

Another cause of premenstrual migraines, and headaches in general, are dips in blood sugar levels, called dysglycemia. This can be reversed by following a low-GL diet and eating little and often, with three main meals and two low-GL snacks a day (see Chapter 7). It is also wise to avoid caffeine, which affects blood sugar balance, and to drink plenty of water, as dehydration can trigger headaches.

Of course, many of these factors overlap. Oestrogen dominance is linked to disrupted glucose balance and magnesium deficiency, and vice versa. Stress can also disrupt glucose balance (see Chapter 4), hence a high percentage of PMS is associated with oestrogen dominance and another sub-set is linked to carb cravings and magnesium deficiency (see Chapter 8).

Finally, managing an overgrowth of *Candida albicans* (see next chapter) has been shown to reduce the frequency and severity of migraine headaches.

Summary

- Eat a low-amine diet, especially if your headaches occur around ovulation, or the midpoint of your cycle.
- Take a high-potency multivitamin, plus 1,000mg of MSM, to assist your body's ability to break down amines, oestrogens and improve methylation.
- Add 200mg of magnesium as a supplement, especially if your headaches are premenstrual.
- Eat a low-GL diet, avoid caffeine and drink plenty of water to avoid dehydration.

CHAPTER 16

Conquering *Candida*

I am indebted to Erica White for her help in writing this chapter.
Candidiasis is the excessive growth of a yeast organism, called
Candida albicans, which is a normal inhabitant of the bowel.
It's the same organism that causes thrush, a common vaginal yeast
infection; however, symptoms of vaginal thrush do not have to be
present to have an overgrowth of *Candida* in the gut. The large bowel
is home to about 2kg (4½lb) of organisms, most of which, in the
right balance, are very important allies for your well-being; however,
given the right conditions, such as eating lots of sugar, opportunistic
organisms such as *Candida albicans* can overgrow, leaving you feeling
generally unwell.

As we have seen in Chapter 6, excessive growth of *Candida* is one
of the contributors to leaky gut, which affects the balance of your
hormones. Addressing any problems in the gut is therefore essential
for hormonal health.

Typical symptoms of *Candida* include: constipation and/or diarrhoea, bloating, allergies, headaches, extreme fatigue, hormone
dysfunction, skin complaints, joint and muscle pain, vaginal and oral
thrush infections, and emotional disorders – many of which mimic
other diseases and are frequently misdiagnosed.

Case Study: *Gina L*

Gina reversed her hormonal health problems by following an anti-*Candida* diet. Here's what she said:

'My life is 100 per cent improved on what it was – even though I still have more improvements to go and the yeast overgrowth needs to be brought under more control. I continue to make steady progress, keeping up the four-point anti-*Candida* plan. Erica White's *Beat Candida Cookbook* was an answer to my prayers.

'Last month I went to see a gynaecologist that I had consulted twice before. Eleven or 12 years ago she diagnosed endometriosis and polycystic ovaries with a large cyst also on one ovary. At the time she wanted to operate and do some procedures on both the uterus and the ovaries, and also to put me on hormones to stop menstruation for an extended period to allow the ovaries to 'rest'. I refused all and asked her to monitor the situation, which she was not particularly happy about.

'I am delighted to tell you that the endometriosis is *gone*, the lining of the womb is normal, and the large cyst and polycystic ovaries have cleared leaving just scars on the ovaries. I am delighted and amazed and am telling everyone who will listen about how amazing nutrition is.'

Is *Candida* your problem?

If you suspect you may have candidiasis check yourself out with the questionnaire overleaf. If you score high it's very important to get yourself properly tested under the guidance of a nutritional therapist (see Resources).

Questionnaire: do you have *Candida*?

	Yes	No
History		
1. Have you ever taken tetracycline or other antibiotics for a month or longer?	☐	☐
2. Have you, at any time in your life, taken other 'broad-spectrum' antibiotics for respiratory, urinary or other infections (for two months or longer, or in shorter courses four or more times in a one-year period)?	☐	☐
3. Have you, at any time in your life, been bothered by persistent vaginitis or other problems affecting your reproductive organs?	☐	☐
4. Have you taken birth control pills for more than two years?	☐	☐
5. Have you taken cortisone-type drugs for more than a month?	☐	☐
6. Does exposure to perfumes, insecticides, cigarette smoke and other chemicals provoke noticeable symptoms?	☐	☐
7. Are your symptoms worse on damp, muggy days or in mouldy places?	☐	☐
8. Do you have athlete's foot, ringworm or other chronic fungal infections of the skin or nails?	☐	☐
9. Do you crave sugar, bread or alcoholic beverages?	☐	☐

Score 2 points for each 'yes' answer.

Total score for History: ☐

	Yes	No

Symptoms

1. Do you often experience fatigue or lethargy? ☐ ☐

2. Do you ever have the feeling of being 'drained'? ☐ ☐

3. Do you suffer from depression? ☐ ☐

4. Do you have a poor memory? ☐ ☐

5. Do you ever experience feeling 'spacey' or 'unreal'? ☐ ☐

6. Do you suffer from an inability to make decisions? ☐ ☐

7. Do you experience numbness, burning or tingling? ☐ ☐

8. Do you ever get headaches or migraines? ☐ ☐

9. Do you suffer from muscle aches? ☐ ☐

10. Do you have muscle weakness or paralysis? ☐ ☐

11. Do you have pain and/or swelling in your joints? ☐ ☐

12. Do you suffer from abdominal pain? ☐ ☐

13. Do you get constipation and/or diarrhoea? ☐ ☐

14. Do you suffer from bloating, belching or intestinal gas? ☐ ☐

15. Do you have troublesome vaginal burning, itching or discharge? ☐ ☐

16. Do you ever experience a loss of sexual desire or feeling? ☐ ☐

17. Do you suffer from endometriosis or infertility? ☐ ☐

	Yes	No
18. Do you have cramps or other menstrual irregularities?	☐	☐
19. Do you get premenstrual tension?	☐	☐
20. Do you ever have attacks of anxiety or crying?	☐	☐
21. Do you suffer from cold hands or feet and/or chilliness?	☐	☐
22. Do you get shaky or irritable when hungry?	☐	☐

Score 1 point for each 'yes' answer.

Total score for Symptoms: ☐

Add up your total score: ☐

Score

If you score above 30 there's a strong likelihood that you have candidiasis. If you score above 20 there's a possibility that you have a degree of candidiasis. I recommend that you see a nutritional therapist and have the appropriate tests to find out if candidiasis is your problem.

What causes candidiasis?

This yeast is not harmful unless it is encouraged to multiply. It flourishes on a diet of sugars in foods such as alcohol, confectionery, processed foods, dried fruits and bread, and also foods high in yeast or fungus, such as mushrooms, Marmite, pickles, vinegar and anything fermented.

Antibiotic therapy, hormone treatments and stress are significant contributors to creating the environment in which this organism can flourish. Indiscriminate use of antibiotics reduces the number of friendly organisms in the gut, creating more room for the unfriendly ones. Hormone treatments and other steroid medications can depress the immune system, enabling the *Candida* organism to take a hold.

Research has shown that *Candida albicans* does not generally convert to a potentially harmful form, in which it does the equivalent of putting down roots, if the gut's immune system is healthy.

Historically, anti-*Candida* diets have focused on 'starving' the organism of fuel required to proliferate, particularly sugars. Dietary sugars are mostly absorbed in the small bowel and, in normal conditions, *Candida albicans* resides in the large bowel. The organism generally accesses its fuel from carbohydrates that form part of the walls of the large bowel and from the breakdown of the bacteria that naturally live in the gut. So, simply limiting dietary sugars is a bit defeatist, as the organism is clever enough to keep itself fed by taking its fuel from our gut membranes.

Restriction of glucose may be helpful, however, as glucose can trigger the change from the normal form of the organism to the more harmful form. Bacteria and other organisms can also use sugars for their survival and so, without testing for the presence of an overgrowth of *Candida albicans* it is not possible to know if a dietary strategy to reduce sugars is specifically targeting this organism.

What are the effects of candidiasis?

When *Candida albicans* changes to a harmful form it develops an extension to itself (a root) called hyphae, which can penetrate the gut membrane contributing to leaky gut (see Chapter 6). In the hyphal form, the organism becomes much more robust and difficult to manage. It also releases toxins (see 'Dealing with die-off' page 164). Rather than just focusing on eradicating the organism, a better strategy is to improve the conditions in the gut that support a healthy balance of gut flora and the production of an important gut immune agent called secretory IgA (SIgA). SIgA is the major antibody in the gut lining from mouth to anus and helps to prevent *Candida albicans* from penetrating the gut membrane. A natural remedy called *Saccharomyces boulardii* has been shown to reduce the incidence of candidiasis when taken during and after treatment for *Candida* (see below) by stimulating the production of the body's own SIgA.

It is possible to test for the level of SIgA in saliva, and some people are genetically low producers. In such instances, low producers need to take more care of their general digestive health. Similarly, there are various tests involving urine, blood, saliva and/or stool samples that can help support a nutritional strategy to address *Candida albicans*, or other imbalances of gut organisms. In particular, it is possible to test for the presence of IgG and IgA *Candida albicans* antibodies in blood and saliva, meaning that your immune system has become hypersensitive and is on the look-out for *Candida*.

Apart from laboratory tests, the questionnaire on page 154 is a good indicator of the likelihood of you having candidiasis. It's important to note, though, that similar symptoms can arise from other organisms in the gut which may not be completely eliminated by an anti-*Candida* programme. There are more comprehensive stool tests that can detect some of the less common invaders of the gut. A nutritional therapist can work with you and recommend the appropriate tests to find out which particular organisms may be contributing to your health problems.

The anti-*Candida* regime consists of five main parts:

1. Diet

Following the Diet for the Good Life, in Chapter 26, is a good fundamental place to start, as it should help on many levels. Prior to independently following restricted regimes I recommend that you work with a nutritional therapist to help identify if an 'anti-*Candida*' strategy is likely to be helpful. Long-term restricted diets, particularly if unfounded, are also associated with health problems, as many essential nutrients may be missed.

The aim of the diet is to massively reduce *Candida*'s sugar supply. This should quickly improve your digestive symptoms and stop fuelling the *Candida*'s growth. All forms of sugar must be strictly avoided, including lactose (milk sugar), malt and fructose (fruit sugar). Xylitol, derived from xylose, the sugar found in cherries, berries, plums and in the fibres of many other fruits and vegetables, is reported to be of value in the control of oral *Candida* infection if used as a substitute for refined carbohydrates.[6] Refined carbohydrates add to the glucose load because they are digested down into glucose, so it is essential to use only whole-grain flour, brown rice, and so on. The simplest guide is to follow a low-GL diet, because this ensures no sugar and only slow-releasing complex carbohydrates. Many people with candidiasis also benefit from the avoidance of yeast (bread, gravy mixes, spreads), fermented products (alcohol, vinegar), mould (cheese, mushrooms) and stimulants (tea, coffee).

Candida often brings on cravings for its favourite foods; at these times steely determination is needed to keep to the diet. Even when *Candida*-related symptoms have completely disappeared, the diet should be maintained for a further year to consolidate the newly corrected balance of gut flora. Before long, a 'sweet tooth' disappears, making it easier to stay on a sugar-free diet. I recommend you read Erica White's *Beat Candida Cookbook*, and follow the recipes, to show that mealtimes can still be an enjoyable experience. Another good book with recipes is the *Body Ecology Diet* by Donna Gates.

2. Immune-boosting supplement programme

A supplement programme is important to boost your immune system so that it can play its role in keeping the *Candida* under control. I recommend you take an all-round comprehensive supplement programme, plus a supplement specifically designed to improve digestion, with both enzymes and probiotics and, during the first month, a supplement designed to support liver function. See Chapter 28.

3. Healing the gut

If the gut is found to be leaky, it can be helpful to supplement butyric acid and glutamine, which are the two major energy sources for the gut wall. Addressing the healing of the gut before actively destroying the *Candida* organism itself usually leads to fewer 'die-off' reactions (see below).

It is worth re-testing at the end of the programme for the presence of *Candida* and the health of the gut wall. In my experience, if the programme does not include nutrients to heal the gut wall, the problem is likely to recur when a more 'normal' diet is resumed.

4. Re-establishing a healthy gut flora

Repopulating the gut with healthy flora is done at the same time as healing the gut. Supplements are needed to carry beneficial bacteria into the intestines and to re-establish a healthy colony. I call it 're-florestation'! The role of these bacteria is to increase acidity by producing lactic acid and acetic acid, and to inhibit undesirable microorganisms that would compete with them for space. Foods rich in prebiotics, which include chicory, Jerusalem artichokes, leeks, asparagus, garlic, onions, wheat, oats and soya beans, help beneficial bacteria to multiply. Prebiotics can be taken after a course of probiotics, such as *Lactobacillus acidophilus* and bifidobacteria, although some probiotics already provide prebotics, the most common one being fructo-oligosaccharides (FOS).

Lactobacillus acidophilus is the major coloniser of the small intestine and *Bifidobacterium bifidum* inhabits the large intestine and vagina; it also produces B vitamins. Other helpful bacteria are the transient *Lactobacillus bulgaricus* and *Streptococcus thermophilus*, which also produce lactic acid as they pass through the bowel. I recommend that prebiotics and probiotics are taken for six months. These friendly bacteria are available as nutritional supplements and are also contained in yoghurt, which is therefore a helpful food provided you have no intolerance to dairy foods. In yoghurt, the lactose (milk sugar) content has largely been converted into lactic acid by enzyme-producing bifidobacteria, which accounts for the sharpness of its taste. You can also get soya yoghurts with added friendly bacteria. The best yoghurts contain *Lactobacillus acidophilus* and bifidobacteria.

To ensure safe passage of these bacteria through the gastric juices, it is necessary to take them in a capsule supplying large numbers of viable organisms in freeze-dried form. Take two capsules daily, at breakfast and dinner, but the dosage can be increased to six daily, or even more, in cases of diarrhoea or illness necessitating antibiotics, which further deplete the friendly flora. An acidophilus cream is a beneficial aid for a vaginal fungal infection.

5. Anti-fungal supplements

Surprisingly, one of the best supplements to tackle *Candida* is a yeast, *Saccharomyces boulardii*. It's a non-colonising yeast, which means that it will never take up residence in your gut; however, as it passes through it stimulates your gut's production of the immune component SIgA (see page 158). Greater amounts of this immunoglobulin make it increasingly difficult for the *Candida* to stick to your gut wall. Some people with *Candida* may be hypersensitive to all yeast, including *S. boulardii*, so taking it could make you feel worse. In this case, you should wait until you've cut all of the yeast out of your diet for about four weeks to reduce your sensitivity and then introduce the *S. boulardii* at very low doses, then increase the doses very gradually. This may mean starting with as little as 1 billion organisms (½ capsule) once daily before building up to the full dose of about 10 billion organisms a day. *S. boulardii* also helps to make the environment of your gut more hospitable to friendly bacteria, so enhancing their chances of taking up residence.

Additional anti-fungal supplements to directly tackle the *Candida* may also be necessary, and can be taken while you are taking the *S. boulardii*, but they should be taken several hours apart so as not to kill off the *S. boulardii* as well. It's generally best not to start any of these additional supplements until you've been on the diet and taking the *S. boulardii* for about a month in order to minimise the 'die-off' reaction (more on this in a minute).

Caprylic acid is one of the most useful anti-fungal agents. It is a fatty acid that occurs naturally in coconuts. Its great advantage is that it does not kill off your friendly flora. As calcium/magnesium caprylate, it survives digestive processes and is able to reach the colon; however, it is usually advisable to wait three months, which allows the dietary restrictions to reduce the activity of the *Candida*, thereby giving the gut wall time to heal and generally improving health. Caprylic acid targets the organism directly in a mass 'slaughter', which causes the release of toxins in what is known as a 'die-off' reaction, as explained below. At this stage the sufferer is more able to tolerate the die-off without feeling too sick. Although this may be slower than targeting the organism with caprylic acid from the start, it usually gives the sufferer a smoother ride.

Olive leaf extract has potent antioxidant and anti-fungal properties[7] and is often used as an anti-*Candida* agent. One of its more active ingredients is called oleuropein, and the potency of extracts is often standardised to the percentage of oleuropein, 6 per cent indicating a good product. It is normally provided as 500mg capsules, which should be taken one, two or three times a day.

Oregano oil is another excellent anti-fungal agent. It also has the advantage of crossing the gut wall into the body so it may be better if you have more body-wide fungal symptoms, such as athlete's foot.

Artemisia is a herb with broad-spectrum anti-fungal properties, useful against a wide variety of pathogens without disturbing the friendly flora. If you have a high score on the *Candida* questionnaire and a history of illnesses that have originated in a hot climate, these are sufficient reasons to suspect a parasite other than *Candida*, and to use a broad-spectrum anti-fungal agent.

Propolis is another natural substance which, according to research at the University of Bratislava, is remarkably effective for all fungal infections of the skin and body.[8] It can be taken as drops and built up gradually – its anaesthetic effect is soothing for oral thrush – and as a cream, for painful muscles.

Aloe vera is gently anti-fungal and is a refreshing mouthwash or gargle, as well as an ingestible aid to digestion. It can be used as an overnight denture soak, in preference to products that are not specifically anti-fungal. Dentures can be an ongoing source of *Candida* re-infection.

Tea tree oil is an anti-fungal agent and, as a cream, can be used for fungal skin conditions. *Candida* is frequently associated with eczema, psoriasis and acne as well as athlete's foot and other fungal skin or nail infections.

Grapefruit seed extract, also called Citricidal, is an antibiotic, anti-fungal and anti-viral agent. The great advantage, however, is that it doesn't have much effect on the beneficial gut bacteria. It comes in drops, best taken two or three times a day, 15 drops at a time, and is also available in capsules.

Other anti-fungal preparations include garlic, goldenseal and pau d'arco. Since these are not nutritional supplements as such, but specific anti-fungal remedies, it is always best to use such remedies for a brief period of time, usually up to three months, under the guidance of a nutritional therapist, having established that you really do have a fungal overgrowth or infection. Improving digestive health, absorption and the balance of gut flora are key to any supplementary programme, as explained above. Some supplementary agents directly 'kill' the organism and can lead to unpleasant die-off symptom reactions, whereas an appropriately staged nutrition programme will help to minimise such reactions.

Dealing with die-off

Thriving *Candida* releases a minimum of 79 known toxins. Dead and dying *Candida* releases even more. A general feeling of toxicity includes aching muscles, fuzzy head, depression, anxiety, nausea and diarrhoea. In specific areas where *Candida* has colonised, there can be an apparent flare-up of old symptoms – sore throat, thrush, painful joints, eczema, and so on. This unpleasant situation is known as die-off, or formally as Herxheimer's reaction.

The art is to destroy *Candida* slowly but surely so that it is not being killed off faster than the body can eliminate the toxins. Initial die-off is usually triggered by the diet, and by vitamins and minerals as they boost the immune system to fight it. These first two points of the five-point plan usually cause more than enough die-off for most people to cope with, and anti-fungal agents should not be added to the regime until this phase is over. By the end of a month the majority of people claim that they feel better than they have for years! That is the time to add the anti-fungal and probiotic supplements to the programme.

Getting started

Most people on caprylic acid start with one medium-strength capsule (about 400mg) daily, without too much difficulty. If after five days they are not battling with die-off symptoms, the dose can be increased to two 400mg, and so on up to six capsules daily. After this, they can graduate to a higher strength capsule (about 700mg) three times daily and increase again if necessary; however, the climb up is seldom straightforward and at some stage there might come a surge of die-off reaction necessitating a drop to a lower level, or even a complete break, while the body eliminates the toxins. This should not be regarded as a setback, but simply a necessary part of the process. Drinking plenty of fluids and taking good levels of vitamin C and B vitamins, as already discussed, will speed up detoxification. Eventually, caprylic acid accomplishes its job; the score on the *Candida* questionnaire will then fall to as low as it can, allowing for 'history' factors, which obviously do not change.

Summary

Thrush is not necessarily an indicator of candidiasis. This skilful organism has evolved over 12 million years and you are very unlikely to 'conquer' *Candida albicans*; however, it is possible to keep it within normal limits in the bowel and in a form that is not harmful to your health.

- Work with a nutritional therapist wherever possible if you think you have candidiasis, as the symptoms are so diverse that they can easily be mistaken for true hormone imbalances. It is especially important to seek expert advice if you are pregnant or considering pregnancy and think that you may have candidiasis.
- Your anti-*Candida* regime is likely to include avoiding sugars and following a low-GL diet, plus nutritional supplements, probiotics and *S. boulardii* to boost your body's immune system.
- Specific anti-fungal remedies, such as caprylic acid, oregano oil and olive leaf extract may also help.

CHAPTER 17

Stopping Cystitis

Cystitis is a common condition where the lining of the bladder becomes inflamed, making urination painful. Most of the time the inflammation is caused by a bacterial infection, in which case it may be referred to as a urinary tract infection (UTI). A bladder infection can be painful and annoying, and can also become a serious health problem if it spreads to your kidneys. For this reason, you should consult your doctor immediately if your symptoms are accompanied by fever, blood in the urine, loin pain, or lower backache.

Although a common cause of cystitis is infection, which can be confirmed by a urine analysis, and hence it is not really related to hormonal imbalances, it is a common female health condition that often overlaps with other hormone-related health problems. Another common cause is candidiasis (see the last chapter) or a food intolerance (see Chapter 6). If there is evidence of infection, for example with *Escherichia coli* (*E. coli*) bacteria, you will probably be prescribed antibiotics. If so, make sure you also take probiotics, but not at the same time, for two weeks after completing the antibiotic course.

If there is no evidence of infection, you may be diagnosed with interstitial cystitis.

Although anyone can get cystitis, including children, adult women are most commonly affected. Most women get at least one attack in their lifetime. For some women cystitis is a rare event, for others it happens four or five times a year. Cystitis is more common in sexually active women, during pregnancy and during and after the menopause.

Common symptoms include an urgent and frequent need to pass urine (often with little or no urine being passed) and a burning sensation and/or a sharp pain when passing urine. Other possible symptoms include blood in the urine, backache, loin pain, lower abdominal aches and generally feeling unwell.

D-mannose – the cranberry connection

Some people report relief from drinking cranberry juice, which is a rich source of D-mannose, a natural sugar. Since most processed cranberry juice has added sugar, why drink sugary cranberry juice when you can get the active ingredient instead?

D-mannose is a naturally occurring simple sugar found in peaches, apples, berries and some other plants. It is a harmless natural sugar, and it is safe for anyone, including young children and pregnant women. It is absorbed into the upper part of the gastrointestinal tract and never reaches the intestines. It therefore doesn't disrupt the normal bacterial growth in that area. Although small amounts of D-mannose are made by our bodies, if we consume a large amount it is promptly excreted into the urine, which is the reason why taking D-mannose helps to heal and maintain a healthy bladder. Also due to the speed at which it is excreted in the urine, it can be safely taken by diabetics. Make sure you buy pure D-mannose supplements, in capsules, with no fillers, additives or preservatives.

Research has shown that E.coli likes to attach to D-mannose, which our body produces naturally as part of the walls of cells. This D-mannose is naturally present in the bladder and the urinary tract, providing the ideal docking ports for the E.coli. In this way, the E.coli can bury themselves into the bladder wall, making them very difficult to get rid of and can lead to repeated attacks of cystitis. The theory is that, by providing a richer supply of D-mannose in the urine, this

167

could persuade the *E.coli* to attach to the free D-mannose instead of the cell wall D-mannose.

Although the cause of interstitial cystitis remains a bit of a mystery, many people report relief by following this strategy:

Diet

- Follow the dietary guidelines in Chapter 26, based on eating low-GL foods and keeping sweet foods to a minimum, because sugar feeds bacterial infections.

- Drink at least eight glasses of filtered or bottled water a day to help flush out unhealthy organisms from the bladder.

- Cranberries and cranberry juice: cranberries contain hippuric acid, which is known to prevent bacteria clinging to the bladder wall and helps to acidify the urine, which can prevent bacteria from adhering to the urinary tract. It is also a rich source of D-mannose. Because undiluted cranberry juice contains higher amounts of active ingredients, it should be chosen over pre-sweetened juice for the best effects; however, this doesn't work for everybody.

- Some people report benefit by making the urine *less* acidic by mixing a teaspoon of bicarbonate of soda with half a pint of water. There are also over-the-counter remedies containing alkalising sodium citrate or potassium citrate, available in solutions or sachets. This too can make it harder for bacteria to thrive.

- Eat organic, live yoghurt every day or take probiotics.

- Avoid all acid-forming foods such as sugar and red meat, and increase alkaline-forming foods such as green leafy veg (see page 332). These foods are all part of the Diet for a Good Life in Chapter 26.

Supplements

- Take 2–4g of vitamin C daily (in 500mg doses throughout the day). Vitamin C helps to acidify the urine. As a result, the bladder is a less appealing environment for harmful bacteria to colonise. Vitamin C also reinforces the body's immune defences.

- Supplement D-mannose, which comes in powder form (it can be mixed into drinks) or capsule form. The dosage depends on the severity of the infection, so use according to the manufacturer's guidelines. It can also be taken at a maintenance dose if you are a regular sufferer.

- Make sure your multivitamin is yeast-free and contains biotin.

- Take *Lactobacillus acidophilus* for at least six weeks – this is especially important for anyone taking antibiotics to treat an infection. Acidophilus helps to maintain a healthy digestive tract. You may also want to try using a probiotic vaginal cream.

Lifestyle advice

- Always wipe from front to back after going to the toilet to prevent bacteria from entering the urethra.

- Use only white, unscented toilet paper to avoid potential dye reactions.

- Avoid potential irritants such as perfumed soaps, bath oils and vaginal deodorants at all times, as chemicals are strongly implicated in this condition. Don't douche.

- Urinate as soon as possible after sex to stop the transmission of bugs into the bladder, and always wash before and after sex.

- If symptoms are acute, avoid intercourse for at least one week, as bacteria can be passed from one partner to another.

- Wear cotton underwear and loose clothing. Avoid tight-fitting jeans, especially in hot weather.

CHAPTER 18

Preventing Polycystic Ovaries

As many as one in ten women suffer from small cysts, follicles less than 1cm (½in) in diameter, that form in the ovary. The presence of these cysts, plus the associated symptoms, is known as polycystic ovarian syndrome, or PCOS for short. According to Verity, the UK charity for women whose lives are affected by PCOS, polycystic ovaries are very common, affecting around 20 per cent of women, although the actual 'syndrome' affects 5–10 per cent of women. PCOS is an increasingly common problem, especially among younger women, and is strongly associated with blood sugar problems and insulin resistance, as explained in Chapter 7. The symptoms, however, are often confused with hormonal problems and therefore not dealt with early.

Ovarian cysts result from an egg failing to develop and be released normally. They can grow to the size of a golf ball and create considerable pain, but sometimes they produce no symptoms at all. After ovulation fails, the developing egg continues to grow under the influence of follicle stimulating hormone (FSH). Each month the rise of FSH is followed by a surge of luteinising hormone (LH), which causes the site of the follicle to swell, stretching the surface of the ovary, causing pain and possibly bleeding at the site. Treatment may involve surgery.

PCOS is also associated with weight gain, excessive body hair, acne, increased facial hair growth, breast pain, depression and mood swings. Yet, because the symptoms are so similar to those of PMS and other hormonal disorders, the condition is often left undiagnosed until symptoms become very severe.

The most common signs and symptoms of PCOS in teens or adult women include:

- Abnormal menstrual cycles

- No periods

- Irregular periods

- Heavy or prolonged bleeding

- Painful periods

- Inability to get pregnant

- Chronic fatigue

- Excess facial hair

- Head hair loss (male-pattern baldness)

- Obesity

- Waist measurement greater than 89cm (35in), or waist bigger than hips (apple shape)

What causes PCOS?

Although there is no one single cause of PCOS, because it is strongly linked with insulin resistance it is very often found in women with diabetes. It is also likely to be, in part, a result of changes in diet, lifestyle and environment, as explained in Part 1.

Women with PCOS are at risk of developing metabolic syndrome – a precursor to diabetes and found in one-third to one-half of all women and adolescent girls with PCOS. They also have decreased insulin sensitivity (insulin resistance), compared with women of similar body weight with normal ovaries. Evidence suggests that insulin resistance, which worsens with weight gain,[9] is the likely link between PCOS and metabolic syndrome,[10] although insulin sensitivity is not always found with PCOS, particularly with non-obese women. Family history seems to be an important factor, as women who have PCOS and a positive family history of type-2 diabetes seem to have a higher risk of abnormal insulin sensitivity and secretion.[11]

The insulin link

The more insensitive or resistant your body becomes to the hormone insulin's attempts to control blood sugar levels, the more the body produces insulin. High levels of insulin appear to stimulate and increase blood levels of androgens (the male hormones) in PCOS and suppress a protein called sex hormone-binding globulin (SHBG), a protein that binds to sex hormones and keeps the levels available in the blood at optimum levels. The use of insulin-sensitising drugs (see below) has been shown to decrease blood levels of insulin in both obese and non-obese women with PCOS, and to simultaneously reduce circulating androgens and to improve ovulation.[12] Another way to lessen your insulin load is to eat a low-GL diet (see Chapter 7).

PCOS causes the ovaries to stop ovulating, which means that the normal cyclic production of oestrogen followed by progesterone either ceases or becomes dysfunctional. Insulin stimulates the ovaries to produce predominantly male hormones, which, in combination with higher insulin and glucose levels, increase weight gain around the waist – a body type that is a risk factor for breast cancer. Signs that the body is being exposed to higher levels of the male hormones include acne, loss of head hair, and an increase in body hair. Lowering insulin levels is crucial for not only treating PCOS but also for resolving most other hormonal imbalances and reducing breast cancer risk.

Depression or mood swings (also associated with insulin resistance, hormone imbalances and being overweight) are also common in women with PCOS. Infertility and miscarriages, common consequences of PCOS, also can be very stressful and depressing. Too much stress may aggravate many aspects of the syndrome, including insulin resistance (as discussed in Chapter 4).

It has been suggested that when zinc is in short supply certain types of cysts can develop, possibly because zinc is required for the growth of the egg. The use of infertility drugs has also been implicated because some of these drugs block oestrogen receptors and increase the output of FSH and LH, even though women are failing to ovulate.

Diagnosing PCOS

There are a number of blood tests that will probably have been performed by your doctor if you have, or are suspected as having, PCOS. An ultrasound may also be performed to confirm the diagnosis.

Blood test results that are generally found in women with PCOS include:

- *High* androgen levels (male hormones, such as testosterone), LH, fasting insulin, prolactin, oestradiol and oestrone, tryglycerides, total and LDL (known as 'bad') cholesterol.

- *Low* levels of SHBG, which are decreased by high levels of insulin, as explained above.

How is PCOS treated?

There are many medications to control the symptoms of PCOS. Doctors most commonly prescribe the contraceptive pill for this purpose. The Pill regulates menstruation, reduces androgen levels and helps to clear acne. Your doctor may also prescribe an insulin-sensitising medication, such as metformin,[13] although some experts believe that this should be prescribed with caution[14] and not 'as a replacement for increased exercise and improved diet'.[15]

A meta-analysis of 13 randomised, controlled trials including 543 women found that metformin has an effect in reducing fasting insulin concentrations, blood pressure and LDL ('bad') cholesterol; however, it was also associated with some unpleasant side effects, including nausea, vomiting and gastrointestinal disturbance, which limited participation levels in some trials. One of the outcomes measured was the 'overall ovulation rate' achieved by metformin alone, or metformin combined with another drug (clomifene). Interestingly, the overall rate of 57 per cent was lower than the ovulation rate achieved with lifestyle improvements that included increased exercise and weight loss.[16] Metformin also interferes with the action of vitamin B_{12} and may raise your homocysteine level (explained on page 149). Make sure you are supplementing vitamin B_{12} if you are on this drug.

A low-GL diet, plus exercise, is a winning formula

Eating a strictly balanced, low-GL diet (see Chapter 7), losing weight, if applicable, and maintaining a healthy weight can improve insulin sensitivity and help lessen the symptoms of PCOS. It is absolutely vital to get your weight under control. Several studies have confirmed the link with obesity and infertility. American researchers demonstrated that obese girls at puberty had up to three times the level of free testosterone than non-obese girls, and high insulin levels.[17] This scenario increases the risk of developing PCOS, and the health risks associated with it. Obesity also affects pregnancy outcomes and risks are increased for both mother and baby.

Dairy products also promote high insulin levels and are best avoided. The essential mineral chromium is required for normal insulin function, helping to reverse insulin resistance just as well as metformin but without the side effects; intakes of 400–600mcg a day help; however, there are not many trials in the context of PCOS.

Following the Diet for the Good Life in Chapter 26 will not only address symptoms of PCOS but also help to minimise the chance of associated conditions, as outlined below.

Stabilising your blood sugar

Controlling your blood sugar levels is key to managing this condition. The net result of stress, or a diet too high in sugar and refined carbohydrates, is an inability to keep blood sugar levels stable, as I have explained in Chapters 4 and 7. The vast majority of women with PCOS show this kind of hormone imbalance. Taking simple steps, like combining protein with carbohydrates and eating healthy snacks to help control fluctuations in blood sugar, can greatly improve how your body handles insulin.

If you have to have sugar, choose xylitol. Foods sweetened with xylitol will not raise your insulin levels, so it is a perfect sweetener for people with diabetes as well as those wanting to lose weight. Avoid all foods sweetened with other sweeteners, especially fructose.

Using xylitol instead of sugar, as well as reducing your intake of high-GL, refined carbohydrate foods, will help to lower the risk not only of PCOS but also of ovarian cysts, fibroids, endometriosis, PMS, hot flushes, weight gain and depression.

Regular exercise helps weight loss and also aids the body in reducing blood glucose levels and using insulin more efficiently. Aim for 20–30 minutes every day or twice this amount every other day.

Natural progesterone

The late Dr John Lee found that supplementing natural progesterone from day 10 to day 26 of the cycle for a few months is often enough to shrink the cysts and no further treatment is required. Taking progesterone from day 10 effectively suppresses ovulation and gives the ovaries time to rest and repair. A nutritional therapist can test your progesterone levels and advise you accordingly. Also read Chapter 24 on the use of natural progesterone.

Associated conditions

As well as the common symptoms listed above, sufferers from PCOS can experience associated health risks, including a higher risk of miscarriage, high cholesterol, hardening of the arteries (atherosclerosis), high blood pressure, heart disease, type-2 diabetes and infertility. In fact, PCOS is the most common cause of female infertility; however, if diagnosed and treated early, risks for these complications may be minimised.

Although PCOS is a complex condition, the good news is that with the right nutritional approach you can reverse it and, in the process, lose weight, improve your skin and overcome exhaustion, depression and mood swings. With a combination of diet, exercise, supplementation and relaxation, many of these problems can be reduced, or even eliminated.

Diabetes and PCOS

Metabolic syndrome, common in women with PCOS, is associated with an increased risk of cardiovascular disease and type-2 diabetes. By the age of 40, up to 40 per cent of PCOS sufferers will have type-2 diabetes or impaired glucose tolerance.[18] Lifestyle changes, as discussed above should reduce this risk. Insulin-sensitising drugs, such as metformin, may also be recommended, although chromium supplementation, as discussed earlier, works just as well and is non-toxic up to 10,000mcg a day.

Diabetes during pregnancy (gestational diabetes)

Gestational diabetes occurs when a woman's ability to process glucose is impaired. The mother's high blood glucose levels can lead to a large baby with immature lungs and problems for the mother and child at delivery. Since PCOS causes high glucose levels, women with PCOS are likely to be screened for gestational diabetes early during pregnancy. A carefully balanced diet and/or insulin injections are generally used to manage the condition. Some doctors allow pregnant women with PCOS to continue taking metformin in pregnancy, whereas others won't prescribe it to women trying to conceive. There is no evidence that it causes birth defects, but the long-term effects on the baby are not known. Chromium, as explained previously, is an alternative. Women and their doctors should discuss the risks and benefits of medications. Women taking medication are usually monitored more closely.

Infertility

As explained in Part 1, a woman's ovaries have follicles, which are tiny, fluid-filled sacs that hold the eggs. When an egg is mature, the follicle releases the egg so it can travel to the uterus for fertilisation. In women with PCOS, immature follicles bunch together to form large cysts or lumps. It is thought that a slight elevation of male hormones (androgens) may inhibit the egg's development, and the egg's failure to mature leads to a lack of ovulation (anovulation) in women with PCOS.

As a result, women with PCOS often don't have menstrual periods, or they only have periods on occasion. Some women with PCOS have periods but do not ovulate. Because the eggs are not released, most women with PCOS have trouble becoming pregnant. They also have a higher rate of miscarriage.

As explained above, women with PCOS may be prescribed fertility drugs, metformin, or steroids (to lower androgen levels) to help ovulation take place; however, it would appear that the use of metformin to improve reproductive outcomes in women is limited. This was the conclusion of an analysis by the highly respected Cochrane Collaboration, which showed that the use of metformin, either alone or in combination with drugs to induce ovulation such as clomiphene citrate, does not increase the chance of having a successful pregnancy.

They concluded that the long-term use of metformin in reducing the risk of developing metabolic syndrome is questionable.[19] Although they state that metformin is still of benefit in improving pregnancy and ovulation rates, there is no evidence that metformin improves birth rates.

Summary

In summary, you can lessen the symptoms of PCOS with drugs, supplements, a strict low-GL diet, exercise and by reducing stress.

Two very good books to read if you have been diagnosed with PCOS are: *PCOS: A Woman's Guide to Dealing with Polycystic Ovary Syndrome* by Colette Harris and Dr Adam Carey, and *PCOS Diet Book: How You Can Use the Nutritional Approach to Deal with Polycystic Ovary Syndrome* by Colette Harris and Theresa Francis-Cheung. Colette Harris is a health journalist who herself suffers from the condition.

For a list of useful websites and organisations, see Resources.

CHAPTER 19

The Hidden Epidemic: Endometriosis

This chapter has been written by Dian Shepperson Mills, founder and lead nutritionist at The Endometriosis and Fertility Clinic.

Endometriosis affects over one hundred million women worldwide and is more common than breast cancer and diabetes. Up to 10 per cent of women in their reproductive years and a quarter to half of all women with infertility have been diagnosed with endometriosis.[20]

Endometriosis is defined as the presence of endometrial-like tissue (the normal womb-lining tissue), but it is found outside the uterus, literally inside the abdominal cavity. This tissue bleeds with the menstrual cycle, and the blood is trapped inside the tummy where it may trigger a chronic, inflammatory pain, as well as poor fertility and reduced quality of life. Endometriosis is found in women from all ethnic and social groups.[21] The profound loss of the ability to live a normal life can have a devastating effect on a woman's confidence and sense of self-esteem. The distress of failing to conceive month after month can be exhausting. Approximately one-fifth of patients with sub-fertility problems may have endometriosis; it also doubles the risk of a premature birth.

Endometriosis is associated with severe period pains, painful intercourse, chronic pelvic pain, ovulation pain, cyclical bowel or bladder-associated symptoms with or without abnormal bleeding, sub-fertility and chronic fatigue. The pain level can be extreme if ovarian cysts burst. Some affected women, however, remain asymptomatic – they may have the disease but they never have any pains.[22]

Getting the correct diagnosis

In 2005 the All Party Parliamentary Group (APPG) at the House of Commons organised an online questionnaire which was answered by 7,500 women, all diagnosed with endometriosis, and showed that it took, on average, more than five years before a doctor would refer a woman complaining of period pain to a specialist gynaecologist. Overall it took an average of nine years to get a complete diagnosis. Altogether 82 per cent of the 7,500 women reported having to take three to four days off work each month, because of severe period pain. Twenty-five per cent of all sick leave in the UK is taken by women because of period pain, yet it is rarely taken seriously. Research reports that as many as half of all menstruating women are affected by period pain, and 10 per cent have severe pain that puts them relatively out of action for three or four days each month.[23]

The APPG is trying to encourage the setting up of Specialist Endometriosis Centres in the same way that specialist cancer centres work. At these centres women will be treated by gynaecologists who specialise in endometriosis operations, and who research and attend endometriosis conferences, keeping up to date with surgical techniques that conserve the organs.[24]

What causes endometriosis?

The endometrium (the inside lining of the womb which rebuilds itself each month), sheds as a menstrual period in a cycle every 28 days. From day 1 to day 14 it is rebuilding itself ready for conception around day 15, when most women ovulate. The endometrium builds up each month in response to oestrogen. This womb-lining layer becomes nutrient-rich, ready to receive the embryo. As the period sheds, some of this blood may drip inside the abdomen via the fallopian tubes. This womb lining may begin 'seeding' itself into 'healthy' tissue inside the tummy over a period of four hours, onto the bowel, bladder and ovaries – the reasons why are little understood. However, it should not be growing there, only inside the womb itself. As this tissue bleeds, the blood becomes trapped inside the tummy's fluids, setting up inflammation, pain and sub-fertility, as it now contains chemicals that should not be there.

Endometriosis is commonly found on the outside of the womb, ovaries, ligaments, bladder and bowel; large blood-filled cysts may form on the ovaries, while adhesions stick organs together. Rarely, it may grow on other organs, such as the lungs, gums, kidneys, diaphragm, stomach and liver.

The four key symptoms of endometriosis

1 Chronic/acute period pains
2 Ovulation pain
3 Pain on intercourse
4 Sub-fertility

Other reported symptoms

5 Abdominal bloating, IBS
6 Bladder pressure, urgency, interstitial cystitis
7 Extreme fatigue
8 Ovary pains, lower back pains
9 Chronic bowel symptoms, rectal bleeding, IBS
10 Low body temperature
11 Recurrent infections, sore throats
12 Immune-system failure
13 Hormone imbalances
14 Pains at all times
15 Low moods, anxiety

Small specks of endometriosis cause enormous pain, yet huge lumps may give no pain.

Approaching your GP

When you go to see your doctor, it really helps to take a list of the main symptoms you are suffering every month. Explaining what the pain is like is another factor. Explain the pain as: pinching, stabbing, wringing, dragging, searing, deep aches, burning, tearing, twinges, backache, left ovary pain or right ovary pain. Does this correspond to the time of the period or when you ovulate mid-cycle? Do your bowel habits change at periods and when you ovulate? Do you become constipated or have diarrhoea before, during or after your period? Explain it all, write it down and go through exactly what happens when and for how many days the pain lasts. Score the pain on a 0–10 scale. Keep a diary. The doctor is more likely to take it seriously if you can show that pain is happening with the period and at ovulation. Some women get pain every day.

Tell your doctor which painkillers you take and how many are needed to stop the pain – or do they not even touch the pain? Ask to be referred to a gynaecologist with specialist interest in endometriosis – be assertive, but not aggressive. Then tell the specialist all the same points. If you are taking the oral contraceptive pill and painkillers during periods but these do not stop period pain, then you must see a specialist. Having a scan may show cysts and if your organs are misaligned, but scans do not show small spots of endometrioisis, only large lumps. It is a great relief to get a diagnosis and know what is causing the pain – and that it is not cancer.

The surgical treatment of endometriosis

Gold-standard diagnosis is done by laser laparoscopy. Pharmaceutical treatments use the oral contraceptive pill to mimic pregnancy, gonadotropin-releasing hormone (GnRH) analogues (artificial copies) such as Zoladex to mimic menopause, or the use of the Mirena coil, as pregnancy and menopause are felt to halt the growth of endometrial tissue. Hysterectomy or removal of the ovaries may be done if the disease is severe, but usually the rogue tissue is just lasered away at laparoscopy or cut out by microsurgery. It should also be the gold standard to conserve the reproductive organs; it would be bad practice to remove the womb and/or ovaries in women where they can be conserved by skilled surgery, where no cancer exists. Research does show that removal of organs does not bode well. It is medically ethical that a patient should be given full information so that she is able to make a proper decision about what happens to her body.

Oxidative stress

Two studies have found a positive association between oxidative stress (explained in Chapter 13) and endometriosis.[25] Having too many oxidants in the body may affect the growth of endometrial tissue. The presence of endometriosis increases oxidative stress, and a diet lacking in antioxidants may contribute to excessive growth of endometrial cells.[26] Significantly, lower levels of vitamin E were found in the peritoneal fluid than in plasma, suggesting that the peritoneal cavity has less antioxidant protection than serum, so the fluid containing the endometriosis might be more susceptible to oxidative stress than serum.[27] Antioxidant nutrients such as selenium, vitamins A, C and E may be supportive, plus proanthocyanidin in berries has an antioxidant effect. Women with endometriosis have lower antioxidant intakes of vitamins C and E, selenium and zinc, and as endometriosis severity intensifies, an even lower intake of antioxidants is present.[28]

Progesterone resistance

Many women with endometriosis have progesterone resistance, which is much like insulin resistance, where the body becomes less responsive to insulin. This is when oestrogen and progesterone become out of balance, particularly when oestradiol, the more growth-promoting type of oestrogen, is not changed into oestrone. Women with endometriosis often show resistance of the endometrium to the effects of progesterone at certain times during the menstrual cycle. This is because there are low levels of a certain enzyme.

Progesterone levels are able to rise 30-fold over the space of 30 minutes, so are difficult to measure accurately. Day 21 is the normal time for a reading to be taken to show ovulation. Low progesterone levels do indicate that an abnormal endometrium is present, and although it does not seem to affect endometrial thickness, it does affect the quality and ability of the endometrium to hold on to the embryo as it tries to implant. Progesterone precursors are magnesium, zinc, vitamin A, vitamin B_6 and amino acids and essential fats; perhaps these nutrients are deficient or poorly absorbed in women with poor levels of progesterone.

Progesterone is produced naturally in the ovary, inside the corpus luteum (see page 8). After the egg has been released from the follicle it seals up and fills with a golden liquid and this produces the progesterone. Progesterone is needed by the body, as it causes the endometrium to shed once a month; it also acts as an antidepressant by calming the nervous system and balancing copper and zinc levels; it protects breast tissue and helps to prevent breast cancer; it acts as a natural diuretic and aids thyroid action; it helps body fat to be used as energy and it normalises blood sugar control; it stimulates bone growth and its effects are needed for a normal menstrual period.

It may be that with all the oestrogenic chemicals we eat and drink (see Part 1), the fine balance of oestrogen and progesterone needed for a healthy menstrual cycle is broken. To bring it back into balance again, eat the best-quality fresh foods you can. Restrict your intake of red meat and dairy foods, and choose organic produce whenever possible. Not only should you avoid sources of oestrogen but you should also greatly limit the much weaker phytoestrogens, which are found in soya, wheat and citrus fruits, as well as in the herbs black cohosh, dong quai and red clover. It may also not be a good idea to have too much folic acid – above 400mcg a day. The herb Vitex agnus castus can help to balance oestrogen and progesterone over three to six months, but must be stopped as soon as you know you are pregnant.

No hormone-influencing herbs should be taken if you are on the Pill or HRT, or the GnRH analogues for endometriosis, as they have effects that might disrupt each other, as would very high levels of vitamins C and E. All supplements are best stopped five days before any operation.

Oestrogen dominance

Endometriosis develops in the presence of excessive oestrogen. Research has found that 79 per cent of a group of monkeys developed endometriosis after having been exposed to certain types of dioxins in their food. The severity of endometriosis found in the monkeys was directly related to the amount of the toxic chemicals, called TCDD, they were exposed to. They showed immune abnormalities similar to those observed in women with endometriosis. TCDD has an oestrogenic effect in the body. According to a World Health Organization report, 'In Belgium the incidence of endometriosis, in women presenting at clinics with infertility, is 60–80 per cent and TCDD concentrations in the breast milk are the highest in the world.'[29] More infertile women with endometriosis had detectable high TCDD levels in serum than the fertile women tested without the disease.

For this reason, women with endometriosis should avoid fatty foods, which may be high in PCBs and dioxins, to reduce their exposure.[30] Oestrogenic pesticides are found in non-organic plant and animal foods so always peel vegetables that are not organic. (For more on how to avoid hormone-disrupting chemicals see Chapter 5.)

As previously explained, the body's clearance system for oestrogen, cholesterol and toxins is the liver. The steroid hormones are broken down in the liver after which they no longer have much hormonal effect. This is key to the management of endometriosis.

Oestrogen has profound effects in the body and on the menstrual cycle. It causes the womb lining to thicken and can prolong menstruation time. It stimulates the nervous system, causing copper levels to increase and zinc to decrease, and it stimulates high levels of the adrenal corticosteroid hormone. In excess it encourages a pregnancy to be aborted. It stimulates breast tissue and has been linked to breast cancer when unopposed at high levels. High oestrogen reduces thyroxine hormone and may produce hypothyroid states. It also causes body fat deposits to increase and impairs blood sugar control, leading to weight gain, as when taking the Pill.

Practise moderation in nutrition

The nutrients that have oestrogenic activity are copper, calcium and folic acid, high levels of vitamin C and E and some essential fats. As with all nutrition, moderation seems to be the key. Diets high in saturated fat are seen to increase concentrations of serum oestrogen.[31] Other research has shown that women who eat meat once a day are up to twice as likely to have endometriosis compared to those who eat less red meat and more fruit and vegetables.[32] Studies have shown that women with the highest intake of red meat increase their risk of endometriosis by between 80 and 100 per cent, while those with the highest intake of fresh fruit and vegetables lower their risk of endometriosis by about 40 per cent. So, reducing consumption of foods that are high in saturated fats and replacing them with fruit and vegetables such as broccoli, cauliflower and cabbage, which contain indoles (see page 188), appears to improve oestrogen metabolism.

Women in Japan have the highest levels of endometriosis in the world, although they have low levels of breast cancer.[33] It is felt that this may be due to the high levels of oestrogenic chemicals, the dioxins, PCBs and phthalates in their diet. It may also be due to the excessive levels of phytoestrogens in the diet from soya and the low levels of vegetables. Soya would also appear to affect fertility. Research at Cincinnati and Auckland zoos showed that the wild-cat breeding programmes did not work when the animals ate a very high level of soya protein in their diet. When two-thirds was exchanged for chicken, the animals fell pregnant naturally. We also know that high levels of peas in the diets of Tibetan men reduce fertility, due to the phytoestrogens contained therein. The moral of the story is to eat pulses in moderation and not to excess.

The role of fibre

Dietary fibre increases the excretion of excess oestrogen from the body. Some fibres such as the lignins found in rye and seeds such as flax and chia are changed by gut flora to form anti-oestrogen compounds, which are protective against cancers.[34] Avoiding the bad saturated animal fats, hydrogenated and damaged 'trans' fats and eating cold-pressed oils is vital. Soluble fibre binds to the oestrogen and inhibits its re-absorption. Good-quality fibre encourages the hormone SHBG, which is a unique transport system for oestrogen. While oestrogen is bound to the SHBG it cannot exert any biological effect within the body.[35] If fibre intake is low, the oestrogen can have a biological effect, triggering the endometriosis implants to grow. A vegetarian, low-fat diet reduces period pain and increases SHBG.[36] Bifidobacteria encourage oestrogen clearance by inhibiting an enzyme known as beta-glucuronidase. This enzyme, when high, encourages the deactivated safe oestrogen to become reactivated so that it can be sent back into circulation (not a good idea if you have endometriosis).

Help from vegetables

The best vegetables to eat are those from the cruciferous family, all rich in B-complex vitamins and magnesium: cabbage, Brussels sprouts, broccoli, cauliflower, kale, turnip, swede, radish, horse-radish, mustard and cress. These contain three unique compounds – indoles, dithiolthiones and isothiocyanates – which influence enzymes that help eliminate excess oestrogen.[37] To help your ovaries and uterus work effectively, make sure that you eat four portions of vegetables every day.

How to reduce pain

Pain can reduce the normal quality of life. Research showed that women with severe pain, infertility and endometriosis had raised levels of PGE2 pro-inflammatory prostaglandins (from arachidonic acid, which is found in high quantities in meat and milk) in their peritoneal fluid (in the abdomen); this is the trigger for the inflammation.[38] Inability to ovulate is clinically called 'luteinised unruptured follicle syndrome' or LUF. In LUF syndrome, women will have the normal sequence of endocrine events and a normal menstrual period, but their ovary will not release the egg. Use of pain-killing non-steroidal anti-inflammatory drugs, NSAIDS, may give rise to LUF. In women with LUF syndrome, steroid hormone concentrations in the peritoneal fluid are much lower after the ovulatory cycle. It is felt that this may facilitate the development of endometriosis.[39]

Some nutrients play a role in relieving pain, including the essential fats, vitamins C, E, K, and some of the B vitamins, DLPA, zinc, selenium and magnesium. Only the natural horseshoe-shaped cisform of linoleic (omega-6) and alpha-linolenic (omega-3) fats are able to contribute to the formation of anti-inflammatory prostaglandins, which reduce pain.[40] So eat raw seeds and buy their oils cold-pressed to use, for example, in salad dressings.

Research looking at the effects of fish oils on endometrial implants showed positive results in that the sites of endometrial tissue shrank when fish oils were fed to rabbits with surgically induced endometriosis.[41] Studies looking at the use of omega-3 fish oils in subjects with severe menstrual pain showed that the oils were effective at reducing pain.[42] Magnesium is known for its relaxing effects on muscle tissue and can help with dysmenorrhoea and lower back pain.[43] Vitamin E can help reduce painful cramps and also reduce blood loss.[44]

Vitamin B_6 (pyridoxine) can have analgesic effects. If B_6 is deficient, the amount of serotonin in the brain decreases and this can lead to depression. Vitamin B_6 may help to relieve the pain associated with premenstrual syndrome. Vitamin B_{12} was shown in three independent trials to have an analgesic effect when injected intramuscularly.[45] When vitamin B_{12} is taken with vitamins B_1 and B_6, they can together produce significant pain relief and reduce inflammation.[46] My recommendation is to try the B vitamins on their own since NSAID painkillers are certainly not ideal for women with fertility problems.

It is known from research that high doses of thiamine (B_1) can suppress pain transmission. There appears to be some relationship between thiamine (B_1) and morphine.[47] A dose of 100mg vitamin B_1 was given for three months to 556 girls with period pain. Eighty-seven per cent felt completely cured, 8 per cent had some pain relief and five per cent showed no effect.[48]

The use of (yeast-free) B vitamins seems to be crucial for women with endometriosis as the regular use of multivitamin supplements may decrease the risk of ovulatory infertility.[49] The conclusion being that a high-potency multivitamin–mineral supplement will increase fertility by supporting ovulation.

Nutritional help

Follow the Diet for the Good Life (Chapter 26) and read Chapters 6, 7 and 16 on food allergies, beating sugar problems and candidiasis. The careful choice of nutritional supplements while you make every effort to improve your diet is the best way to improve your reproductive health. Harvard University and the American Dietetics Association both advise that a multivitamin–mineral should be taken each day.[50] Research at the University of Leeds suggests that women taking a multivitamin capsule every day may double their chance of getting pregnant, as it is felt that better quality ova are produced by the ovary.[51]

Choose supplements that are hypoallergenic and free from yeast, wheat gluten, lactose, sugar and dairy. Consult a doctor before you try to get pregnant. Also, seek advice from a nutritional therapist (see Resources).

The basis for a good supplement programme for endometriosis is:

- A daily multivitamin–mineral (look for one containing only 2,000iu vitamin A)

- Magnesium citrate 200mg
- Bioacidophilus 16 billion viable organisms
- Pesticide-free omega-3 fish oil 1,000mg

Optional extras are:

- Slippery elm 300mg – to soothe and heal the gut membrane
- Chromium polynicotinate 100mcg – to balance blood sugar
- Zinc citrate 20mg – for additional immune support
- Cold-pressed omega-6 evening primrose oil 1,000mg

Endometriosis – the natural approach

The following case study describes the natural procedure that helped Mary, who suffered with painful endometriosis for several years.

Case Study: Mary

Mary's periods began when she was 12 years old; they were always heavy and painful, so bad that at night she had to sleep on towels. She was eventually diagnosed with polycystic ovaries at 25 years of age. By then she was plagued by severe back pains during periods and was unable to sleep. Two years later a laparoscopy was done, but it showed nothing. The pain was so bad that Mary was unable to work. She sought a second opinion. A year later another operation showed a large lump of endometriosis inside the bowel. She was placed on pseudo-menopause drugs for six months to stop her periods and shrink the lump. After six months, however, it was still there, so a bowel operation was undertaken to remove it. Two years later the symptoms returned with bleeding from the bowel, so another bowel operation was done to remove a section of it and the endometriosis lump, which was now the size of a golf ball.

After the operation she was so ill she could not get out of bed and a third bowel operation was done with a blood transfusion.

Mary and her husband wanted to have a family, but the doctors said that this was unlikely from the state of the endometriosis and her bowel. Mary was very ill and could not work or do much in a day. She read my book (*Endometriosis: A Key to Healing and Fertility Through Nutrition*) and came to see me. We had to work on the GI tract first so we looked for imbalances in gut flora and food intolerances. I prescribed anti-inflammatory omega-3 oils and probiotics. Mary was advised to exclude wheat-based foods from her diet for one month. When reintroduced it caused bloating and Mary's periods became more painful. A gluten sensitivity blood test was positive so now wheat products were avoided. Hair mineral analysis showed high copper levels so we used zinc to chelate the copper. We used antioxidants to reduce the inflammation and changed the diet to include cooked vegetables, as raw ones caused problems. Stewed fruits and fish were accepted. Slowly but surely Mary's bowel began to function normally again and she was able to introduce more foods. After a few months Mary fell pregnant and gave birth to a baby girl. Two years later I worked with her again and Mary gave birth to a baby boy. Now Mary is very careful with her diet. Her periods are fine unless she eats the wrong foods.

How effective is the natural approach?

In a recent research trial involving 198 women with diagnosed endometriosis who had visited The Endometriosis and Fertility Clinic, using the approaches referred to in this chapter, those who had reported sub-fertility had a 52 per cent success rate in falling pregnant, 86 per cent reported pain reduction, and 26 per cent of the group who had not reported fertility problems fell pregnant.[52]

Dian Shepperson Mills has researched the relationship between endometriosis and diet for ten years. She works closely with physicians in Europe and North America, and has given lectures worldwide.

Her research interests also include fertility, polycystic ovaries and premenstrual syndrome. Dian is:

- Founder and lead nutritionist at The Endometriosis and Fertility Clinic

- The Chair of the Nutrition Special Interest Group for the American Society of Reproductive Medicine (ASRM)

- Trustee of the Charity Endometriosis SHE Trust UK (www. shetrust.org.uk)

- Governor of the Institute for Optimum Nutrition

- An advisor to the International Endometriosis Association USA

For more information, read Dian's book *Endometriosis: A Key to Healing and Fertility Through Nutrition*, co-authored with Michael Vernon (see Recommended Reading).

CHAPTER 20

How to Prevent Breast Lumps and Cancer

Many women experience benign cysts or lumps in their breasts. Symptoms are tender breasts and movable cysts, which are usually near the surface. The problem usually progresses until the menopause and then subsides. It is associated with too much oestrogen, particularly oestrone and oestradiol, which are extremely active stimulants of breast tissue.

Food and drinks containing the chemical methylxanthine (found in tea, coffee, cola and chocolate) have been shown in several studies to aggravate the problem. Although most cysts are benign, they can indicate an increased chance of developing breast cancer.

Help from vitamins

Vitamin A has been shown to help reduce breast pain and, in one study, reduced breast cyst masses by at least 50 per cent in five patients out of ten.[53] Vitamin A (retinol) is a fat-soluble vitamin and is more readily toxic than water-soluble vitamins, because it can be stored in the body. Women aiming to become pregnant need to be particularly careful about how much vitamin A they consume, and should not exceed 3,000mcg a day. Beta-carotene is converted to vitamin A in the body although this reaction requires zinc. Taking vitamin A as beta-carotene is considered a safe alternative because the body doesn't convert more than it needs; however, it is generally best to get some retinol as well. Retinol is usually extracted from fish oils but there is also a vegetarian version used in supplements called retinyl palmitate.

Several studies supplementing vitamin E up to 450mcg have been associated with remissions.[54] Evening primrose oil (EPO), which contains the essential fatty acid gamma-linolenic acid, or GLA, has also been shown to reduce breast pain, tenderness and cyst size (1,500mg twice a day).[55] Borage and blackcurrant seed oils are more concentrated sources of GLA than EPO, requiring fewer capsules to be taken. A low-salt diet also helps to reduce breast tenderness and swelling.

Minerals that help

Iodine deficiency is also linked to the development of breast cysts. Iodine is a key nutrient required for a normally functioning thyroid gland. Thyroid hormone deficiency has widespread effects on the body, including the menstrual cycle. Selenium, zinc and iron are also necessary nutrients for normal thyroid function, as are the amino acids phenylalanine and tyrosine. Seaweeds, including nori, kelp and dulse, are good food sources of iodine. Kelp is also a good supplementary source.

Iodine and selenium deficiencies, and the importance of having adequate amounts for normal thyroid function, are well established. It has been suggested that a combined deficiency of iodine and selenium may enhance the development of breast cancer. Selenium is an essential mineral for the activity of a major antioxidant enzyme called glutathione peroxidase, as well as being essential for enzymes used in the manufacture of thyroid hormones. When these enzymes are not functioning efficiently it can contribute to increased free-radical load and can lead to damaged DNA, which is associated with breast cancer. Increased levels of antioxidants, on the other hand, are associated with a reduced risk of breast cancer. Research suggests that iodine itself might act as an antioxidant. Japanese women and men have a lower incidence of breast cancer, and their diet is rich in seaweed. Rates of breast cancer increase in Japanese women when they emigrate and start to consume Western-style diets.

Follow the Diet for the Good Life as described in Chapter 26 and consult a medical practitioner experienced in the use of natural progesterone if you are considering using this hormone.

Preventing breast and other hormone-related cancers

According to Cancer Research UK, more than 45,000 women were diagnosed with breast cancer in the UK during 2006, which equates to 125 women every day. Breast cancer is currently the most common cancer in women in many countries worldwide, including the UK and the USA. We have seen more than a 50 per cent increase in incidence in the UK over the past 25 years. For every ten women diagnosed with breast cancer, eight of them are over fifty. The average risk of developing breast cancer during one's life is one in ten, and its incidence is going up, not down, unlike that for many other cancers.

Other female-related cancers include cervical cancer, the second most common, endometrial (the lining of the womb) cancer and ovarian cancer.[56] Taken together, these three cancers result in 9 per cent of all new cases of cancer in a year. Cervical cancer is primarily caused by an infection of the human papilloma virus (HPV). If you'd like to find out more about these cancers read my book *Say No to Cancer*.

However, survival rates have significantly improved in the last three decades, particularly if cancer is diagnosed early. Recent statistics show that eight out of ten women with breast cancer survive beyond five years, compared with five out of ten in the 1970s.

Although death rates from breast cancer are declining, around 12,000 women and 90 men still die from breast cancer each year, with the highest percentage of deaths in women over 70; however, 1,300 women under 50 are likely to die from breast cancer each year in the UK alone. After lung cancer, breast cancer is now the second most common cause of cancer death in women in the UK.

The good news is that, by understanding the risk factors involved and the nutrients that help prevent breast disease, you can not only reduce your chances of getting it in the first place but also reduce your risk of recurrence.

Accepted risk factors

- **Family history** Women with a mother, sister or daughter with breast cancer. Risk increases by 80 per cent.
- **Obesity** increases the risk in post-menopausal women by up to 30 per cent.
- **HRT and the Pill** HRT, if used for five years or longer increases breast cancer risk by 35 per cent, and oral contraceptive pill use increases the risk by about 25 per cent.
- **Alcohol** As little as one alcoholic drink a day may increase the risk by 12 per cent.

The risks with synthetic hormones

Synthetic hormones are strongly linked to the development of breast cancer. There is a 50 per cent greater risk in women who took the Pill before the age of 20.[57] With regard to HRT, the *New England Journal of Medicine* reported that, 'Studies over a six-year period have shown that the longer HRT is taken there is a fourfold increased risk of developing breast cancer.'[58] Progestogens (synthetic progesterone) also assist the development of blood vessels which may encourage the spread of cancer. The risk of HRT is now well known and has led to a medical reluctance to prescribe it. Nowadays, contraceptive pills also use a lower dose of synthetic hormones, which have not been conclusively linked to an increased risk. Even so, natural birth control is a better option, especially for those in a stable relationship and with a stable monthly cycle.

Other contributory factors

Even though many women with breast cancer are surviving more than five years following diagnosis, I believe that women are poorly informed about other potential risk factors for developing breast cancer. Many women are aware that there is a real risk of developing breast cancer, although unclear on what factors are involved and how to minimise their risk.

Eight out of nine breast cancers occur in women without a family history of breast cancer. The environment versus genes debate continues, although research on twins indicates that environment is more important than genes. A study involving 45,000 pairs of twins found that cancer is much more likely to be caused by diet and lifestyle choices – things we can change – than by genes. Identical twins, who are genetically the same, had no more than a 15 per cent chance of developing the same cancer. This suggests that the cause of most cancers is about 85 per cent environmental – that is, down to factors such as diet, lifestyle and exposure to toxic chemicals. This study found that diet, smoking and exercise accounted for 58–82 per cent of cancers studied.[59]

With so many changes in our diet, environment and lifestyle since the beginning of the 20th century, it is difficult to pinpoint the factors that contribute towards breast cancer. Having children later in life is associated with a higher risk, as is not having children, possibly because of the lack of extra progesterone that is present during pregnancy, as explained in Chapter 1 (breast cancer tends to occur where there is oestrogen dominance). Smoking has also been linked to the development of breast cancer. Other factors that have been shown to correlate with an increased risk include rapid growth and a greater adult height, a high body mass, weight gain in adulthood, consumption of alcohol, the total fat intake, consumption of dairy and/or meat, a high intake of animal proteins, and exposure to DDT residues as well as other environmental chemicals, particularly phthalates.

Eating plenty of fruits, vegetables, fibre and carotenoids (from orange foods such as carrots and sweet potatoes) is considered to be protective, as is physical activity. Less conclusive, however, although data is accumulating, is the evidence for the protective role of vitamin C, isoflavones, complex carbohydrates and lignans, a group of chemicals found in plants and particularly in flax and sesame seeds (see Part 5).

The oestrogen link

Three in every four breast cancers are oestrogen positive, meaning their growth is stimulated by oestrogen. Oestrogen acts like a key turning the lock, stimulating a cancer cell to divide and grow. Sixty-five per cent of breast cancers are reported to be sensitive to both oestrogen and progesterone; that is, both hormones can contribute to cancer growth. If cells have 'receptors' for one or both hormones the cancer is considered to be hormone-receptor-positive. Oestrogen receptivity is generally considered more important in terms of predicting response to drug treatments that target hormone receptors. Health outcomes improve when the cancer is responsive to both oestrogen and progesterone.

Breast cancer tends to be most prevalent when oestrogen dominance is likely; that is, during the five to ten years before the menopause. It is more likely to occur when oestrogen levels are high and progesterone levels are low. When women under 40 have their ovaries removed (the ovaries being the primary site for the production of oestrogen in pre-menopausal women) the incidence of breast cancer is significantly reduced.[60] Men treated with oestrogens for cancer of the prostate also show an increased incidence of breast cancer.[61] Xenoestrogens are increasingly being recognised as a likely link in the growing incidence of breast cancer.

The fat factor

Cancer Research UK supports a link between too much dietary fat, particularly saturated fat, and the risk of breast cancer. This was based on a study that examined the association of dietary fat, or fat-containing foods, with a risk of breast cancer.[62] This finding was independent of the known association of obesity with breast cancer risk.

It is a complex cycle, in that high body mass is associated with an increased risk: large numbers of fat cells produce more oestrogen, which in turn raises the susceptibility to accumulating more fat. Fatty tissue is also an ideal storage site for toxins such as pesticides, phthalates and organochlorines.

The so-called beneficial omega-3 and omega-6 oils also need to be used with care, as they are prone to oxidation and therefore should never be exposed to high heat, as in frying. The balance between the two oils is also important in terms of risk. Current evidence cannot exclude the possibility of a small increased risk of a high intake of linoleic acid, a member of the omega-6 family of fats, with breast, colon, rectal and prostate cancer in humans. Modern diets have a propensity to be too high in omega-6 fats compared with omega-3, as omega-6 fats are used in processed foods such as cakes, biscuits and buns and are frequently used to fry foods such as crisps and chips. So, it is better to eat more oily fish and flax seeds, or supplement a pollutant-free omega-3 essential fat supplement (see the Diet for the Good Life in Chapter 26).

Which foods and nutrients help prevent breast disease?

As we have seen throughout this book, some foods have beneficial properties whereas others cause problems in the body and eventually illness.

Eat the right high-fibre, low-GL carbohydrates and avoid sugar

Eating too much sugar and refined carbohydrates promotes high insulin levels, which stimulate the growth of breast cells.[63] Also, too many carbohydrates, which promote weight gain and obesity, is a risk factor for breast cancer. To put this in context, a woman smoking accounts for 30 per cent of the cancer risk whereas being significantly overweight accounts for 20 per cent of risk. High sugar and high-GL diets clearly promote breast and other cancers, as has been shown in many studies – this was discussed in Part 1.[64]

Both healthy breast cells and breast cancer cells have receptors for insulin, although research has shown that breast cancer cells have more of these receptors than healthy cells. Studies have shown that if insulin levels are high at the time of diagnosis with breast cancer, then the prognosis is less positive. Once insulin has attached to the receptor, it will encourage the cell to divide and multiply, encouraging the tumour to grow.

Sufficient dietary fibre – that is 35g daily – helps to bind used-up oestrogen and eliminate it, helping to reduce the likelihood of it being reactivated and reabsorbed. Good sources of dietary fibre are wholegrains, pulses, vegetables and fruit. Animal produce contains none; however, the best fibres are soluble fibres found in oats, flax and chia seeds. Make it a point to eat these every day.

Why milk is a four-letter word

Another major promoter of insulin that is strongly linked to breast cancer is milk. Almost three-quarters of the world's population live in the equatorial zone between the tropic of Cancer and the tropic of Capricorn, where cow's milk is not generally used as a staple food and a diet rich in plant food is depended upon. There is little incidence of breast cancer in those areas.

Professor Jane Plant, in her book *Your Life in Your Hands*, fully discusses the potential perils of dairy products and hormone-related cancers, including breast and prostate cancer. Professor Plant recovered from breast cancer herself and strongly believes that removal of dairy products was pivotal to her recovery.

She reports that milk and meat from dairy animals have a significant amount of the hormone prolactin and a factor called insulin-like growth factor-1 (IGF-1), as described in Chapter 3, and that the levels have increased as a likely result of modern agricultural trends in dairy farming.

Pre-menopausal women and men who have higher levels of IGF-1 in their blood have a higher risk of breast cancer, and men with higher levels appear to also have an increased risk of prostate cancer. Professor Plant also reports that cell culture studies have shown that IGF-1 and prolactin promote the growth of breast and prostate cells in the laboratory.

If you are considering largely avoiding dairy products as a preventative measure, it is important to eat more seeds, nuts, beans and root vegetables, which are good sources of calcium. Also, many non-dairy milks are calcium enriched. A good multivitamin–mineral supplement should provide 200mg. Testing for levels of IGF-1 is also an option to explore with your nutritional therapist. A low level equates to a low risk.

Increase antioxidant foods and nutrients

The activity of free oxidising radicals, which damage cells, is a critical factor in the development of most cancers. Fat oxidises in breast (and other) tissue, increasing its susceptibility to cancer, so it is advisable to take the full range of antioxidant nutrients. Although it used to be accepted that a high intake of fruit and vegetables would be cancer protective, a study published in the *Journal of the National Cancer Institute*[65] showing a marginal benefit of eating five servings of fruit and vegetables a day, has got everybody thinking. Some would argue that five servings are not enough. In fact, this study showed a 12 per cent decrease in cancer risk by eating seven servings a day, which equates to fruit with breakfast, two fruit snacks and two servings of vegetables with each main meal. Others would say we should be looking at specific anti-cancer foods. I recommend you eat the foods with highest antioxidant ratings, generally foods with a strong green, yellow, orange and red colour; for example, there is good evidence that tomatoes, high in lycopene, are protective against breast and prostate cancer.

Another way to boost your antioxidant status is to supplement critical antioxidants, including vitamins A, C and E, and the minerals zinc, selenium and manganese (see the chart in Chapter 28 for dosage levels).

Many amino acids, the building blocks of protein, also act as antioxidants. So, ensuring an adequate intake of protein is also important. Melatonin, derived from the essential amino acid tryptophan is, for example, a potent antioxidant. Research has shown melatonin to slow the rate of breast cancer and this was related to melatonin's role in sleep. Many individuals with cancer suffer from sleep problems, and nurses who often work night shifts have high rates of breast and colon cancer. See the section in Chapter 13 on insomnia on page 126 for ways to help you get more sleep.

Similarly, glutathione is a major antioxidant found in the cells, and a low level of its reduced form compared to its oxidised form is a marker of cell toxicity. Glutathione, derived initially from the essential amino acid methionine, is made up of three non-essential amino acids, cysteine, glycine and glutamic acid. By non-essential this means the body can make them and, as indicated above, if there is enough folate and vitamins B_{12} and B_6, the body should be able to convert methionine to glutathione. Vegetarian diets can be low in methionine, particularly if little dairy, nuts and seeds are eaten.

The non-essential amino acid taurine, which is found primarily in fish and meat, can also be in short supply in vegetarian diets. Taurine is another major antioxidant and is made in the body from cysteine. Vitamin B_6 is needed for this conversion.

Whether you are a meat eater, vegetarian or vegan, what is important is to ensure that you achieve the right nutrient intake from whatever your dietary preference might be. To have sufficient antioxidants, this would mean ensuring adequate protein and a good intake of vegetables and fruit (see Diet for the Good Life in Chapter 26).

However, I think that controlling your blood sugar and insulin levels, by avoiding sugar and cutting right back on milk, will prove to be more preventative than simply increasing the fruit and vegetables you eat, so don't put all your eggs in the antioxidant basket. It is just one piece of the equation for hormone-related cancers.

Vitamin D is vital

A deficiency in vitamin D is increasingly correlated with various cancers and other chronic illnesses. Research reported in 2008 has also demonstrated poorer survival rates if people were found to be vitamin D deficient at the time of diagnosis.[66]

Several teams of researchers have found that adequate levels of vitamin D lower the chances of developing breast cancer. Low levels of vitamin D in serum have been correlated with breast cancer disease progression and spread of cancer to the bones,[67] and studies suggest that increased intake of vitamin D reduces the risk of breast cancer in pre-menopausal women.[68]

Scientists at Manchester University reported that women with advanced breast cancer that had spread to their bones were less likely to die of the disease when they had high amounts of active vitamin D in their blood.[69]

And a team of cancer prevention specialists at the University of California, San Diego, found that women with the highest level of vitamin D in their blood (up to 130 nmol/L) had a 50 per cent lower risk of breast cancer than those with the lowest level of 32 nmol/L.[70]

'The results were very clear,' said co-author Dr Cedric Garland, 'the higher your level, the lower the risk.' To have a blood level that would cut your risk by 50 per cent, the researchers said that you would have to take 50mcg (2,000iu) daily and also spend 10–15 minutes in the sun. In fact, Dr Garland has estimated that 600,000 cases a year of breast and colorectal cancer could be prevented by an adequate intake of vitamin D.[71]

The B vitamins

B vitamins are involved in breaking down oestrogen and clearing it from the liver. Vitamins B_{12}, folate and B_6 are critical nutrients used in the manufacture of agents that detoxify oestrogen, including sulphur, glutathione and compounds called methyl groups. They are also vital for a process called methylation and keeping your homocysteine level down. A high homcysteine level equates to an increased risk of cancer. Ensuring your diet is rich in B vitamins, as described in the Diet for the Good Life, is critical to hormonal balance.

Summary

The best way to prevent breast lumps and to lower your risk of breast cancer is to:

- Eat a low-GL diet, high in fibre, especially soluble fibre in oats, flax and chia seeds.
- Minimise your intake of all dairy products, having more fish and vegetarian sources of protein.
- Eat lots of antioxidant-rich fruit and vegetables, and supplement antioxidants.
- Ensure you get plenty of vitamin D from a combination of sun, seafood and supplements. You need to supplement 15mcg a day.
- Ensure you get plenty of B vitamins, both from eating a wholefood diet and making sure your daily multivitamin provides around 20mg of B_6, 200mcg of folic acid and 10mcg of B_{12}. If your homocysteine level is high you may need more.
- Control your weight through a combination of diet and exercise.

CHAPTER 21

Preventing and Reversing Osteoporosis

Osteoporosis is the silent thief that robs your skeleton of up to 25 per cent of its bone mass by the time you reach 50. It is now a serious epidemic in Britain. Bones become porous, or osteoporotic, due to the progressive loss of minerals, mass and density, and this can result in fractures. It is reported that one in two women, and one in five men, will suffer a fracture after the age of 50. If current trends continue, hip fractures might increase from 46,000 in 1985 to 117,000 in 2016. It is estimated that the cost by 2020 of treating all fractures resulting from osteoporosis in post-menopausal women will be £2 billion.

Yet skeletal material dating from between 1729 and 1852, unearthed during the restoration of Christ Church, Spitalfields, in London, showed significantly less bone loss in women then than today, despite our supposedly better diet. Investigators found no sign of menopausal change in the unearthed bones. So, although osteoporosis is connected to the hormones, this information suggests that some aspect of modern living doesn't suit our skeletons.

The role of ovulation

Women are more at risk than men of developing osteoporosis. The female hormones oestrogen and progesterone are protective to women's bones, just as the male hormone testosterone is protective to men's. But, from the age of 35, women regularly fail to ovulate, minimising their production of progesterone, the major hormone for bone strength. Women at most risk of developing osteoporosis are those that have had an early menopause (before the age of 45), either naturally, or surgically by removing the womb and one or both ovaries.

Major well known risk factors

Early menopause

Anorexia

Bulimia

Over-dieting

Over- or under-exercising

Heavy intake of alcohol and drugs

Many missed periods

Previous fracture from slight injury

Significant corticosteroid use

Losing several inches in height

Having a close relative with brittle bones

History of heavy cigarette smoking

Osteoporosis is mostly a 'silent' disorder and a fracture is often the first indication of a problem. Loss of height, back pain, tooth loss and a bent posture are indicators of osteoporosis, particularly after the age of 50.

A balance of hormones

The interplay of hormones is fundamental for preventing osteoporosis. Oestrogen works by removing old damaged bone, and when oestrogen levels decline at the menopause bone loss is accelerated. Progesterone is the bone builder, as it works on bone cells that rebuild new bone to replace the old. The stress hormone cortisol, when chronically elevated, can contribute to bone loss. The balance of parathormone (the hormone that regulates calcium levels in the body) and calcitonin (the hormone that lowers blood calcium) help to control calcium balance between the blood and bones. Thyroid hormones, testosterone and growth hormone also affect bone health.

Osteoporosis is a slow, progressive disease: bone loss starts in most women from the mid thirties. It does not happen overnight with the last menstrual period. Children and young adults are generally building bones, but between the ages of 30 and 40 the balance between bone growth and bone loss is about equal, and after 50 bone growth decreases and bone loss increases. Developing, supporting and maintaining bone health is a lifelong commitment.

The HRT question

Treatment strategies have largely been focused on HRT, bisphosphonate drugs (such as Fosamax), and calcium and vitamin D supplementation. Although the Women's Health Initiative trial showed a small decreased risk of hip fracture,[72] there is now a substantial body of evidence that HRT should not be recommended to women to prevent or treat osteoporosis, and that the risks outweigh the benefits. It seems that bone mass is only preserved in those who take HRT for seven years or more[73] and, even when you take it for that long, bone mineral density rapidly declines once you stop taking it. Following a European-wide review of the balance of risks and benefits of HRT, it is no longer recommended as first choice of therapy for prevention of osteoporosis, according to advice from the Medicines and Healthcare Products Regulatory Agency (MHRA) in 2003.[74] HRT does, however, remain a treatment option for those who cannot use other osteoporosis prevention therapies or for whom other therapies have been shown to be ineffective, although the decision must be made with care.

Younger women who use short-term HRT will probably gain little or no protection against fracture beyond the age of 70, according to one study.[75] At 75, the women's bone mineral density was found to be only just over 3 per cent higher than that of women who had never taken HRT. So, unless you are prepared to take HRT for life, it is unlikely to protect you against osteoporosis – and the longer you take it, the greater your risk of developing breast and womb cancer. (See 'Beyond calcium – bone-friendly minerals', page 218, for ways of building bone density nutritionally.)

Eighteen European specialists reviewed the data on HRT and osteoporosis. No long-term benefits were identified. Hip fracture risk was as great for women who stopped HRT as those who had never used it. Protection from HRT is lost within five years of stopping. Furthermore, many women cannot tolerate HRT and stop within a year of using it. Other women may trial many forms of HRT before finding one that suits them.

The conclusion of the European specialists was: 'For healthy women without menopausal symptoms the benefit–risk analysis of HRT for the prevention of osteoporosis is not favourable'.[76] Officially, doctors in the UK are now told that the risks outweigh the benefits, and not to prescribe it for osteoporosis prevention. But it is still commonly prescribed for this reason in other parts of the world.

Fosamax

Many women with digestive problems cannot take Fosamax and it is associated with many side effects, including oesophageal irritation and ulceration, bone and muscle pain. Intravenous Fosamax is linked with a horrendous condition called osteonecrosis of the jaw that results in deterioration and death of the jawbone. Fosamax also increases risk of atrial fibrillation, and one long-term study revealed that it raises the risk of stress fractures in the bones of the legs. So where does this leave us? Specialists say there is an urgent need to find replacement therapies.

Is natural progesterone an answer?

Bones have two kinds of cell: osteoblasts which build new cells, and osteoclasts which get rid of old bone material, such as calcium. Oestrogen, which influences osteoclast cells, doesn't actually help to build new bone. It only stops the loss of old bone. Progesterone, on the other hand, stimulates osteoblasts, which actually build new bone.[77] In this study (below), using natural progesterone cream increased bone density four times more than taking oestrogen.

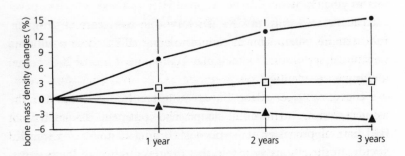

The effects of natural progesterone ●, oestrogen □, or no hormone supplement ▲ on bone density

In the time leading up to the menopause, most women start to have cycles in which ovulation doesn't occur (known as anovulatory cycles). After the menopause, ovulation never occurs. If no egg is released, no progesterone is produced (because progesterone is only made in the ovary sac once the egg is released); however, the body does continue to produce small amounts of oestrogen. Scientists are now starting to think that it is the relative excess of oestrogen to progesterone – creating, in effect, a progesterone deficiency – that precipitates osteoporosis, rather than the deficiency in oestrogen. This would explain why bone loss commonly starts from the age of 35, long before the actual menopause. In the pre-menopausal years, anovulatory cycles (in which no progesterone is produced) become increasingly common. Loss of bone mass density is known to occur in women who have such anovulatory cycles.[78]

Improve your diet before using hormone therapy

As mentioned earlier, diet and lifestyle strategies should precede the use of hormone therapy, whether natural or synthetic. Applying natural progesterone when all the building blocks for bone health are not in place is a band-aid approach. If, for example, calcium is deficient in the diet or poorly absorbed due to low levels of stomach acid or a leaky gut, relying on progesterone as a bone builder is somewhat missing the point.

Having said that, the late Dr John Lee used natural progesterone with his patients for 20 years and reported excellent results and no known serious side effects. Dr Lee reported in the *Lancet* that giving nature-identical progesterone, as a transdermal skin cream, was four times more effective than oestrogen HRT, with none of the associated risks.[79] However, two placebo-controlled studies did not find natural progesterone applied according to the recommended standard instructions to be effective in preventing bone loss in post-menopausal women.

Professor Cooper, from Southampton University, reported following their study that there was no indication the creams did any harm, and there were some indications they could be beneficial in terms of reducing severe menopausal symptoms, such as hot flushes and night sweats.[80]

Natural progesterone, which is prescribable as Pro-Juven, doesn't increase breast cancer risk and may even help to prevent it. As previously mentioned, natural hormones should only be used under the supervision of a medical practitioner experienced in their use.

Understanding osteoporosis

It is important to understand that osteoporosis is not a calcium deficiency disorder – it is a disorder where calcium is lost from bone. Ninety-nine per cent of calcium in the body is in bone. Simply replacing calcium and giving vitamin D that aids calcium being deposited in the bone is linear thinking in terms of managing this devastating and largely preventable disease. Up to 4 per cent bone loss a year can occur by the time a woman reaches her late sixties. Many women are now working beyond 60 and are seeking healthy active retirements.

Dairy products are a good source of dietary calcium and have long been promoted to women as a dietary intervention for the prevention and management of osteoporosis. As explained in Chapter 20, however, almost three-quarters of the world's population live in the equatorial zone where cow's milk is not a staple food but who eat a diet rich in plant foods. There is little incidence of osteoporosis in people living there. By comparison there is a high incidence of osteoporosis in Sweden, where the intake of calcium-rich foods is high.

Harvard Medical School researchers reported that drinking lots of milk and eating calcium-rich dairy foods may not help women avoid bone fractures in later life and may, in fact, increase the risk. The 12-year study, which involved over 120,000 women throughout the US, found that women who drank two or more glasses of milk per day actually had a 45 per cent higher risk of hip fractures and a 5 per cent higher risk of forearm fractures than women who drank less.[81]

Many nutrients have been shown to be important for bone health, including calcium, magnesium, phosphorous, boron, zinc, vitamins D, C, K, A and B_6, antioxidant nutrients and protein. Calcium and phosphorous are the two major bone minerals.

The way the body absorbs and handles calcium in the body is very complex. Let's take a look at why just taking additional calcium is only part of the answer.

Less well-known risk factors

Too much protein

Inappropriate levels of stress

Poor intake of specific nutrients

Poor use of specific nutrients

Poor absorption of specific nutrients

Too much salt

Too little stomach acid

High use of stimulants and fizzy drinks

High intake of phytates

Too much sulphate

Too much protein

One of the most significant, yet less well-known risk factors for osteoporosis, according to a World Health Organization research survey, is excessive protein consumption.[82] This is for two main reasons. Protein is digested in the presence of high levels of acid (hydrochloric acid, or HCl) in the stomach; and women, particularly those over 50 years of age, often produce insufficient levels of this. HCl is also vital for releasing minerals from food, so low levels can lead to poor absorption of minerals, including calcium, magnesium and zinc, all of which are vital for bone health.

The second problem is that foods that are high in protein create strong acids in the body, which has to work very hard to neutralise them. It does this by calling on body reserves of what are known as alkalising minerals, most significantly calcium. To maintain life, the blood has to be kept very slightly alkaline, and the body will do this at all costs, even if it means using calcium from the bones.

The Inuit – who suffer the highest rates of osteoporosis – have a classic high-protein diet: plenty of seal meat and fish, with very few fruits and vegetables. Fruits and vegetables contain acids, but they are weak and very easy for the body to dispose of. Red meat, chicken, fish, eggs and dairy produce are all high protein foods. The trend towards eating low-fat dairy foods may be protective to your blood vessels, but not as kind to your bones. As soon as the fat content of a food is lowered, the percentage of protein increases. So high intakes of cottage cheese and low-fat yoghurt may not be such a good idea after all. As mentioned earlier, a high percentage of the world's population do not eat dairy products; however, if you eat little or no dairy products then it is essential to get good levels of calcium from other foods, including nuts, seeds and dark green leafy vegetables.

What the studies tell us

The Nurses' Health Study, conducted in the US and analysed by the Harvard School of Public Health, found that women who consumed 95g (3¼oz) of protein a day, as compared with those who consumed less than 68g (2¼oz) a day, had a 22 per cent greater risk of forearm fractures.[83] In another study, eating more than 80g of protein a day, which is equivalent to bacon and eggs for breakfast and a steak for dinner, was found to increase the risk of osteoporosis.[84]

This happens because protein is made of amino acids, and protein-rich foods therefore generate more acid in the body. Because the body cannot tolerate substantial changes in the acid pH of blood, it neutralises or 'buffers' this effect through two main alkaline agents: sodium and calcium. When the body's reserves of sodium are used up, calcium is taken from the bones – a finding that has been confirmed by 'metabolic ward' studies in which people are kept in a controlled environment, fed precise diets and measured for their calcium loss. Such studies have found that a negative calcium balance is created when 95g of protein is consumed while a person eats 500mg of calcium. The calcium intake must be raised to 800mg before calcium balance is achieved – that is to say, when the calcium entering the body is the same as the amount leaving. And the more protein you eat, the more calcium you need. According to a report in the *American Journal of Epidemiology*, an 11-year study of 40,000 elderly Norwegians also found an increased risk of hip fractures among those eating high amounts of non-dairy protein (meat/fish/eggs), as well as among those who had either a high coffee or low calcium intake.[85]

The fact that high-protein diets lead to calcium deficiency is nothing new. Dr Shalini Reddy from the University of Chicago conducted a six-week study on ten healthy adults eating a low-carb diet. Volunteers lost an average of 4kg (9lb) over the course of the study – that's 680g (1½lb) a week. That's the good news. The bad news was that the acid excretion in the urine, which is an indication of acid levels in the blood, rose by 90 per cent in some volunteers. There was also a sharp rise in the amount of calcium excreted in the urine during the low-carbohydrate, high-protein diets, and even the 'maintenance' diets for these regimes, despite only a slight decrease in calcium intake. This means the people were losing calcium from the body. Also, urinary citrate – a compound that inhibits kidney stone formation – decreased, implying an increased risk of kidney stone formation.[86] According to Dr Reddy, 'Consumption of a low-carbohydrate, high-protein diet for six weeks delivers a marked acid load to the kidney, increases the risk of stone formation, decreases estimated calcium balance, and may increase the risk of bone loss.' These studies all suggest that such high-protein diets may increase the risk of bone loss over the long term. Of course, we are going to have to wait a while to find out, but I'd rather you weren't the guinea pig.

Can calcium supplementation help?

Research is also beginning to show that if you eat a high-protein diet, no amount of calcium supplementation can correct the imbalance. In one study, published in the *American Journal of Clinical Nutrition*, subjects were given a moderately high protein diet (12g nitrogen) and a very high protein diet (36g nitrogen) plus 1,400mg of calcium.[87] The overall loss of calcium was 37mg per day on the 12g nitrogen diet and 137mg per day on the 36g nitrogen diet. The authors concluded that, 'high calcium diets are unlikely to prevent probable bone loss induced by high protein diets'. The negative effects of too much protein have been clearly demonstrated in patients with osteoporosis. Some medical scientists now believe that a life-long consumption of a high-protein, acid-forming diet may be a primary cause of osteoporosis.[88]

Of course, this begs the question as to whether eating a lot of dairy produce (high in both protein and calcium) would be protective or contribute to osteoporosis risk. Diane Feskanich, the director of the study involving 120,000 women described on page 214, said, 'I certainly would want women to have adequate calcium in their diets, but I would not rely on that as the prime prevention against osteoporosis.' There is no clear pattern of evidence that drinking milk prevents osteoporosis.

Poor absorption

Many factors can contribute to poor absorption of minerals, besides too little stomach acid. The small intestine is lined with thousands of minute structures called villi, which waft about, maximising the body's ability to absorb nutrients. Foods rich in gluten – wheat, rye, oats and barley – can blunt the villi, decreasing the surface area available for absorption. High intakes of dairy produce can also aggravate the gut membrane, leading to poor absorption. Another major factor known to interfere with good absorption is an overgrowth in the gut of the yeast organism *Candida albicans* that is responsible for causing thrush (see Chapter 16). Diets rich in phytates, found in wheat and soya products, can bind to important minerals in the gut – such as calcium, magnesium and zinc – impairing their absorption.

Too much stress

Just like too much protein, too much stress makes the body leach calcium from the bones. Stressors include caffeine, nicotine, drugs and physical or emotional pressure. Every time your body is stressed, a red alert signal goes out into the body. Whenever this happens, calcium is moved out of the bones into the blood to help prepare the body for the perceived danger. A stressful job, relationships, and/or relying on tea, coffee, chocolate and cigarettes to see you through the day will almost certainly rob your bones of calcium. To add insult to injury, the calcium is not adequately returned to the bones, as the body is hardly ever able to perceive that the emergency is truly over during the day. The level of calcium in the blood is very tightly regulated, and so if it is not returned to the bone the body may 'dump' calcium on artery walls, in joint tissue or as part of a painful gall or kidney stone. Stressed people often show a high level of calcium in their hair, which is another method that the body uses to 'dump' calcium.

Sub-optimum nutrition – the modern curse

For most people, sub-optimum nutrition is the rule not the exception. It can occur simply through just not eating enough food; but in the Western world it is more likely to be caused by eating foods that are high in calories, but not nutrients: predominately refined foods, alcohol and confectionery. A limited diet that repetitively uses the same foods is likely to be one that is unbalanced and unable to provide all the nutrients needed for health, including bone health. It is sometimes an excess of a particular nutrient that causes the problem, in combination with low levels of other nutrients.

Getting the right balance for calcium

Calcium needs a balance of phosphorous and magnesium to build bone effectively. Typical 'junk food' diets are rich in phosphorous, which disrupts this balance. Dairy produce is rich in calcium, but low in magnesium, which is needed to absorb and use calcium properly in the body. Nuts, seeds and green leafy vegetables are rich sources of both. Reducing salt could also help, as too much salt causes a loss of calcium from the body. Other minerals for bone health include boron, which helps prevent the loss of calcium and magnesium in the urine, and manganese, which helps new bone to be laid down. Vitamin D, the sunshine vitamin, is vital for the absorption of calcium and phosphorous, and it also helps to stop them being lost in the urine. Zinc, vitamins A, B$_6$ and C are all important for connective tissue that acts as a support for bone.

Beyond calcium – bone-friendly minerals

The story sounds good. Your bones are made of calcium, so the more calcium you have, the stronger your bones; however, research has shown mixed results from supplementing calcium. Similarly, some trials have found an increased – not decreased – risk of fractures in people with a high milk intake.

Vitamin D is also needed for your body to utilise calcium, and a meta-analysis of five trials involving patients with corticosteroid-induced bone mass loss showed that this combination of nutrients was effective.[89] However, not all trials have tallied with this finding. A study involving more than 3,000 women at risk of osteoporosis, found no protective effect from giving 1,000mg of calcium plus 800iu of vitamin D (as cholecalciferol).[90]

Another study, published in the *New England Journal of Medicine*, found a mild improvement in bone mass density, but no significant reduction of risk of a hip fracture from 1,000mg of calcium and 400iu of vitamin D.[91] Personally, I still recommend that you supplement calcium (500mg) and vitamin D (400iu). But it is best to do so by taking a bone-friendly formula that also provides magnesium (250mg), silica (30mg) and boron (1mg) – all of which are needed for good bone health.

Other important bone nutrients

Nutrient	Best Food Sources
Zinc	Nuts, seeds and whole grains
Manganese/boron	Unprocessed foods
Silicon/copper	Unprocessed foods
Vitamin A	Yellow and deep-green vegetables
Vitamin C	Berries, potatoes, most fruits and vegetables
Vitamin K	Cauliflower and green vegetables
Vitamin B_6	Fruits, vegetables and whole grains

Other beneficial nutrients

Increasingly, vitamin K has been shown to be important for bone health. It helps urinary calcium loss and facilitates the binding of osteocalcin (a calcium-binding protein) to hydroxapatite crystals, helping to create the right balance of bone mineralisation. Although we take in vitamin K from food, the gut bacteria also make a type of vitamin K that we can store in the liver. Antibiotic therapy, stress and poor digestive function can all upset bacterial balance in the gut, leading to poor manufacture of vitamin K.

Antioxidant nutrients, including vitamins A, C and E, zinc and selenium are important, because free radicals are formed when bone is being broken down. As mentioned earlier, when oestrogen levels fall, the rate of bone breakdown is increased, leading to more free radicals being produced.

Certain plant foods contain phytochemicals, which have hormone-like activity. Cultures whose diets are rich in soya and/or wild yam, which both contain such phytochemicals, show little evidence of osteoporosis. Most interesting is the role of a group of naturally occurring hormone-like substances called isoflavones (a type of phytoestrogen) found in soya. These seem to enhance bone-building and prevent the breakdown of bone. Ipriflavone, a derivative of these naturally occurring isoflavones, has been extensively tested and has proven, in over a dozen trials, to increase bone density and decrease bone loss, when given with either calcium, oestrogen HRT or vitamin D, significantly more than when these are given alone.[92]

The homocysteine connection

One interesting discovery is the link between homocysteine (see page 65), low B_{12} levels and bone and joint health. Over the last five years there have been more and more studies linking high homocysteine and low B_{12} levels to increased risk of fractures, osteoporosis and decreased bone mass density, particularly in women. Homocysteine is now thought to damage joints[93] and other tissue directly. It looks as if homocysteine actually damages bone by encouraging its breakdown and interfering with the collagen matrix, which is what holds bone together. Collagen is made from vitamin C, which is yet another reason why I recommend a daily intake of 1g taken twice a day.

A number of studies suggest that having a high level of homocysteine in your blood may weaken bone and increase the risk of fractures.[94] One of these was a very large study (involving 2,268 men and 3,070 women) by Dr Clara Gjesdal and her colleagues at the University of Bergen in Norway. Known as the Hordaland Homocysteine Study, it showed that elevated homocysteine and low folate levels were associated with reduced bone mineral density (BMD) in women, but not in men.[95] When it was fracture risk that was being evaluated, two surveys from 2004 found a doubling to quadrupling in the incidence of fractures in people with high blood levels of homocysteine.[96]

Dr Markus Herrmann, from the University of Sydney, Australia, and colleagues from Germany and Italy reviewed a total of 28 studies and concluded that high homocysteine levels (and possibly B-vitamin deficiencies) have a detrimental effect on bone quality, because they stimulate the cells that clear out old bone (osteoclasts). Since there is no direct effect on the bone-*building* cells (osteoblasts), old bone ends up being cleared away faster than new bone is produced.[97]

It is not yet clear if it is the homocysteine itself which is causing the damage to bone and increased fracture risk or whether homocysteine levels are just reflecting low levels or deficiencies of either folate or B_{12} – nutrients that *do* have a direct effect on bone.[98] Some studies suggest that low folate levels influence BMD and/or fracture risk,[99] whereas others implicate B_{12}.[100] Patients with a type of anaemia, called pernicious anaemia (caused by lack of B_{12} in the blood), have decreased BMD at the lumbar (lower) spine, and in comparison with the general population they have almost double the risk of hip fracture.[101]

Dr Rosalie Dhonukshe-Rutten, from Wageningen University in the Netherlands, has shown that low B_{12} is associated with low BMD in adolescents and that frail elderly women with a B_{12} deficiency were seven times more likely to have osteoporosis than women with normal B_{12} levels. Older women, but not men, with low BMD had significantly lower vitamin B_{12} levels than older women with higher BMD.[102] This is because B_{12} has a direct effect on bone-building cells and also stimulates an enzyme involved in the process of forming new bone called alkaline phosphatise (ALP). Another of her studies showed that high homocysteine and low B_{12} were significantly associated with less bone strength, increased bone turnover and a three times higher risk of fractures in men and women; however, the impact of low B_{12} was more severe in women than men, whereas high homocysteine was more associated with fractures in men.[103]

Not many studies have been carried out to see what effects supplementing homocysteine-lowering nutrients has on BMD and fracture risk; however, since stroke increases the risk of subsequent hip fracture by two to four times, one Japanese study followed 433 stroke patients, aged 65 and over, for two years to see if treatment with folate (5mg) and vitamin B_{12} (1,500 mcg) would have any effect. The combined treatment of folate and B_{12} was found to be a safe and effective way of reducing the risk of hip fracture in these patients.[104]

A low level of oestrogen, which is very common in postmenopausal women, also appears to raise homocysteine and increase osteoporosis risk. Theoretically, increasing oestrogen could help lower homocysteine.[105] This has been shown in some preliminary studies,[106] but not in others. Until more is understood about how homocysteine and oestrogen are related, I am reluctant to recommend oestrogen HRT as a means to lower homocysteine, for two reasons. One is that it is less effective than the nutritional strategy to lower homocysteine; the other is that it carries an increased risk of breast and uterine cancer. Natural progesterone HRT (not to be confused with synthetic progestins used in most HRT preparations) does not have these associated risks. But no one has yet investigated whether this lowers homocysteine.

Because B vitamins lower levels of homocysteine, supplementing vitamins B_6, B_{12} and folic acid, plus trimethylglycine (TMG), could be a good idea. As many as two in five people over 60 are B_{12} deficient, if tested. The lowest level that corrects B_{12} deficiency is 500mcg a day. While fish, meat, eggs and milk all contain B_{12}, only milk and fish consumption are linked to increasing blood B_{12} levels, possibly indicating that these foods have more bioavailable B_{12}. Even so, you are unlikely to get more than 3mcg of B_{12} from your food. Most B_{12} experts think that we could all benefit from a daily intake of 10mcg which is the minimum I'd recommend in a good multivitamin.

The importance of exercise

Good weight-bearing exercise, such as walking briskly on a regular basis, is a fine way to help keep calcium in the bones. For osteoporosis prevention, follow the exercise programme given in Chapter 26, page 300; however, if you already have osteoporosis, you will need a gentler programme (see 'Exercise if you have osteoporosis' opposite) as your bones will be too fragile to resist the stresses and strains which are beneficial in stimulating bone growth in more robust individuals. Having said that, it is important that you take regular gentle exercise to maintain physical function and also to prevent further deterioration.

Exercise if you have osteoporosis

The following forms of exercise are recommended for people with osteoporosis.

- 10 minutes of walking daily
- Hydrotherapy and aqua aerobics
- T'ai chi

The latter two are great for improving balance safely.

Whether preventing or living with osteoporosis, you can definitely benefit from regular exercise. By becoming more active in your daily life and at least taking time out to walk for 10 minutes a day you should definitely feel a difference in your health within six weeks. Get pleasure from your chosen activity – if you don't like it, you won't do it! So make sure you find an activity that suits you; have fun and try something different from time to time.

Osteoporosis prevention and reversal plan

Prevention is far better than looking for a cure and, according to the work of the late Dr Lee, osteoporosis is a reversible disorder. It appears that, even for someone in their seventies, the condition can be reversed. The human body responds marvellously to being provided with the correct raw materials needed for health. If hormone replacement therapy is still needed, consider natural progesterone as opposed to oestrogen HRT. The combined supplementation of vitamins and minerals, plus hormones, has not only proven more effective in restoring bone density but is also more effective in retaining it once HRT is stopped.[107] Whether or not the complete approach recommended in this book – including diet, low stimulant intake, exercise and supplements – can replace HRT has yet to be put to the test.

Here's what to do:

1. Don't consume more than 40g (1½oz) of protein a day. This is not usually a problem for vegetarians, who should aim to have two servings daily of a protein vegetable food, such as lentils, beans or tofu. For a meat-eater this means meat certainly no more than once a day and, ideally, no more than three times a week. (For recommended portion sizes see page 301.)

2. Supplement a bone mineral formula. This should include 500mg of calcium, 350mg of magnesium, 10mcg of vitamin D, 2mg of boron, 10mg of zinc, plus vitamin C, 40mcg of vitamin K and B vitamins.

3. Consider using natural progesterone cream. If pre-menopausal, check your hormone levels and, if oestrogen-dominant, use natural progesterone. If post-menopausal, use it anyway. Your doctor can prescribe it. In case of difficulty, or for information, contact the Natural Progesterone Information Service (see Resources).

4. Take regular exercise.

5. Eat plenty of wholefoods.

6. Eat plenty of nuts, seeds and yellow and green vegetables. Rely on seeds and nuts for minerals, not dairy products. Dairy products, especially cheese, are high in protein and oestrogenic hormones and low in magnesium. A heaped tablespoon of ground sesame, sunflower, flax or pumpkin seeds will give you significant amounts of calcium, magnesium and zinc, plus essential fats.

7. Eat a varied diet that includes some soya milk, tofu and wild yam.

8. Reduce animal protein to the minimum. Eat fish rather than meat. Fish is preferable because it provides more anti-inflammatory essential fats and fewer oestrogenic hormones.

9. Avoid 'junk foods', fizzy drinks and stimulants, such as coffee.

10. Limit alcohol.

11. Test your homocysteine and, if high, take a high-strength homocysteine formula providing at least 500mcg of B_{12}, plus folic acid, B_6 and other homocysteine-lowering nutrients.

12. Seek advice from a professional nutritional therapist to check out complicating factors like candidiasis, digestive function and individual supplement requirements.

Tests for osteoporosis risk

To assess your risk of osteoporosis, your GP can recommend a BMD scan or a nutritional therapist can recommend a simple urine test.

Bone mineral density (BMD) scans

Two very good techniques are available that give reliable and accurate readings. BMD scans can be requested through your medical practitioner or paid for privately. Dual photon absorptiometry (DPA) is 96–98 per cent accurate for the hips and spinal column. Dual energy X-ray absorptiometry (DEXA) is also 96–98 per cent accurate but does use low-dose X-rays. These detect osteoporosis at moderately advanced stages.

Pyrilinks-D

This is a urine test that measures deoxypyridinoline (DPD), a crosslink of collagen found in bone. This test enables your medical practitioner or nutritional therapist to identify and monitor your risk of bone loss. DPD is a specific marker for bone resorption; that is, how quickly old bone is cleared. The test is non-invasive and convenient, and can demonstrate response to therapy as early as one month in. Pyrilinks-D is said to identify bone loss early in menopause. Results of a 22-month study involving elderly and pre-menopausal women with elevated Pyrilinks-D values showed double the risk of hip fracture.[108] Pyrilinks-D values combined with BMD scans predict risk even more accurately.

Genetic testing

It is now possible to test for genetic variations in genes that are involved in bone breakdown, inflammation and collagen formation as well as how calcium and vitamin D_3 regulate bone metabolism. More personalised preventative and therapeutic nutrition strategies can be designed based on findings from genetic testing. The benefit of this type of genetic testing is that diet and lifestyle modifications can generally help reduce risk and/or progression.

It is important to remember that osteoporosis is a complex condition. It is very much a case of detective work to identify the underlying factors in each individual. For best results I recommend that you work with a nutritional therapist and your medical practitioner.

PART 4

∾

BALANCING YOUR HORMONES NATURALLY

In this part I explain in detail how oestrogen and progesterone work in the female body and how being deficient in progesterone causes your hormones to become unbalanced. Although there are a number of health risks connected with the use of synthetic hormones, they are nevertheless most frequently chosen by doctors for hormonal problems. This is in spite of research and growing numbers of women reporting benefits after using natural progesterone. This section explains all you need to know about this natural alternative and lists the tests you can take to see whether your body is deficient in certain hormones. A nutritional therapist or doctor can then prescribe a natural approach that will be suitable for you.

CHAPTER 22

Oestrogen and Progesterone in Detail

Mainstream medicine has made a strong case for prescribing synthetic hormones, not only for use in contraception, but also for use in a variety of female hormone-related conditions – from heavy or painful periods to PMS, and infertility to menopause. In the 1990s it was predicted that in 15–20 years time three in four women would be taking HRT, which was at that time touted as the answer to the menopause *and* as a potential anti-ageing elixir. Several decades after the inception of synthetic hormones, however, we are beginning to understand how they can undermine, rather than promote, the balance of women's hormones.

The myth of the safety of HRT started to unravel at the beginning of the 21st century when a major trial, involving more than 27,000 women (the US government-sponsored Women's Health Initiative), revealed an increased risk of breast cancer and strokes from blood clots in women taking HRT. In fact, the trial was cut short due to significant increases in both cardiovascular problems, such as heart attacks, and breast cancer. However, the findings did indicate that HRT might offer protection against osteoporosis (see Chapter 21). The trial's author, Dr Valerie Beral, estimated that 'the use of HRT by women aged 50–64 years in the UK over the previous decade had resulted in an estimated 20,000 extra cases of breast cancer'.[1]

This study predicted that a reduction in prescriptions for HRT would result in a decrease in breast cancers, which is exactly what happened. Following this study, the number of prescriptions for HRT more than halved in both the US and the UK. Research published in 2009 showed that breast cancer incidence has fallen in line with that prediction.[2] The result of this, according to a recent report in the *British Medical Journal*, is 1,500 fewer cases of breast cancer each year in the UK.

How the female hormones work

In order to see why synthetic hormones may give rise to health problems, it is necessary to understand how the two major female sex hormones, oestrogen and progesterone, work. Hormones are messengers made in one part of the body, and released into the blood to affect specific distant organs. To respond to the changing needs of the body, an intricate system controls their continuous production, breakdown and disposal.

To maximise reproductive ability, the body produces a balance of oestrogen and progesterone. They are similar in structure and closely interrelated in many ways, with generally opposite effects, but each helps the other by increasing the sensitivity of target organs.

Oestrogen

As has been explained elsewhere, oestrogen is primarily produced by the ovaries, although from the menopause onwards fat cells and the adrenal glands become the primary producers of this hormone. (This explains why it is important to keep your adrenal glands healthy and to maintain a comfortable weight to ease the transition to menopause.)

It is oestrogen that creates the bodily changes in girls and that stimulates ovulation (as explained in Chapter 1). It also prompts the laying down of fat stores during pregnancy, ensuring that during a famine, the pregnant woman will have energy reserves to use.

Progesterone

In 1929, three years after oestrogen had been identified in the urine of menstruating women, progesterone was identified in the corpus luteum (the sac in the ovary from which an egg has been released). Modern science now enables us not only to identify hormones but also to begin to understand how they exert their effects in the body.

As we saw in Chapter 1, progesterone is the only hormone in the body produced in relatively large quantities, especially during pregnancy. Although such large amounts of the female hormone are present in the last three months of pregnancy – 30 times more than normal – this does not influence the gender of the growing child: baby boys do not turn into baby girls, for example.

Progesterone is made initially by the corpus luteum of the ovary during the latter half of the menstrual cycle. It is made from cholesterol, which is produced mainly from the carbohydrates and fats in your diet.

Progesterone plays a pivotal role in the synchrony of other steroid hormones: from it the body makes the three major oestrogens as well as testosterone, the stress hormone cortisol, and other corticosteroids, plus aldosterone (which helps control water balance in the body). The production and conversion of progesterone into other hormones is critical for hormone balance. A low cholesterol level can therefore affect the balance of these hormones, and it may also affect the manufacture of vitamin D.

During pregnancy, progesterone maintains a healthy endometrium, ensuring that the developing baby is well nourished throughout. The corpus luteum continues to make progesterone to support the growing foetus until the placenta is mature enough to take over production. It does this by facilitating the transfer of nutrients from mother to the developing embryo and helping to suppress any immune rejection of the baby.

Progesterone has a variety of other important biological effects, including:

- Helping the body to burn fat for energy

- Reducing anxiety and lifting the mood by acting as a natural antidepressant

- Maintaining an even weight via the control of water balance and promoting efficient thyroid function, thus improving metabolism

- Preventing the blood from clotting inappropriately

- Keeping the correct balance of zinc and copper in the body

- Maintaining proper oxygen levels within cells (an important factor in the prevention of cancer)

- Protecting against fibrocystic breast disease and breast cancer

- Protecting against endometrial cancer

- Counteracting the harmful effects of excess oestrogen

- Stimulating new bone formation

- Preventing cyclical migraines

- Supporting a normal sleep pattern

- Restoring normal sex drive

The limited functions of progestogens

The synthetic progesterones, known as progestogens, are not capable of providing the full range of progesterone's functions. They fit the progesterone receptor sites, blocking the ability of the natural hormone to carry out its functions. Because progestogens are stronger and more potent, they are also more difficult for the body to deactivate and break down. So, even if progesterone is produced in adequate amounts, it may not be able to exert its full effects in the competing presence of synthetic hormones. Similarly, xenoestrogens (the hormone disrupters explained in Chapter 5) can block the action of the natural hormone and scramble its message.

Are you progesterone deficient?

For hormones to work well, they need to be in balance. In modern times this appears to be a difficult condition to fulfil. The insidious competition from synthetic hormones (mainly oestrogens) and xenoestrogens is often too much of a challenge for the body to deal with and can lead to oestrogen dominance (see box below) and/or underproduction of progesterone.

Problems associated with oestrogen dominance in women

- **Breast cancer** is strongly linked (see Chapter 20).
- **Endometrial growths and cancer** of the lining of the womb are thought to be caused by unopposed oestrogen (see Chapter 19).
- **Polycystic ovaries** are strongly linked (see Chapter 18).
- **PMS** is strongly associated with hormonal imbalance and produces a multitude of symptoms that can be similar to those associated with excess oestrogen (see Chapter 8).
- **An underactive thyroid gland**, through the effect of oestrogen interfering with thyroid hormone reception (see Chapter 14).
- **Blood sugar levels** Symptoms are similar to oestrogen dominance, PMS and thyroid problems. The hormones insulin and glucagon and the stress hormone cortisol are all involved in the control of blood sugar levels. Stress hormones are made from progesterone in the body, so low levels can adversely affect how we cope with stress (see Chapters 4 and 7).

cont ▶

Other health problems associated with oestrogen dominance
Accelerated ageing, allergies, breast tenderness, depression, fatigue, fibrocystic breast disease, fibroids, headaches, infertility, irritability, memory loss, miscarriage, osteoporosis, reduced sex drive and water retention.

In addition to this, women make more oestrogens relative to progesterone from their mid thirties onwards, as they increasingly do not ovulate with every menstrual cycle. Some research suggests that anovulatory cycles are endemic among women in industrialised countries.

The effect of this is that little progesterone is produced and the body is exposed to a relative excess of oestrogen throughout the month (see illustration 'Risk factors of insulin resistance and associated diseases' on page 31). Sub-optimum nutrition, stress and too much exercise can all contribute to anovulatory cycles; however, it is xenoestrogen exposure that is considered to be the most potent factor involved.

It is often possible to detect an anovulatory cycle due to a change in pattern and heavier, longer or shorter periods. You can also test for this with an ovulation kit (see Resources).

Because of the regular occurrence of anovulatory cycles before the menopause, oestrogen levels become increasingly out of balance, leading to the symptoms of oestrogen dominance. The pituitary gland responds by releasing higher levels of follicle stimulating hormone (FSH) and luteinising hormone (LH), which in turn can lead to a further increase in production of oestrogens.

Oestrogen dominance can also occur in ovulatory cycles, especially if they are longer than normal. The first half of the cycle is usually 14 days but can last up to six weeks or more. The second half of the cycle is more constant – usually between 10 and 16 days. Oestrogen dominance is more likely to arise in the second half of an ovulatory cycle, as progesterone is present for a shorter period of

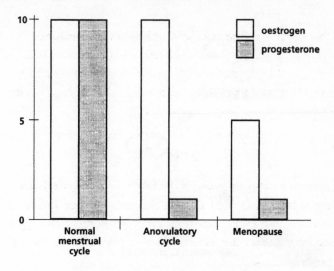

Oestrogen and progesterone ratios

time in relation to oestrogen. This creates a longer period of oestrogen unopposed by progesterone.

What happens when progesterone levels decrease?

Unfortunately, the body can adapt to low progesterone levels by making more oestrogen via an alternative biochemical pathway through the production of another hormone called androstenedione, which has some masculinising effects if this pathway is activated for too long. (Men make most of their oestrogen in this way.) After the menopause, androstenedione and a similar hormone called androstenediol become the major intermediaries in the production of oestrogen in the body.

Cholesterol is converted to a hormone called pregnenolone, which is either made into progesterone or another hormone called DHEA (dihydroepiandrosterone). From DHEA, the body is able to

235

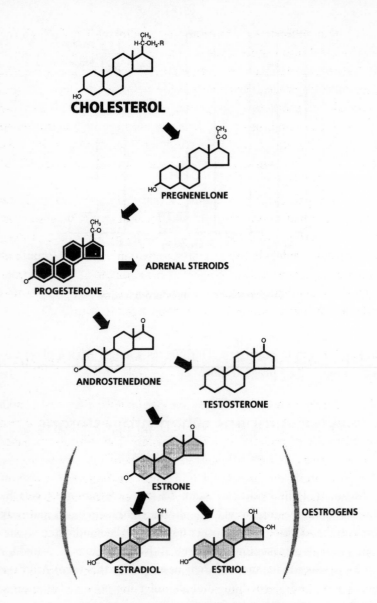

How hormones are made from cholesterol

make either androstenedione or androstenediol, either of which can be converted into testosterone or oestrogens (see illustration opposite). If oestrogen is made this way, there is a tendency for testosterone to be formed instead (particularly if the receptor sites for oestrogen are filled with synthetic oestrogens or xenoestrogens). This can lead to unwanted symptoms such as hair loss on the scalp and unwanted hair on the legs and face. These symptoms plus obesity, as we have seen, are three key symptoms of polycystic ovarian syndrome (PCOS) (see Chapter 18).

At menopause, the production of oestrogen in the body falls by only about a half to one-third pre-menopausal levels. Progesterone, however, decreases to a 120th of baseline levels, yet it is oestrogen that has more widely been prescribed to treat menopausal symptoms and protect against osteoporosis and heart disease. With environmental and synthetic hormone exposure too, it is little wonder that progesterone has a hard task keeping oestrogen in check.

The fate of oestrogen and progesterone

After oestrogen and progesterone have completed their tasks, they are taken in the blood to the liver, where they are deactivated and passed to the digestive tract for elimination. This constant production and break down, in response to the body's continual needs, is what controls the balance of hormones. An optimum supply of nutrients, including some B vitamins, helps ensure that the process runs smoothly. Low levels of magnesium reduce the liver's ability to deactivate oestrogen; a deficiency of vitamin B_6, which works synergistically with magnesium, has the same effect.

As previously discussed in Chapters 2 and 3, oestrogen, in the wrong form or quantity, can become toxic to cells. Thus, your body rapidly breaks it down. In order for oestrogen and its metabolites to be detoxified they must be combined with compounds called methyl groups, glutathione and sulphate. Important nutrients to support these processes include the amino acids methionine, cysteine, glycine and glutamate, as well as magnesium, iron, B_{12}, B_6, B_2 and folate. A major route for oestrogen detoxification is by binding with a compound called glucoronide in the liver. This process is known as glucoronidation, a very important detoxification 'pathway' which is dependent on the nutrient calcium-d-glucarate, found in apples, Brussels sprouts, broccoli, cabbage and beansprouts.[3] Other foods found to help this process include garlic, onions, carrots and garden cress.

Salvestrols – the hidden factor in fruit that breaks down hormones

An enzyme in the liver, called CYP1B1 (pronounced 'sip-one-be-one'), converts oestrone and oestradiol to oestrogen metabolites called 4-hydroxyoestrone. This form of oestrogen has been described as 'oestrogen on fire' as it can readily damage DNA; however, the next step completes the breakdown of the hormones by binding 4-hydroxyoestrone to methyl groups, requiring B vitamins and the antioxidant glutathione. Without an adequate supply of methyl groups and/or glutathione, excess 4-hydroxyoestrone metabolites can damage DNA. See Chapter 25 to find out how you can test for oestrogen metabolites, including 4-hydroxyoestrone.

CYP1B1 is found in many human cancers, including those of the bladder, brain, breast, colon, ovaries and uterus. But don't think of it as 'bad'. Some researchers believe that CYP1B1 is in fact a tumour-specific rescue enzyme because, if it is provided with a stream of 'weapons' derived from food, it causes the enzyme to unleash an array of chemicals that are lethal to cancer cells. The researchers have termed these potent food-derived agents salvestrols. There are compounds in fruits and vegetables that the CYP1BI enzyme converts into something toxic only to cancer cells. (If you'd like to find out more about this, read my book *Say No to Cancer*.) So, the very same process that protects you from excess oestrogen metabolites could also help to protect you from cancer. The problem is that we don't eat enough of these salvestrols in our modern-day diet, partly because we don't eat enough fruit and vegetables, partly because non-organic food tends to contain fewer, and partly because salvestrols tend to be found in bitter-tasting foods, which we tend to eat less of. Tangerines, dark red grapes and cranberries are good sources. For other good food sources, see the Diet for the Good Life in Chapter 26. An alternative is to supplement salvestrols (see Resources).

The importance of fibre

Adequate soluble fibre in the diet, from foods such as oats, flax and chia seeds, as well as aubergine and okra, also helps to bind sex hormones excreted into the digestive tract, aiding their elimination. Too little fibre encourages their reactivation and reabsorption into the circulation. Soluble fibres, such as fructo-oligosaccharides (FOS), selectively stimulate the beneficial bacteria in the gut known as bifidobacteria. A beneficial balance of these inhibits an enzyme that is capable of reactivating oestrogen. FOS is present in small quantities in the diet and is also available as a supplement.

The more plant fibre you eat the higher your blood levels of sex hormone-binding globulin (SHBG) are likely to be. The more SHBG you produce, the less 'free' oestrogen there is available to the oestrogen-sensitive tissues. The balance of bound to unbound hormone very much dictates the activity of a hormone, and the right nutrition helps to keep that balance healthy.

Post-menopause, SHBG levels naturally diminish; this is probably how the body frees up oestrogen as levels decline. Oestrogen is important for bone health and this may be nature's mechanism to help conserve bone; however, if a woman is over-exposed to oestrogen-like molecules, such as xenoestrogens from the environment, or oestrogens from dairy products, this may work against her by increasing circulating levels of the unbound, active hormone. Coupled with poor elimination, perhaps from compromised liver detoxification, oestrogen dominance is exacerbated.

See Chapter 25 for details of hormone testing and the significance of levels of SHBG.

Redressing the balance

It is important to realise that oestrogen is a vital hormone for human survival. It is the imbalance of oestrogen to progesterone, and not excess oestrogen per se, that is thought to be responsible for many of today's female health problems. What is becoming increasingly evident is that even small amounts of oestrogen metabolites can be toxic if there are insufficient resources in the body to bind with them and make them safe, including methyl groups, glutathione and sulphate (see earlier discussion on page 237).

Fifty years ago, when man-made chemicals were first used in industry, little thought was given to their potential effects on reproduction. At that time more concern was focused on whether they were likely to be carcinogenic. Only now are we realising that the by-products of man-made, industrial chemicals are capable of wreaking havoc with hormone balance in all species.

We are unlikely ever to understand the complexity of hormonal interaction in its entirety, but the measures for maintaining and improving health presented in this book are sound. To correct the imbalance between oestrogen and progesterone there are two possible approaches:

1. Ensure optimum nutrient intake and the healthiest possible lifestyle, including a reduced exposure to pollutants.

2. As 1, plus, where indicated, the application of natural progesterone, guided by a doctor experienced in its use.

It is clear that optimal nutrition and a sensible lifestyle are key components in addressing the problem of oestrogen dominance. Part 5 details how you can optimise your nutrient intake by paying particular attention to the Diet for the Good Life in Chapter 26.

Synthetic hormones

In the last 40 years, synthetic varieties of hormones have been promoted as the answer to a whole spectrum of women's health problems, but there are more natural ways to balance hormones. I believe that it is virtually impossible for synthetic hormones to restore the natural hormone balance in the body. At best they can simulate some of the actions of natural hormones, but usually at a price. I am sure that women would not take the risk of using the synthetic forms if they knew the implications for their health and that of their children, especially if they are also aware of the unavoidable exposure to environmental oestrogen-like substances.

Female hormones, natural or synthetic, are potent substances that have widespread effects. Synthetic forms of oestrogen and progesterone (progestogens) are commonly prescribed and synthetic progestogens are very similar in structure to natural progesterone; however, although the body accepts and uses them, and they lock into the same receptor sites in cells, they may convey a different message. What is more, this effect is made worse because synthetic hormones act in the body for longer than natural hormones and the body has difficulty metabolising them and disposing of them.

The two most popular forms of synthetic hormones are the contraceptive pill and HRT. These uses are not without their problems, as the next chapter explains.

The Pill and HRT – Exploding the Myths

With hindsight, it is likely that history will record the widespread prescribing of synthetic hormones to women – that is, the contraceptive pill and HRT– as one of medicine's biggest ever bungles. Whatever the purpose of these treatments, their effect is to disrupt the natural balance and interaction of oestrogen and progesterone in the body.

The contraceptive pill

Controlling fertility has been a major preoccupation for a long time. Back in the 1960s the time was ripe for effective contraception. Venereal diseases were being treated effectively, and constraining religious beliefs were being eroded. There was no longer the same social pressure to regulate women's sexuality. The market expanded rapidly, filling the coffers of the pharmaceutical industry.

One of the myths about the Pill is that it is a problem-free form of contraception; however, one early researcher, Dr Ellen Grant, author of *The Bitter Pill*, was shocked when synthetic hormones were not withdrawn from the market due to their known serious side effects. The Pill is certainly a highly effective contraceptive, but it also creates problems, including depletion of many vital nutrients, difficulty for some women in re-establishing a normal menstrual cycle or conceiving after stopping it, raised blood pressure, risk of fatal blood clots, and a higher risk of certain types of cancer. The more recent lower dose Pill has somewhat mitigated these risks but not eradicated them.

How the Pill works

The Pill works by suppressing a woman's natural hormones and interfering with the natural balance of oestrogen and progesterone. The production of luteinising hormone (LH) is inhibited, preventing ovulation; cervical mucus becomes hostile to sperm; the lining of the womb is altered so that an egg has difficulty embedding in it; and the hormonal state of pregnancy is simulated. The Pill stops proper menstruation; bleeding – better termed withdrawal bleeding – only occurs each month when the hormones are not taken for seven days.

How the Pill is made

The hormones in contraceptive pills are made in pharmaceutical laboratories. Progestogens are most commonly manufactured from natural progesterone-like substances found in foods such as soya.

The known risks of the Pill

The risks are similar for both the 'combined' and the 'mini' Pill. The combined Pill – a combination of synthetic oestrogen and progestogen – is considered to be more potent. It should not be given to women who have ever suffered from blood clots, liver disease, high blood pressure, obesity, known or suspected breast or any other hormone-related cancers, or vaginal bleeding of unknown cause. Taking the combined Pill increases the risk of coronary artery disease, particularly in women who smoke. Some women with a history of epilepsy, migraine, asthma or heart disease find their symptoms get worse while taking the Pill. Progestogen-only pills are sometimes recommended for women who have problems with the combined Pill.

Signs to stop taking the mini Pill (which contains only progestogen) are visual problems, headaches or migraines, or if there is any serious unexplained illness. If you are taking any type of oral contraception it is advisable to contact your doctor immediately if any of the following occur: blood in the urine, dizziness or nose bleeds, fainting, migraines or unusually severe headaches, numbness or tingling, pregnancy, severe or sudden chest pain, coughing up blood, visual disturbance, yellowing of the skin.

Side effects of taking the Pill

Nausea, vomiting, headache, breast tenderness, weight changes, lowered sex drive, depression, blood clots, changes in skin colour, high blood pressure, loss of periods, irregular bleeding.

It should be understood that, although this is very rare, the Pill (particularly the combined Pill) can be life-threatening. It can lead to a fatal blood clot that ultimately blocks the blood supply in the lungs. Studies in Britain indicate that a woman who is on the Pill is twice as likely to experience a fatal blood clot as a non-Pill user.[4]

Lesser known risks of the Pill

Synthetic hormones can affect the way the body uses many nutrients. The balance of these in the body is essential for ensuring the precise synchrony of hormones as well as for countless other functions.

Vitamin A

Because excessive levels of vitamin A have been found in the blood of women on the Pill,[5] supplementing vitamin A (over and above that found in a multivitamin) is not advisable while taking the Pill, but it is important to ensure a good dietary intake.

After stopping the Pill, however, supplementing vitamin A is important, because the Pill elevates blood levels of the vitamin by mobilising reserves in the liver, so stores may well need replenishing. The high level of vitamin A found in the blood of Pill users may be partly why it helps skin problems like acne, and why stopping the Pill often brings about skin problems even in women who had not suffered from them before.

Vitamin C

Following concerns that vitamin C increases the 'potency' of oestrogen, by raising oestradiol in the blood, one group of researchers cautioned Pill users against taking vitamin C supplements. A thorough investigation into such processes showed, however, that 1g of vitamin C daily does not have this effect.[6] Even if vitamin C did potentiate oestrogen, the body would compensate by producing less.

The B Vitamins

The essential metabolism and elimination of synthetic hormones is a process that requires methylating B vitamins – including B_2, B_6, B_{12}, folic acid and choline, so it is wise to supplement these in a multivitamin or B complex.

Vitamin K

While using the Pill, avoid supplementing vitamin K (over and above that found in a multivitamin), as it is involved in blood clotting (and the risk of blood clots is increased by synthetic hormones); however, dietary intake of vitamin K, from green vegetables and cauliflower, for example, need not be restricted.

Note Supplementing vitamin K should also be avoided if you are taking blood-thinning drugs.

Copper, zinc, manganese and iron

Higher levels of copper in the body are associated with Pill use. Since copper increases the amount of oestrogen in the body, high copper levels may increase the risks associated with oestrogen dominance. Copper also competes with zinc, which is required at every step of the reproductive process. It is best not to supplement copper unless supplementing ten times as much zinc. On the other hand, too much zinc can also deplete iron and manganese. As Pill-takers usually lose less blood at the monthly bleed than in normal menstruation, extra iron supplementation may not be needed. Unless tests show an iron deficiency, taking more than the 10mg of iron found in a good multivitamin should not be necessary. For manganese, 3–5mg is sufficient. So an ideal daily supplement might provide 15mg of zinc, 10mg of iron, 3mg of manganese and 1.5mg or less of copper.

When effectiveness is reduced

Some combined pills are taken for 21 days followed by a 7-day break. Other preparations are taken every day, and include a week of Pills that contain no hormones. Taking the Pill in this way minimises the risk of forgetting, which adds to the reliability of this method of contraception. The effectiveness of the Pill can, however, be reduced if you suffer from diarrhoea and vomiting, or you are taking certain medications, including antibiotics, sedatives, anti-arthritic drugs and anti-epileptic drugs.

The mini Pill must be taken every day, at the same time, to maintain good contraceptive cover. A delay of only three hours can result in a loss of protection. Its effectiveness is high, but lower than that of the combined Pill.

Hormone replacement therapy (HRT)

HRT is available in pills, patches and implants, and there are around 50 preparations to select from, so your doctor will usually assess which one to give you largely according to risk and convenience. Some women take several years to find one that suits them. Some never find the right one. The most common reasons for discontinuing HRT are unwanted side effects and weight gain, and one-third to two-thirds of women discontinue it within the first two years.[7]

HRT has been recommended to prolong women's active sex lives after the menopause and, ever since its introduction, figures have been manipulated to infer a variety of benefits, including stronger bones and protection from heart disease, as we have seen.

Women are also told that HRT is a 'complete cure' for the menopause, and indeed for some it does relieve symptoms such as hot flushes, vaginal dryness and loss of libido. There are several other problems, however, in its chequered history which make it a high-risk drug to take, especially for any length of time; see the box below.

The chequered history of HRT

The first version of HRT was produced in the 1940s, and was derived from pregnant mares. In the 1950s, oestrogen replacement therapy was being prescribed to women on a large scale as an aid to easy and successful pregnancy, to help with 'women's problems' as a contraceptive, and eventually as a 'miracle cure' for any female reproductive problem, even prophylactically to prevent miscarriage. By the 1960s, pharmaceutical companies developed the argument that the menopause was a medical condition and that HRT could relieve its adverse effects and return women to their younger sexual selves. In the 1970s, however, it was seen that menopausal women on HRT had an increased chance of endometrial, or womb, cancer, with the increased chance ranging from 200 to 1,500 per cent, depending on how long the woman had been taking it.[8] The drug companies' answer to this was to

cont ▶

add progestogen to oestrogen in HRT. There was also a drive by some doctors and pharmaceutical companies to get women to have their uteruses removed so that they could continue to take 'safe' doses of oestrogen.[9] In 1977, three doctors reported the growing incidence of endometrial cancer in relation to exogenous oestrogen.[10]

Adding progestogens to HRT did reduce the risk of endometrial cancer, but did not eliminate it entirely,[11] and there was still a risk for two years after stopping oestrogen implants. In the 1980s, a flow of studies linked HRT to a variety of conditions (including endometrial and breast cancers, and cardiovascular problems), the evidence for which became undeniable in the 1990s.[12] Doctors also began to find a rare vaginal cancer in young women whose mothers had taken DES (the first synthetic oestrogen), and it was eventually taken off the market. Later research also showed that the women who had taken DES had a slightly increased risk of breast cancer,[13] and thousands of 'DES sons and daughters' had cancers and malformations of the genitals.

Also in the 1980s, a series of studies showed that synthetic human hormones had the capability to produce cancer, thrombosis and cardiovascular problems. (Although the fact that HRT could cause cancer had been known by manufacturers since the 1950s in any case.) A British study published in the *British Journal of Obstetrics and Gynaecology* in 1987, which followed 4,544 women for an average of 5½ years, showed that breast cancer risk was 1.5 times greater in HRT users, while the risk of endometrial cancer nearly trebled.[14] In 1989, a study involving 23,000 Scandinavian women showed that taking HRT for longer than five years doubled the risk of breast cancer.[15] It also revealed that adding progestogens to cut down the womb cancer risk raised the risk of breast cancer.

In the 1990s more studies highlighted the risks of taking HRT: in 1995 a study showed that women in their sixties who had been on HRT for five or more years increased their risk of developing breast cancer by 71 per cent.[16] Overall, there was a 32 per cent increased risk among women using oestrogen HRT, and a 41 per cent risk of those using oestrogen combined with synthetic progestin, compared to women who had never used hormones.

cont ▶

Another study, following 240,000 women for eight years, found that the risk of ovarian cancer was 72 per cent higher in women given oestrogen.[17] Studies continued in 1997,[18] 1998,[19] 2002,[20] 2003,[21] and 2004,[22] confirming the risks of breast and ovarian cancer, strokes and blood clots through taking HRT.

More recently, in 2005 the Million Women Trial was reported in the *British Medical Journal*, which said 'We estimate that 20,000 women have contracted breast cancer due to HRT,'[23] and in 2009 the *New England Journal of Medicine* stated that 'A 50% drop in use of HRT in the US has stopped 1,000 breast cancer cases a year.'[24] A study in 2010 shows that there is double the risk of death from breast cancer in post-menopausal women on HRT.[25]

How HRT is made

Unlike the Pill, which mainly uses the synthetic oestrogen ethynyl estradiol, most oestrogens used in HRT are so-called 'natural'; that is, taken from a pregnant mare's urine or the ovaries of pigs. Dr Marilyn Glenville writes in her book *Natural Alternatives to HRT*, 'Not all the oestrogens in the mixture are natural to humans and some can behave like the synthetic ethynyl estradiol, which tends to affect liver metabolism by producing changes in blood clotting and blood fat levels.' Furthermore, an official investigation by a representative of the World Society for the Protection of Animals reported that the mares were not kept in acceptable conditions. The synthetic pro-gestogen used in HRT is the same as that in contraceptive pills.

The known risks of HRT

Generally, the side effects of HRT are similar to those associated with taking the Pill (see page 244). Taking oestrogens by mouth is associ-ated with nausea, vomiting, bloating and abdominal cramps. Oral oestrogens go to the liver first to be broken down, so it becomes difficult to know how much will end up in the blood.

HRT via a skin patch by-passes the liver, giving a higher level of oestrogen in the blood, but may be associated with a localised discoloration of the skin.

Increasingly popular are oestrogen implants: pellets are inserted under the skin during a minor operation. Although they should last for six months, frequently women return three to nine weeks later, complaining of recurring menopausal symptoms. Implants are associated with an addiction to oestrogen, and it has been suggested that women who gain such tolerance to oestrogen have psychiatric problems and also require larger than normal amounts of oestrogen.

Professor Howard Jacobs, of the Middlesex Hospital in London, suggested that it may be the continual saturation of the oestrogen-sensitive cells that makes them lose the ability to respond accordingly; they become oestrogen resistant, in much the same way as they might become resistant to insulin. It is also indicated that early use of oes-trogen, in the Pill, may set the stage for an increased need for HRT.

Does HRT work at all?

HRT– originally called 'oestrogen replacement therapy' – works by replacing the depleted oestrogen levels that occur at the menopause. It is thought that low levels are responsible for the increased risk of heart disease and osteoporosis as well as many of the symptoms of menopause (hot flushes, vaginal dryness, depression). The oestrogen-only preparations were, however, soon linked to an increased risk of endometrial cancer, as we have seen, and are no longer recommended for women who still have their wombs. Instead, such women are pre-scribed a combination synthetic progestogen/oestrogen treatment.

For a moment, let's put aside the considerable risks of cancer and circulatory disease that women take when using HRT, and let's ignore the horrendous side effects that some women on HRT experi-ence – which can include heavy or irregular bleeding if taken before the cessation of periods, water retention, weight gain, PMS-type symptoms and nausea. Aside from these, just how effective is HRT as a treatment for menopausal symptoms, which is the main reason women choose to use it?

Hot flushes and night sweats are often cited by women as the worst of the menopausal symptoms. As a meta-analysis published in 2004 shows, there have been 24 good-quality trials of HRT for symptom relief, involving over 3,000 women,[26] and they show that it comes up trumps. HRT reduces hot flushes or night sweats by 74 per cent compared to placebos, although quite a few on HRT in these trials dropped out because of the side effects. Placebos themselves were also quite effective, reducing reports of hot flushes or night sweats by 50 per cent, showing how important placebo-controlled trials are in this area. So, the difference is actually a 24 per cent reduction in symptoms.

'It's a big dilemma,' says hormone-specialist Dr Marion Gluck, author of the book *It Must Be My Hormones*. 'Do you get the relief from menopausal symptoms like hot flashes, night sweats, disrupted sleep, irritability and risk something much worse, or do you just have to put up with them?'

If you don't have menopausal symptoms, it really isn't worth taking HRT. That's the conclusion of a 2004 review assessing the benefits versus the harms of HRT in the *British Medical Journal*. It concludes: 'HRT for primary prevention of chronic diseases in women without menopausal symptoms is unjustified. Women free of menopausal symptoms showed a net harm from HRT use.'[27] If you are concerned about osteoporosis, research is showing that changes in diet and exercise are a lot more effective, and certainly safer, than HRT.

The danger of using synthetic hormones doesn't just lie in the subtle differences in their chemical structure and effect, but also in the amounts given and their balance with other hormones. The amounts of hormones in the Pill or conventional HRT treatment can be many times higher than the body would naturally produce. Women vary a lot in the amount of oestrogen they make. Some women are naturally low oestrogen producers, making 50–200mcg a day. Others make up to 700mcg a day. HRT provides an oestrogen dose of between

600 and 1,250mcg a day. For most women, this is just too high. Oestrogen produced by the body is balanced with progesterone but, if this balance is lost, oestrogen unopposed by progesterone becomes a health problem.

The natural alternatives

Fortunately, you can help balance your hormones naturally. The main way is through lifestyle changes and specific foods, nutrients and herbs, which can lessen the severity of menopausal symptoms, and improve bone health safely and effectively. Exercise is also a key balancer of hormones. We've looked at these in previous chapters. But if you'd still like to go down the hormonal route, there are natural, or bio-identical, hormones available. The next chapter explains what these are, how they differ from non-bio-identical hormones, and why many women are now using them as a safe and effective alternative to HRT.

CHAPTER 24

Bio-identical Hormones – A Safer Alternative

I would like to thank Dr Tony Coope, GP and health writer on the informational website www.bio-hormone-health.com, for his help in writing this chapter.

Natural hormones are essential substances that help to keep us fit and healthy when they are in balance. Cells all over the body 'recognise' natural hormones and therefore, when in balance, they respond to them appropriately.

As we have seen, progesterone is a key hormone from which oestrogens, and other hormones, are made; and almost everything in the body is ultimately made from the food we eat. To make nature's hormones work best, it is therefore sensible to provide your body with the best possible raw materials. Part 5 of this book shows you how to do this.

Addressing the problem of oestrogen dominance through an optimum diet and lifestyle alone may, however, not be enough for some women. In certain instances, it is appropriate to correct a hormone deficiency by supplementing a bio-identical one – derived from a natural source such as soya or wild yam – which has been converted in the laboratory to exactly the same structure as the body would have made for itself. Such a hormone is called a natural, or bio-identical, hormone because it has exactly the same chemical structure as that produced by the body.

Where an actual disease state associated with oestrogen dominance has already been diagnosed, such as fibroids or fibrocystic breast disease, the case for supplementing a naturally derived hormone is even stronger, especially if hormone tests have confirmed oestrogen dominance. Combining natural hormone supplements with an optimised diet and lifestyle increases the chances of such health problems resolving; however, I recommend hormone testing to assess the need for natural hormones (see Chapter 25).

How bio-identical hormones are made

Several years after progesterone was identified, it was realised that large amounts were also produced in the placenta, and human placentas were soon the major source of progesterone used in experimental work. In 1939 it was found that sapogenin, in the sarsaparilla plant, could be converted into a progesterone-like compound. Soon afterwards diosgenin, a substance in wild yam, was converted in the laboratory into progesterone, in exactly the same form as the body produces.

By the early 1950s, thousands of plants were found to contain active oestrogen- and progesterone-like substances, called phytoestrogens and phyto-progesterones, which have been explored earlier in this book. The major modern source of diosgenin is the soya bean. The body cannot convert diosgenin into progesterone itself. This has to be done in a laboratory, albeit from a natural food.

From these raw materials it is possible to produce not only body-identical progesterone (also called 'natural' progesterone) but also synthetic forms of progesterone (progestogens), oestrogen and the male hormone testosterone. The manufacture of altered forms is easy and cheap and, because they are not natural, they can be patented for great profit. Despite early and continued success by some physicians using natural progesterone for PMS, threatened miscarriage and ovarian cysts, research into natural hormones declined in the face of competition from synthetic, patentable and more profitable forms.

cont ▶

This turned out to be a serious problem because only the exact natural progesterone molecule can trigger a precise set of instructions that maintain pregnancy, bone density, normal menstruation and other 'acts' of the hormonal dance that occurs in every woman. Natural progesterone also has, even at levels considerably higher than those produced by the human body, remarkably little toxicity.

Yet almost without exception, every contraceptive pill or HRT prescription, be it a pill, patch or injection, contains synthetic progestogens (also called progestins) – altered molecules that are similar to, but different from, genuine progesterone. They are like keys that open the lock but don't fit exactly – consequently generating a wobble in the body's biochemistry.

The HRT dilemma

Given that the dangers associated with synthetic hormone replacement therapy are now well recognised, the idea of a form of HRT containing hormones that are identical to the ones your body produces naturally has been generating a lot of interest. The ones you get in regular HRT are similar to the real thing but they have been slightly altered. Could that be the source of the problem?

'Replacing the oestrogen that your body is no longer producing with the versions found in conventional HRT is like replacing parts designed for a Chevy with those made for a Mercedes,' says Dr Jonathan Wright, Medical Director of Tahoma Clinic in Washington, USA, and a long-time advocate of bio-identical hormones. 'They may be roughly the same, but with both engine parts and biology, very precise measurements matter.'

The idea of bio-identical hormones has been attracting a lot of attention in the US, especially since actress Suzanne Somers, previously best known for her role as a ditzy blonde in the 1980s sitcom hit *Three's Company*, published a best-seller on their benefits.[28] However, claims that they are safer or more effective have been dismissed as 'marketing' by the US drugs authority, the FDA. Some bio-identical hormones are approved by the FDA and are available on prescription but not all (see the chart below).

Bio-identical oestrogens and micronised (finely ground in the laboratory for better absorption) progesterone have been made into a range of products. Commercially available bio-identical oestradiol comes in several forms, including pill, patch, cream and various vaginal preparations. Micronised progesterone comes in a capsule or as a vaginal gel.

The delivery method is important. Bio-identical oestradiol in pill form is converted in the liver to oestrone, the weaker bio-identical oestrogen. But, given in a patch, it enters the bloodstream as the original oestradiol. Creams, gels and lotions applied to the legs or arms can also deliver it directly to the bloodstream, although it's less certain how much is absorbed.

When oestrogen is taken as a pill, because it is first processed through the liver, it stimulates proteins associated with heart disease and stroke, such as C-reactive protein, activated protein C, and clotting factors; however, if a transdermal patch is used, the liver is not involved and, even at the same level of blood concentration, these effects do not occur.

Bio-identical hormones

Type/source	Brand name(s)	Preparations
17 beta-estradiol/plants (micronised)*	Estrace, others	pill
	Alora, Climara, Esclim, Estraderm, Vivelle, others	patch
	Estrogel	transdermal gel
	Estrasorb	topical cream
	Estrace	vaginal cream+
	Estring	vaginal ring+
	Femring	vaginal ring
Estradiol acetate	Vagifem	vaginal tablet+

Type/source	Brand name(s)	Preparations
Medroxyprogesterone acetate (MPA)	Prochieve 4%	vaginal gel
Micronised* progesterone USP	Prochieve 4%	vaginal gel

*Particles are made smaller for better absorption.
+For vaginal symptoms only.

In the UK, the situation is typically much more low key. There's been far less publicity about bio-identical hormones, although a small but growing number of women have been taking them. Several brands are available on the NHS; however, most GPs are reluctant to prescribe them, usually saying there is no evidence that they work, which is not true.

Are synthetic hormones bio-identical?

So what exactly does it mean to say that a hormone is bio-identical? As explained on page 24, there are three types of oestrogen in the body – oestradiol, oestrone and oestriol – found in very different proportions. Oestriol is the weakest, and pre-menopausal women normally have lots of it; it makes up about 90 per cent of the total amount. The next most abundant is oestradiol, the most potent one, at around 7 per cent, followed by oestrone at 3 per cent. But in regular HRT, the oestrogen part doesn't come in anything like those proportions.

One of the most common brands is one called Premarin, which comes from the urine of pregnant mares. Not only are the proportions different from human hormones but it also contains extra horse oestrogens. Oestrone shoots up from being the least to the most abundant at 75 per cent; next comes oestradiol which, together with two other horse oestrogens, makes up between 6 and 15 per cent. And finally there is 5 to 19 per cent of another horse hormone called equilin. Even in hormones that are molecularly very similar, the difference in effect can be huge. One way of summing up the difference between men and women would be that it is the difference between early exposure to testosterone or oestrogen. But the oestrogen oestradiol is actually more like testosterone than it is like Premarin. Yet women are advised that Premarin is a suitable replacement for oestrogen.

Why progesterone is key

The progestogens (called progestins in the US) are synthetic, similar but non-identical versions of the hormone progesterone. Because progesterone is a natural substance and cannot be patented, it is generally not profitable for a pharmaceutical company to obtain a licence to produce it as a medicine (this process can cost millions of pounds). But if that natural substance is slightly changed it can then be patented and licensed; however, such a substance is no longer 'natural' to the body. Even a tiny change from the natural hormone can result in considerable side effects.

During menopause the amount of progesterone in your body drops more dramatically than oestrogen, to almost zero. Non-identical progestogen is added to regular HRT to reduce the risk of womb cancer, which exists from oestrogen alone.

You can get an idea of how big the difference is between bio-identical progesterone and progestogen from their effect on pregnancy. Progesterone is the hormone that the body makes to support pregnancy[29] – it's used as part of infertility treatments, while progestogen raises the risk of miscarriage. According to NHS Direct, other side effects include breast tenderness, headaches, mood-swings and depression. The main, although rare, side effect of progesterone is mild sleepiness.

Examining the evidence for bio-identical hormones

So are the identical versions of these hormones safer and more effective? It's an attractive idea that makes sense, but what's the evidence?

Studies have shown that they can help relieve hot flushes and vaginal dryness, but as yet, few large studies have investigated the differences among the various hormones and methods of administration. More research is needed to further understand these differences and compare the risks and benefits. At the moment, there is no big trial comparing the two, but there are plenty of people who find that regular HRT just doesn't agree with them, quite apart from the possible long-term risks of taking it, whereas a switch to bio-identical HRT (BHRT) transforms them.

Case Study: *Sharon*

Sharon, an advertising executive with two teenage children, knew her husband was losing patience with her wild mood swings.

> 'Starting the menopause was hell. My GP suggested antidepressants, but I knew I wasn't depressed. I just wasn't myself any more.'

It was then that Sharon heard about hormone-specialist Dr Gluck:

> 'The first thing she did was to listen to me. I felt that everyone else was trying to offer me a ready-made solution. She then did something else that, oddly, no one else had done, which was to measure what my hormone levels actually were.
>
> 'It turned out that my oestrogen level wasn't too bad but that I had almost no progesterone, so my oestrogen wasn't being balanced. She explained that progesterone affects a brain chemical called GABA (which is targeted by tranquillisers), which is why it has a calming effect.'

Sharon was given a progesterone cream to rub in, and within six weeks the mood swings had gone and she was functioning normally again.

Apart from using bio-identical hormones which, she says, are gentler and better tolerated, hormone-specialist Dr Marion Gluck also treats the individual patient rather than offering a similar combination to everyone. 'Some need more oestrogen or progesterone but I check other hormones like testosterone which is vital for a woman's sex drive, and thyroid, low levels of which can result in fatigue and depression.'

But this approach gets very little support from most NHS GPs, who may point to a few small studies that have found no benefit from using progesterone. The official advice is that providing you have as low as possible a dose of regular HRT and don't stay on it for any longer than five years, your risks of any problems are very low.

'There is absolutely no evidence that bio-identical hormones are any safer,' says Dr Sarah Jarvis, speaking for the Royal College of GPs. But the official view of the Royal College would be thought curious in France, where both progestogens and progesterone are widely used. Because of this, there is much more research carried out on the difference between them. In the UK, progestogens are only included in HRT to stop cancer developing in the lining of the womb. But French studies suggest that progesterone has all kinds of other benefits, almost none of which come from progestogens.

Dr Tony Coope has found great benefits in his patients using bio-identical HRT and adds, 'It is always rather rash in Medicine to claim "There is absolutely no …" anything, and sure enough, a recent meta-analysis[30] from the USA found that "patients reported greater satisfaction with HRT containing bio-identical progesterone compared with those that contain a synthetic progestin"; and in addition that "bio-identical hormones are associated with lower risks, including those of breast cancer and cardiovascular disease, and are more efficacious than their synthetic and animal-derived counterparts".'

Lessons from France

'There is evidence that progesterone has beneficial effects on the breast tissue, on blood vessels and for strengthening bones,' says Dr Michael Schumacher of the Kremlin-Bicêtre hospital in Paris, 'although more research needs to be done. Many of the benefits of progesterone come from the fact that while oestrogen stimulates cells, progesterone calms them down.'[31]

As a result, one striking claim for progesterone is that it might lower your risk of dementia. In the brain, oestrogen and progesterone combine to protect cells, while progestogens reduce this protective effect. 'There is strong evidence that the ageing nervous system remains at least to some extent sensitive to the beneficial effects of progesterone,' says Schumacher.

While the Women's Health Initiative (WHI) study showed that combining progestogens with oestrogen slightly raised the risk of strokes and breast cancer, Schumacher's work explains how progesterone can lower these dangers. 'Oestrogen combined with progesterone could make for a safe and effective form of HRT,' he says, 'although such an option may not be very attractive for the pharmaceutical industry.' The reason for this, as I have already explained, is that progesterone is not patentable, precisely because it is a natural substance, and so it won't be a big money spinner.

The claim that progesterone may protect against breast cancer has been backed up by a large ongoing French study of 54,548 menopausal women, comparing what happens to those who take progesterone in their HRT with those who get progestogen. The latest report has found that after eight years, while those on progestogens have a raised risk of breast cancer, those on progesterone don't.[32]

As a result of this research, there has been a change in prescribing in France. 'After the WHI study, many women had stopped taking oestrogen pills,' says Dr Virginie Ringa of the French Institute for Health and Medical Research, Le Kremlin-Bicêtre, Paris. 'Now they are using an oestrogen patch together with oral progesterone. But it is true that none of this has been tested in large clinical trials.'

Can progesterone reduce stroke risk?

Meanwhile in the US, Dr Schumacher's claim that progesterone can protect blood vessels and cut down the risk of strokes has just been supported in two small trials at Texas University. Researchers gave a progesterone cream or a placebo to 30 post-menopausal women for eight weeks. Not only did the cream improve their symptoms but there was also no rise in various markers in the blood that make strokes more likely, such as inflammation and a tendency to form clots.[33]

'We also found similar beneficial results when we gave a cocktail of individualised bio-identical hormones to 75 patients and compared the results to regular HRT,' says Dr Kenna Stephenson, Assistant Professor of Family Medicine at The University of Texas Health Center. The women were tested after a year. The results were reported at the American Heart Association annual meeting in November 2008.[34]

'Last year the FDA issued an alert on the dangers of bio-identical hormones, yet our 12 month data would suggest that they are safe and effective for peri/post-menopausal women when high quality creams are used,' says Stephenson.

The call for more research

Evidence like the above doesn't completely prove the case for bio-identical hormones and everyone agrees there needs to be more research. So will the big trials that doctors are demanding now be run? The depressing truth is that it's unlikely without strong consumer pressure. Calls for such research are not new.

Thirty years ago an editorial in the *Journal of the American Medical Association* asked how long clinicians will have to wait for proper clinical trials on the benefits of oestriol, the weakest of the oestrogens. 'Enough evidence has been accumulated,' it said, 'that we may say that it is safer than oestrone and oestradiol.' The trials have still not been done.[35]

What to do if HRT is not working for you

If you are unwilling to wait and HRT isn't working for you, what can you do? You can go to a private doctor who specialises in hormones, like Dr Gluck. The Natural Progesterone Information Service has a growing list of doctors prescribing bio-identical hormones (see

Resources). As well as prescribing bio-identicals, these practitioners will check the state of your hormones in general using a salivary hormone test.

Dr John Moran, who works in London, explains that this is useful because the level of one hormone can affect the working of another. 'Oestrogen, for instance, needs to be balanced by testosterone or you are likely to see an increase in inflammation,' he says. 'Low levels of progesterone may affect thyroid function.'

Another fan of bio-identical hormones is Dr Shirley Bond. In most cases, she finds there is both a deficiency in oestrogen and a relative oestrogen dominance due to very low progesterone. Because the body can make oestrogen from progesterone if it needs to, her first option is to use a transdermal progesterone cream.

'I often start with a 3 per cent progesterone cream, giving the equivalent of 20 to 40mg per day in the second half of the menstrual cycle,' she says. 'If there's no menstrual cycle, then I recommend three weeks on progesterone and one week off.' Hormone expert Dr John Lee (author of *What Your Doctor Didn't Tell You About the Menopause*), used to say that progesterone was good for sweats and hot flushes. Dr Gluck says,

I don't find that it always works on its own. Some women do better with a combination of progesterone and isoflavones – a red clover supplement, for example.

If that doesn't do the trick, then I give Utrogestan, which is a progesterone pill, combined with Hormonin. Hormonin is a combination of oestradiol, oestrone and oestriol, which are the three types of oestrogen that a woman's body produces. This is much more sophisticated and safer than giving just oestradiol. As soon as it starts working, I reduce the oestrogen dose to half a Hormonin tablet per day, or even a quarter-tablet per day. In fact, I like to get the dose as low as possible.

When the oestrogen dose is low enough, I switch from the progesterone pill to a cream (which provides less progesterone). Occasionally, I'll add the herb black cohosh in combination with a soya-based phytoestrogen-rich vaginal gel.

One of the most common complaints of peri- and menopausal women is a loss of sex drive. After the menopause, sex can become more painful due to vaginal dryness and thinning of the vaginal mucosa. A soya-based gel can help[36] as can an oestriol-based cream such as Ovestin.

Topping up testosterone

Dr Bond recommends a soya-based gel for women who are having problems with sex drive or vaginal dryness. Recent animal research confirms that this does have an effect. 'If that doesn't work, I recommend Ovestin, which is an oestriol cream,' she says. 'This is a gentler form of oestrogen than oestradiol, and I always advise using it in conjunction with progesterone cream.'

Testosterone deficiency is a common cause of lack of sex drive, in both men and women, the only difference being that men tend to make and need more of it. It's a hot topic in the medical journals. Two recent studies have found benefits with greater effect at higher doses, although that has to be balanced by the greater risk of unwanted hair growth.[37] Dr Bond and Dr Gluck often recommend testosterone for women. 'I think it can be very important, especially for women who have lost their sex drive. It can help with libido,' says Bond. 'I may recommend Testogel, a transdermal testosterone cream designed for men, but women should use less than the full dose. I don't like testosterone implants. They often deliver too much testosterone, which can make women too aggressive.'

What is available on the NHS

If regular visits to a private doctor are not a financial option, then bio-identical hormones are available on the NHS, so ask your doctor about them. The oral progesterone used in France – called Utrogestan in the UK – is now licensed in the UK for treating the menopause. And so are patches or creams containing bio-identical oestradiol, which is then absorbed directly through the skin; brands include Estrogel and Estraderm. Hormonin will give you the three oestrogens in a bio-identical form. Doctors can also prescribe Pro-Juven, a transdermal progesterone cream, as an unlicensed medicine.

I strongly recommend you first get your hormone balance tested, which is explained more in the next chapter, and find a good medical practitioner with plenty of experience in using bio-identical hormones (see Resources). The very first step is to do all you can to balance your hormones by following a hormone-friendly diet, lifestyle and daily supplement programme.

The purpose of bio-identical hormone therapy is to replace those hormones in which you are deficient by taking them in the identical form at a dose consistent with what a healthy body would produce naturally – not in high doses or synthetic forms. With judicial use many women report considerable benefits with little risk of adverse effects.

Natural hormones – how and when to use them

The subject of exactly how and when to use natural hormones depends on a person's hormonal deficiencies; however, since I have mostly concentrated on health issues related to oestrogen dominance throughout this book, here is some guidance on the different forms of bio-identical progesterone available and those conditions it may be helpful for. In some instances, a natural source of oestrogen is necessary to manage resistant hot flushes and vaginal dryness; however, oestrogen supplementation is not advisable for women with diabetes, varicose veins, a high blood-fat level, high blood pressure, fibrocystic breasts, fibroids, obesity, a history of breast cancer, endometrial cancer, ovarian cancer or any clotting disorders. Your doctor will only prescribe oestrogen or testosterone if your test results and/or your symptoms warrant them.

I strongly recommend that you only consider natural hormone supplementation under the guidance of a doctor familiar with its use and a nutritional therapist who can optimise your diet and lifestyle (see Resources). The best way to identify whether you would benefit is to have your levels checked (see Chapter 25). Avoid being tempted to self-supplement, as hormones, natural or otherwise, should be used with care and are only available on prescription in the UK. Many natural hormones are available over the counter in the US and some other countries, but I do not recommend that you self-prescribe them.

If your own doctor is unwilling to prescribe a natural hormone for you, a list of doctors who are able to do this can be found by contacting the Natural Progesterone Information Service (see Resources).

The progesterone pill called Utrogestan, now available in the UK, is a body-identical progesterone. It can be synthesised in a laboratory from diosgenin, which is found in wild yams, but it is quite different from wild yam extract, which does not contain progesterone and is not effective – as was found in 2001 – against hot flushes.[38]

Progesterone is given in amounts equivalent to those normally produced by a woman who is ovulating (between 20 and 40mg a day) and, unlike oestrogen or synthetic progestogens, it has no known cancer risk – in fact, as the late Dr John Lee discovered over a decade ago, quite the opposite.[39]

Since the body can make oestrogen hormones from progesterone, as well as the adrenal hormones and testosterone, which are important for sex drive, a natural progesterone patch is more likely to prevent oestrogen dominance while maintaining your libido. It may also be good for the other menopausal symptoms. In one double-blind trial from 1999, some 83 per cent of women on progesterone found that it significantly relieved or completely arrested menopausal symptoms, compared to 19 per cent on the placebo.[40] As effective as HRT without the risks, it also has the pleasant side effect of improving skin condition and reducing wrinkles, according to a study published in 2005.[41] If given with oestradiol (see 'Inside story: oestrogens', in Part 1, page 24), it works better at relieving symptoms compared to oestradiol plus progestogens and is better for you.[42]

Dr Lee's website, www.johnleemd.com, gives the full story on the use of natural progesterone, as do his excellent books, *What Your Doctor May Not Tell You about Menopause* and *What Your Doctor May Not Tell You about Breast Cancer*.

Forms of natural progesterone

Natural progesterone can be taken orally, as a cream rubbed into the skin, by injection, under the tongue, vaginally or rectally.

Oral 200mg daily of micronised (finely ground in the laboratory for better absorption) progesterone is considered a physiological dose.

Transdermal creams Commercially available creams might contain up to 450mg progesterone per ounce. Prescriptions can be formulated up to 900mg per ounce. Formulation of progesterone cream is not supervised by the FDA in the US, making standardisation difficult to establish.

Between ¼ to ½ teaspoon twice daily is generally recommended, but the efficacy will vary depending on the dose provided in the cream.

Delivering hormones through the skin has been considered by some as a breakthrough, as it is associated with fewer side effects. Compared with oral progesterone, the delivery of the cream is considered superior because it supplies a relatively continuous release of the hormone. Application of the cream may also have local benefits, as when applied directly to breast tissue, where a significantly high level of progesterone has been demonstrated. Oral progesterone has to be metabolised by the liver first before entering the bloodstream, with significant loss of the original dose.

If using natural progesterone, it is recommended that the cream be massaged into the skin until it becomes well absorbed. It can be applied to any area of the body, but it is best absorbed where the skin is thinner – in places such as the neck, chest, breast, lower abdomen, inner thighs, wrists, palms and inner arms. A regular rotation of the cream to different parts of the body is helpful to ensure maximum absorption and to reduce any localised reaction to the cream. A few women have reacted to some added components in the cream.

Injection An intramuscular injection of progesterone is rapidly absorbed and is reported to give the most consistent levels of progesterone in plasma. Levels remain elevated for up to three days, although this is not considered a practical solution for frequent use.

Vaginal Vaginal suppositories supplying natural progesterone have been available since the 1970s and used to help manage problems with miscarriage and some types of infertility. Some doctors also use a vaginal application for a number of women with PMS.

Some women do not find vaginal or rectal (see below) application acceptable. Placing the suppositories high enough into the vagina can be a problem and can contribute to vaginal discharge when they liquefy at body temperature. Itching, discharge and yeast infections may also arise with vaginal preparations. As a result, newer, non-liquefying preparations have attempted to remove these unwanted side effects and, more recently, a sustained-release gel has been manufactured.

A dose of 100mg progesterone trans-vaginally has been shown to quickly increase the level of progesterone in the blood, peaking at around four hours. Vaginal gels have been shown to help protect the endometrium even when the blood level of progesterone is relatively low. This suggests a direct benefit to the uterus when administered vaginally. In combination with oestriol this also helps vaginal dryness.[43]

Rectal Rectal suppositories were developed to help avoid the side effects of vaginal gels. Data is variable with regard to the impact on blood levels of progesterone using this form of delivery.

Sublingual (under the tongue) Lozenges formulated to use under the tongue have been reported as not damaging the oral membranes. Sublingual progesterone has been used to help alleviate PMS and to counteract the stimulating effects of oestrogen in menopausal women taking oestrogen replacement. Sublingual application is likely to be preferable to oral, as it will be absorbed directly into the blood, without being passed through the liver first.

When to use natural progesterone

Premenstrual syndrome (PMS)

Natural progesterone cream can help reduce symptoms associated with PMS. The cream is used in a way that would simulate the natural menstrual cycle (see illustration 'The normal menstrual cycle' on page 9). Read Chapter 8 for further guidance on PMS.

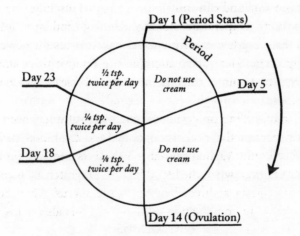

Using natural progesterone cream for PMS

The usual dosage is as follows, but this should be confirmed with your doctor when the prescription is written:

An eighth of a teaspoon to a quarter teaspoon twice daily on days 14 through to 23 of the menstrual cycle, depending on the strength of the cream you are using.

A quarter teaspoon to a half teaspoon twice daily on days 24 through to day 1 (the start of your period), depending on the strength of the cream you are using.

Currently the data is sparse, demonstrating the efficacy of natural progesterone for relieving PMS, and long-term studies on safety have not been conducted. Although it has not yet been approved by the FDA for use in treating PMS, it is however considered by those familiar with its use in this condition to be a very safe and effective treatment.

Dr Tony Coope, a colleague of Dr Shirley Bond, writing for the website Bioidentical Hormone Health, is particularly interested in the similarities in the patterns of symptoms, both physical and emotional, between PMS, postnatal depression (PND) and mental disturbance, and the menopause, suggestive of a common hormonal mechanism within these three conditions.

With 12 years' experience of bio-identical hormones, Dr Coope believes that very few women should have to suffer the disruptive symptoms of PMS, to remain long term on antidepressant or anti-psychotic medication or, in extreme cases, to have to resort to total hysterectomy to resolve this complex condition. Dr Katharina Dalton and Dr John Lee, he says, laid the foundations, and now we have high-quality hormonal, nutritional, herbal and emotional approaches available. (For further discussion of these issues, visit www.bio-hormone-health.com.)

Menopause

Women respond to the menopause differently, some with mild and some with acute symptoms, so each one's requirements for progesterone will vary.

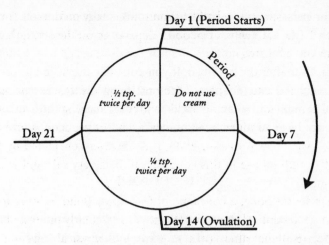

Typical prescribed use of natural progesterone cream for the menopause

Research supports the application of natural micronised progesterone to protect the uterine lining from oestrogen's stimulating effects and it is without the side effects associated with synthetic progestogens, as discussed above. Micronised progesterone is generally prescribed rather than commercially available.

Persistent vaginal dryness and hot flushes

Natural progesterone cream, used vaginally, has been very successful in treating vaginal dryness. Insert ¼–½ teaspoon daily in addition to your usual application, or as instructed by your health practitioner.

For hot flushes, use extra natural progesterone cream for immediate relief of symptoms – ¼–½ teaspoon every 15 minutes for one hour following the hot flush.

For persistent menopausal symptoms, progesterone oil is more effective. For hot flushes, place 2–5 drops of the oil under the tongue and retain it for five minutes. Repeat the dose every 10–15 minutes for the hour after the hot flush. If you don't like the taste, the oil may also be rubbed into the soles of the feet. If you use this method, apply the oil at night and wear old socks to prevent staining the bedclothes. (Chapter 13 gives more detail on dealing with the menopause.)

Osteoporosis

It is a good idea to determine the extent of your bone loss before starting treatment with natural progesterone cream and then to check yearly whether the situation has improved. See Chapter 21 for further guidance on osteoporosis.

Although two placebo-controlled studies did not find natural progesterone applied according to the recommended standard instructions to be effective in preventing bone loss in post-menopausal women, there are several ways in which progesterone should help support bone health:

1. By the stimulation of osteoblasts in the formation of new bone.

2. In stress-induced osteoporosis. Data suggests that progesterone binds to stress-hormone receptors in bone-building cells.

3. In reducing the loss of calcium in the urine.

The suggested dosage for prevention and treatment of osteoporosis is as follows:

Use a cream that contains 20mg progesterone per ¼ teaspoon or equivalent. Rub ⅛–¼ teaspoon of the cream into the skin twice daily from days 7 through to the end of the cycle, as indicated opposite, or according to your health practitioner.

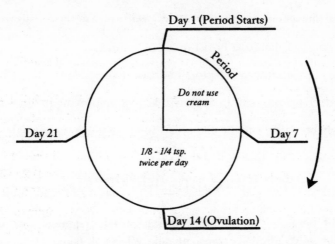

Using natural progesterone cream for osteoporosis

More trials are needed on the efficacy of progesterone for the prevention and management of osteoporosis. What has been shown is that when the luteal phase of the menstrual cycle is shorter in premenopausal women, leading to a decrease in the total progesterone produced in each cycle, the incidence of osteopenia (where bone mineral density is lower than normal) is greater. Osteopenia is considered by many experts to be a precursor to osteoporosis.

Breast disease

Although the literature remains controversial, progesterone appears to have several mechanisms by which it could protect against breast cancer. Progesterone appears to:

- Activate an enzyme that converts the more potent form of oestrogen – oestradiol – to the less potent form, oestrone.

273

- Activate an enzyme that combines oestrone to oestrone sulphate.

- Encourage glandular breast tissue to mature.

- Suppress oestrogen receptors in breast tissue.

- Reduce the production of growth factors, improving prognosis.

- Help breast cells to die and breast tissue to return to normal.

Are there any side effects?

'Natural' progesterone, as found in transdermal creams, is reported to have only minimal, transient side effects if taken as recommended. Some women report temporary, incidental 'spotting' in the first three months of use. If you experience any persistent spotting or breakthrough bleeding this should be reported to your doctor. Likewise, seek help if you experience headaches or other progressive symptoms.

During the first few months of use, symptoms of oestrogen dominance, including breast tenderness, breast swelling and weight gain, may be experienced. This is because oestrogen and progesterone are closely interrelated, and although they generally oppose one other, each helps the other by making target organ cells more sensitive. In time, however, when sufficient progesterone has been absorbed through the fatty layers of the skin, this effect should cease.

The ability of oestrogen and progesterone to make the cells of a target organ more sensitive has given cause for concern because, during the first three months of use, progesterone could theoretically promote a cancer by stimulating oestrogen-sensitive target organs like the breast or uterus.

Some studies that appear to indicate that progesterone is carcinogenic under closer scrutiny have either used progestogens (synthetic progesterone) or very high levels of progesterone, well above that which the body would naturally produce.

Similarly, it has been claimed that progesterone suppresses the immune system. Undoubtedly, progesterone has a localised immunosuppressive effect in the womb during pregnancy to prevent any immune rejection of the baby, which contains its father's 'foreign' proteins; however, research generally indicates that, during pregnancy, the overall effect of the increased production of progesterone is to enhance the function of the immune system.[44]

One research paper indicates that progesterone is protective to breast tissue, as described on page 273.[45] The late Dr John Lee hypothesised:

> When oestrogen and progesterone receptor testing of breast cancer cells is done, it is generally the rule that progesterone receptors are not found unless plenty of oestrogen receptors are present. Oestrogen stimulates the emergence of progesterone receptors. Since oestrogen stimulates cell proliferation (which is not desirable in cancer cells) and progesterone inhibits proliferation in favour of cell maturation, it would seem wise to supply the needed progesterone.

It has been Dr Lee's experience that, in a minority of women, symptoms of breast tenderness, breast swelling and weight gain do not respond to progesterone creams well, even after six months of use. Many more do, however, especially when combined with optimum nutrition.

If you take thyroid medication, be sure to consult your doctor, because progesterone increases thyroid activity, so you may require a lower dose of medication.

Working with your doctor

Natural (or bio-identical) progesterone, although under-researched, seems to help many women without the associated risks of non-bio-identical progestogens. Backed up with simple diet and lifestyle changes, as well as herbal and dietary supplements, the chances are that you'll achieve an equivalent result, but sleep easy without the risk of problems in the future. As a nutritional therapist, I cannot stress enough the importance of diet and lifestyle in the prevention and management of illness.

Your own doctor may not be aware of the science behind natural progesterone, and they may not know that they can prescribe it. The Natural Progesterone Information Service (NPIS) produces an information pack for doctors (see Resources), so it is best to go armed with this information. If your doctor is not familiar with, or interested in, these more natural approaches, the NPIS can refer you to a doctor who is.

CHAPTER 25

Testing for Hormone Imbalances

There are many ways in which laboratory tests can help to build a picture of hormonal imbalances. As you will realise from reading earlier chapters, the body uses various strategies to balance hormones. This chapter focuses on the tests that provide direct, or indirect, insights into how the body is managing oestrogen.

There are many tests that can give useful insights into the balance of oestrogen in the body, enabling your nutritional practitioner to design a more targeted nutritional therapy programme. I have selected those tests that I consider to be the most useful.

Nutritional therapists and nutritionally orientated doctors can work with you, taking into account the results of the tests detailed here. Many of the tests described are not easy to access on the NHS and would most likely need to be paid for privately. This may prove prohibitive for some people. Following the general guidelines for diet and lifestyle (see Part 5) remains the best strategy for improving hormonal balance; however, testing helps to personalise recommendations and provides a means of monitoring progress.

Saliva hormone tests

Hormones generally work in harmony with each other and an imbalance in one hormone can contribute to imbalances in others. It is possible to test the following hormones using saliva: oestrogen, progesterone, testosterone, DHEA, cortisol and melatonin.

The benefit of using saliva is that it better reflects the amount of 'free' hormone; that is, the amount available to have an effect on hormone-sensitive tissues. Blood measures the amount of hormone that is in circulation, including that which is 'bound' and hence unavailable for the body to use effectively.

The 28-day saliva test for oestrogen, progesterone and testosterone. This test involves collecting 11 saliva samples throughout the month to help build up a picture of the balance of these hormones at different times in the month. This test is particularly helpful for women having difficulty conceiving, as it will show whether ovulation has occurred that month, or whether it has occurred earlier in the cycle than normal. Some women are prone to miscarriage, and this can be caused by problems in the second half of the cycle, the luteal phase. Progesterone is the pregnancy hormone and needs to be produced in adequate amounts following ovulation to maintain the pregnancy. Some women produce too little progesterone over this period. The test will provide insights into the balance of oestrogen to progesterone over the month and help to identify whether you are oestrogen dominant. It is possible to be progesterone dominant, although this is relatively uncommon compared to oestrogen dominance. This test only measures the quantity of oestrogen and not whether potentially harmful metabolites are being produced in excess amounts. Depending on the reason to test, it can be helpful to combine this test with an oestrogen metabolite test. (This test is available through a health practitioner.)

One-day oestrogen progesterone ratio This test is particularly helpful for menopausal women and helps to guide the use of HRT, including bio-identical hormones, and may give insights into imbalances that contribute to menopausal symptoms.

One-day DHEA and cortisol test This test measures DHEA and cortisol at four different times over one day. Helping to restore stress-hormone balance as a priority strategy can help to rebalance other hormone imbalances. Understanding a stress hormone imbalance can start to unravel imbalances underpinning anxiety, depression, cognitive decline and chronic fatigue as well as blood glucose imbalance and obesity. Ongoing stress can also undermine the immune system, leading to frequent colds, infections, allergies and cancer. The impact of chronic stress on sex hormone balance can be profound.

Sex hormone-binding globulin (SHBG), testosterone and insulin test

The amount of 'free' oestrogen available to oestrogen-sensitive tissues will largely be determined by how much of the total is bound to the protein SHBG. Measuring SHBG involves a blood test and is frequently recommended by doctors and nutritional therapists to help understand hormone balance, enabling appropriate treatments to be recommended for women at different times of life. The amount of SHBG produced will be influenced by age, food and environment.

When measuring SHBG, it is also worthwhile including blood insulin levels and testosterone by blood or saliva test. This trio of tests is a cost-effective and valuable insight into hormonal imbalances. (These tests are available through a practitioner.)

Oestrogen metabolites test

As discussed in previous chapters, it is not just the total amount of 'freely circulating' oestrogen that can disrupt hormonal balance, but the type of oestrogen. Even small quantities of unbalanced oestrogen metabolites are associated with an increased risk of breast cancer, prostate cancer and osteoporosis.

This urine test, suitable for women and men, can be done at home and the results sent to your doctor or nutritional therapist, enabling them to design an appropriate support programme. You will be sent a kit with full instructions on how to collect the urine sample to send to the laboratory. This test helps give a practitioner a more in-depth understanding of your hormone balance, both in the menstruating years and after the menopause. (This test is available through a practitioner.)

The menstruating years

Researchers have shown that high fat production and high insulin levels can decrease the level of SHBG (which is sometimes tested by endocrinologists). As explained in Chapter 18, high insulin and low SHBG in blood is frequently found in women with polycystic ovarian syndrome (PCOS).

Since SHBG binds both oestrogen and testosterone, the consequence of low levels of SHBG from puberty to the menopause may be too much freely circulating oestrogen and testosterone.

Maintaining a 'healthy' weight through appropriate diet and exercise should support hormonal health at different times of life. Obesity has been linked to most types of cancer. Diets that provide a good balance of protein to carbohydrate at each meal and snack, plus stress management and exercise are all useful strategies for managing good levels of SHBG. Although data is somewhat conflicting, phytoestrogens have been shown to help stimulate the production of SHBG (see the Diet for the Good Life in Chapter 26).

Researchers now suggest that SHBG could be a useful early assessment for liver function well before symptoms of hormonal imbalance arise. Low levels of SHBG indicate sub-optimal liver function, and a repeated measurement of SHBG could be used as a way of monitoring the effectiveness of dietary interventions towards improving liver function.

Post-menopause

After the menopause the level of SHBG generally declines, allowing a higher level of free oestrogen. As explained earlier, this hormone is needed to inhibit the breakdown of bone. The resulting increase in oestrogen then continues to support tissues such as bones and the brain for longer.

The level of testosterone also declines after the menopause but remains high relative to oestrogen. Testosterone converts to oestrogen as can be seen in the illustration 'How hormones are made from cholesterol' on page 236, and it is reported that, post-menopause, this increases oestrogen locally in tissues like bone, without a similar increase in the blood.

As long as the level of oestrogen is in balance with progesterone, and the type of oestrogen is a 'healthier' form, the supporting oestrogen levels after the menopause should be positive.

Detoxification challenge test

As explained in previous chapters, hormones, other chemicals naturally produced in the body, food, medicines and environmental pollutants are all processed by the liver in order to be rendered 'harmless', and then eliminated from the body, mainly through urine and the stool.

This combined urine and saliva test measures the two phases of liver detoxification, Phase I and Phase II. Phase I can be likened to the garbage can in that it processes all rubbish whether generated within the body, or taken into the body through food and environment. The toxic metabolites are then handed on to a 'Phase II detoxifier', the majority of which require amino acids for their production. Many other nutrients are needed to support both these phases, including vitamins and minerals.

This test, which is available through a practitioner, can be conducted at home and the samples sent to the laboratory. The results will reveal how each of these phases is functioning and which 'path-ways' in the liver, if any, require nutritional support.

Homocysteine

Although homocysteine is a vital compound in the body (see page 65), high levels can indicate shortages of B_6, B_{12} and folate. To assess homocysteine levels, it is now possible to do a simple fasting blood test via a finger prick at home to send on to the laboratory.

Thyroid hormones

An underactive thyroid gland is not an uncommon health problem (see Chapter 14). When assessing thyroid hormone function it is important to have a full thyroid screen which involves measuring the following in the blood: unbound levels of T4 and T3, reverse T3, total thyroxine, TSH and thyroid antibody levels, so that a properly targeted nutritional support programme can be designed.

It is possible to measure T3 and T4 in urine over a 24-hour period, which is thought to be a good indicator of a mild case of underactive thyroid, called 'thyroid dysfunction'. Blood tests might not prove sensitive enough to pick up mild cases.

Urinary pyridinoline (PYD) and deoxypyridinoline (DPD)

Osteoporosis is now a serious epidemic in Britain. High levels of PYD and DPD in urine can indicate a rapid rate of bone loss. (This test is available through a health practitioner.) Testing for osteoporosis was explored in Chapter 21.

The tests at a glance

Test	What it measures	When it might be useful
28-day saliva test for oestrogen, progesterone and testosterone (11 samples throughout the month)	Levels and balance of each of these hormones	For women having difficulty conceiving, as it will show whether ovulation has occurred that month, or whether it has occurred earlier in the cycle than normal
One-day oestrogen progesterone ratio		For menopausal women with symptoms who are considering using BHRT
One-day DHEA and cortisol (four samples throughout the day)		To restore stress hormone balance – for those with anxiety, depression, cognitive decline and chronic fatigue, blood glucose imbalance, under-functioning immune system and obesity
Sex hormone-binding globulin (SHBG), testosterone and insulin (blood and saliva)		A cost-effective and valuable insight into hormonal imbalance for women and men

cont ▶

Test	What it measures	When it might be useful
Oestrogen metabolites (urine taken at home and sent away)	Main three types of oestrogen (oestradiol, oestrone and oestriol) and oestrogen metabolites – shows levels and ratios of protective versus more harmful metabolites	Recommended for women at risk of oestrogen-dependent cancers, women recovering from hormone-related cancers and other disorders relating to high oestrogen levels. To direct a nutritional strategy to improve ratios of protective to more harmful oestrogens and oestrogen metabolites
Detoxification challenge test	How well Phase I and Phase II detoxification are functioning	A good indication of which Phase/pathways need to be supported nutritionally
Homocysteine		Can show up shortages of B_6, B_{12}, folate and magnesium, cysteine, glutathione and sulphur, major Phase II detoxifiers, so helps determine both liver function and antioxidant status
Thyroid hormones (blood)	Unbound levels of T4 and T3, reverse T3, total thyroxine, TSH and thyroid antibody levels	An underactive thyroid gland is not an uncommon health problem. Results of this test will enable a properly targeted nutritional support programme to be designed
Urinary pyridinoline (PYD) and deoxypyridinoline (DPD)	High levels of PYD and DPD in urine can indicate a rapid rate of bone loss	To test for osteoporosis risk

Summary

If you have menstrual irregularities, or are post-menopausal and have menopausal symptoms, check your oestrogen and progesterone levels with a hormone saliva test, or opt for one of the more general tests above (see Resources). Most imbalances can be corrected with a combination of the right diet and nutritional supplements plus, in some cases, natural or bio-identical hormones. Your health-care practitioner may recommend these tests to help personalise your plan for restoring your hormone balance. The best place to start is by following the Action Plan for Hormonal Health, explained in Part 5.

PART 5

YOUR ACTION PLAN FOR HORMONAL HEALTH

In this Part you'll find out how to put all the pieces together and create your own action plan for balancing your hormones naturally. The three essential pieces are: balancing your diet, taking herbal phytonutrients and taking the right nutritional supplements. Your ideal personal health programme depends on the particular health issues that you want to resolve.

CHAPTER 26

Diet for the Good Life

The 'perfect' diet is one that provides every single cell in the body with the best supply of nutrients – it is the foundation of health.

Theoretically, it is hard for hormonal balance to be achieved without the rest of the body processes and systems benefiting as well. Nutrients required for hormonal health have multiple roles to play in the body, helping to support immunity, detoxification, digestion, absorption, energy production, mood and sleep as well as helping the body to repair. The converse is also true – that supporting immunity, detoxification, digestion, absorption, energy production, mood and sleep are essential for hormone balance.

The preceding chapters in different ways demonstrate how important nutrients are to support these processes; for example, antioxidants, amino acids, beneficial fats, the roles of individual vitamins and minerals, the balance and types of carbohydrates and sugars in the diet.

The focus of the Diet for the Good Life is to support hormonal health and, in so doing, it should help all the body processes to function more optimally, potentially giving rise to health benefits beyond this expectation. Although the preceding chapters have discussed hormonal problems, the basis of the Diet for the Good Life could equally be used to alleviate many health problems.

The basis of this diet is to eat plenty of complex low-GL carbohydrates, balanced with moderate amounts of protein, plus sufficient essential fats, a minimum of saturated fats and plenty of water. The foods recommended also provide an alkaline-forming diet and give you good levels of vitamins and minerals, both consistent with optimal health. Later in this chapter you'll see that there are five menu plans to enable you to put the basic principles of this diet into practice.

First, I describe the different food groups, vitamins and minerals, and talk about what you should be drinking.

Fats

There are two kinds of fat: saturated (which is hard, as in butter) and unsaturated (which is liquid, as in flax oil). It is not essential to eat saturated fat, nor is it advisable to eat too much. The main sources are meat and dairy products. There are also two kinds of unsaturated fats: monounsaturated, of which olive oil is a rich source, and polyunsaturated, found in nut and seed oils and, particularly, in oily fish. Being *mono*unsaturated, olive oil is close to saturated; for example, it becomes solid in the fridge. Olive oil also contains a small amount of omega-6.

Certain polyunsaturated fats, called linoleic and linolenic acid, or omega-6 and omega-3 oils, are vital for the brain and nervous system, immune system, cardiovascular system and skin. A common sign of deficiency of these substances is dry skin. The Diet for the Good Life provides a balance of these two essential fats. Pumpkin, flax and chia seeds are rich in linolenic acid (omega-3) while sesame and sunflower seeds are rich in linoleic acid (omega-6). Linolenic acid is converted in the body into DHA and EPA, the most potent omega-3s, which are also found in mackerel, herring, kippers, salmon and tuna. These essential fats are easily destroyed by heating or exposure to oxygen, so it is important to have a fresh daily source and not to use sesame or sunflower oil for cooking. It is better to use butter (in moderation), coconut oil or olive oil for cooking, as saturated fats generate less harmful oxidants on heating.

Although fish, particularly the oily variety, is a good source of omega-3 fats, it is also worth considering that many fish are polluted with PCBs and possibly mercury. PCBs tend to accumulate up the food chain, and store in fat, and are more likely to be concentrated in oily fish. Mercury is also higher in larger oily fish, generally in higher concentrations in fish bigger than salmon, such as tuna, swordfish and marlin although, in truth, this does depend somewhat on the species and where it is caught; for example, yellow fin tuna is low in mercury, whereas blue fin tuna tends to be much higher. For purists, you can opt for a purified omega-3 fish oil supplement, free from PCBs and mercury. Arctic cod and halibut are among the least polluted fish.

Processed foods often contain hardened polyunsaturated fats, known as 'hydrogenated' or 'trans' fats. These are worse for you than saturated fat and are best avoided. They are generally found in cakes, biscuits and buns and other processed foods. Checking food labels carefully and following the Diet for the Good Life will limit your intake of these foods.

Protein

There are 22 amino acids (which are components of protein) and these are the building blocks of the body. As well as being vital for growth and the repair of body tissue, they are used to make hormones, enzymes, antibodies and neurotransmitters, and they help to transport substances around the body. Both the quality of the protein you eat (determined by the balance of these amino acids) and the quantity you eat, are important.

The best-quality protein foods, in terms of amino acid balance, include eggs, meat, fish, poultry, soya, nuts, seeds, beans and lentils, particularly when combined with whole grains. Animal protein sources tend to contain a lot of undesirable saturated fat, whereas vegetable protein sources tend to contain additional beneficial complex carbohydrates and are less acid-forming than meat. It is best to limit red meat to one or two portions a week (poultry can be eaten for four to five portions a week) and also look for organic sources, which should have a lower saturated fat content. It is difficult not to take in adequate protein from any diet that has three meals a day, whether that is a vegan or vegetarian diet or one that includes meat. Many vegetables, especially 'seed' foods, such as runner beans, peas, corn and broccoli (the heads are the seeds) contain good levels of protein and help to neutralise excess acidity, which can lead to loss of minerals including calcium (see Chapter 21 for more about osteoporosis and protein intakes).

Ideally, each meal and snack should provide a reasonable balance of protein and carbohydrate, with roughly equal portions of protein and starchy carbohydrates, such as potatoes, pasta and rice. At least half your meal should be fresh vegetables. The menu plans that follow have taken into account the balance of protein with each meal to maximise hormonal balance and there's something for everyone – meat-eaters, vegans and vegetarians or for those following special diets.

Carbohydrates

The main fuel for the body is carbohydrate, which comes in two forms: 'fast-releasing' as in sugar, honey, malt, sweets and most refined foods, and 'slow releasing' as in whole grains, vegetables and most fresh fruit. The latter foods also contain more complex carbohydrate and/or more fibre, both of which help to slow down the release of sugar. The more slow-releasing the carbohydrate, the lower the 'glycemic load' on the body; in other words the lower the effect it has on the blood sugar levels. This can be measured as a food's GL score. Typically, you don't want to have a meal with more than a score of 15 GLs – or 10 GLs if you want to lose weight. How to achieve this is explained in Chapter 7. Fast-releasing carbohydrates tend to give a sudden burst of energy, followed by a slump, whereas slow-releasing carbohydrates provide more sustained energy and are therefore preferable. Refined foods like sugar or white flour lack the vitamins and minerals needed for the body to use them properly and are best avoided. The perpetual use of fast-releasing carbohydrates can give rise to complex symptoms and health problems.

Some fruit, such as bananas, dates and raisins, contain faster releasing sugars and are best kept to a minimum by people with glucose-related health problems. Slow-releasing carbohydrate foods – fresh fruit, vegetables, pulses and whole grains – should make up two-thirds of what you eat, or around 70 per cent of your total calorie intake.

Fibre

Rural Africans eat about 55g (2oz) of dietary fibre a day – compared to the UK average intake of 22g (¾oz) – and have among the lowest incidence in the world of bowel diseases such as appendicitis, diverticulitis, colitis and bowel cancer. The ideal intake is not less than 35g (1¼oz) a day. It is easy to get a good intake of fibre – which absorbs water in the digestive tract making the food contents bulkier and easier to pass through the body – by eating whole grains, vegetables, fruit, nuts, seeds, lentils and beans on a daily basis. Fruit and vegetable fibre helps to slow down the absorption of sugar into the blood, thereby helping to maintain good energy levels. Oat fibre, and the fibre found in flax and chia seeds, is soluble fibre, which is particularly good at preventing constipation and the putrefaction of foods, which are underlying causes of many digestive complaints. Soluble fibre also helps to eliminate excess cholesterol. Refined diets that include a lot of meat, eggs, fish and dairy produce will undoubtedly lack fibre.

Water

Two-thirds of the body consists of water, which is therefore our most important nutrient. The body loses 1.5 litres (2¾ pints) of water a day through the skin, lungs, gut and via the kidneys as urine, ensuring toxic substances are eliminated from the body. We also make about 300ml (½ pint) of water a day when glucose is 'burned' for energy. Therefore, the minimum water intake from food and drink is more than 1 litre (1¾ pints) a day and the ideal intake is around 2 litres (3½ pints) a day.

Fruit and vegetables consist of around 90 per cent water. They supply it in a form that is very easy for the body to use, at the same time providing the body with a high percentage of vitamins and minerals. One to three pieces of fruit, and six to eight portions of vegetables, amounting to about 1kg (2lb 4oz) of these foods, can provide 1 litre (1¾ pints) of water, leaving a daily 1 litre (1¾ pints) to be taken as water or in the form of diluted juices, or herb or fruit teas. Tea and coffee in excess can contribute to water loss in the body, so include no more than two cups of tea or coffee daily and, to aid a restful night's sleep, avoid drinking any after 3.00 p.m. Green tea does contain caffeine but it is rich in the amino acid l-theanine which helps to reduce anxiety and should aid sleep.

Alcohol

A high intake of alcohol not only puts pressure on the liver's resources to detoxify but can also inhibit the absorption and use of many nutrients in the body. The liver is one of the key organs for controlling and balancing hormones, as this is where excess hormones can be removed. If the liver is over-taxed by a poor diet and alcohol, this elimination will not occur. Many people enjoy alcohol in moderation, and in the menus I have included one unit of red wine. Aim to have no more than four units of alcohol in a week (not all in one go) and consume them alongside a main meal to lessen the 'sugar' effects of the alcohol; however, for migraine sufferers, red wine in particular can make migraines worse. Many women with hormonal problems tolerate alcohol poorly, particularly after the menopause. You might need to make a decision to stop alcohol if you find it makes your problems worse. After a period of time reconstructing your diet, lifestyle and supplement programme, you might find you tolerate alcohol a bit better. Drink water after alcohol to aid detoxification.

Vitamins

Although vitamins are needed in much smaller amounts than fat, protein or carbohydrate, they are no less important. They 'turn on' enzymes, which in turn make all the body processes happen. Vitamins are needed to balance the hormones, produce energy, boost the immune system, make healthy skin and protect the arteries; they are vital for the brain, nervous system and just about every physical process. Vitamins A, C and E are antioxidants, which means they slow down the ageing process and protect the body from cancer, heart disease and pollution. Vitamins B and C are vital for turning food into mental and physical energy. Vitamin D, found in milk, eggs, fish and meat, helps to control calcium balance and a deficiency is increasingly linked to many chronic illnesses. Vitamin D can also be made in the skin in the presence of sunshine. The B and C vitamins are richest in living foods: fresh fruit and vegetables. Vitamin A comes in two forms: retinol, the animal form found in meat, fish, eggs and dairy produce, and beta-carotene, which is found in red, yellow and orange fruits and vegetables. Vitamin E is found in seeds, nuts and their oils, and helps to protect essential fats from going rancid.

Minerals

Like vitamins, minerals are essential for just about every body process. Calcium, magnesium and phosphorus help to make up the bones and teeth. Nerve signals, vital for the brain and muscles, depend on calcium, magnesium, sodium and potassium. Oxygen is carried in the blood by an iron compound. Chromium helps to control blood sugar levels. Zinc is vital for all body repairs, renewal and development. Selenium and zinc support the immune system. Brain function depends on adequate magnesium, manganese, zinc and other essential minerals. These are but a few out of thousands of key roles that minerals play in human health.

We need large daily amounts of calcium and magnesium, which are found in vegetables such as kale and cabbage and in root vegetables. They are also found abundantly in nuts and seeds. Calcium alone is found in large quantities in dairy produce. Fruits and vegetables also provide large amounts of potassium and small amounts of sodium, which is the correct balance. All 'seed' foods – which include seeds, nuts, lentils and beans, as well as peas, broad beans, runner beans, whole grains and broccoli – are good sources of iron, zinc, manganese and chromium. Selenium is abundant in nuts, seafood, seaweed and seeds, especially sesame.

Maintaining the right acid–alkaline balance

As mentioned earlier in the chapter, the foods that are recommended for optimum health – and therefore hormonal health – are the basis of what is known as an alkaline-forming diet. When foods are metabolised by the body, a residue is left that can alter the body's acidity and alkalinity. Depending on the chemical composition of the metabolised foods (known as 'ash') the food is called acid-forming or alkaline-forming. The correct balance in our bodies is one that is not too acid; however, this is not the same as the immediate acidity of a food. Oranges, for example, are acid due to their citric acid content, but citric acid is completely metabolised so the net effect of eating an orange is to alkalise the body, and therefore oranges are classified as alkaline-forming.

As previously explained, protein is made of amino acids, and is acid-forming. Foods such as fruits and vegetables are high in potassium and magnesium. These foods, as well as seeds and nuts, are high in calcium. They have a more alkaline effect on the body because the minerals they contain are alkaline. Your body can, and does, compensate, keeping the blood at the right pH; however, excessively high acid-forming diets are not good for you. By eating plenty of fresh fruit and vegetables on a daily basis, you will ensure that your diet is more alkaline-forming. Roughly 80 per cent of our diet should come from alkaline-forming foods, and 20 per cent from those that are acid-forming. The table in Appendix 3 shows which foods are which. This is not a comprehensive list of all foods because not all foods have been analysed but it gives you a pretty good idea.[1]

Organic food

Unadulterated organic whole foods have formed the basis of the human diet through the ages. Only over the last 50 years or so has the human race been subjected to countless man-made chemicals found in food and the environment.

One major requirement for health is to eat foods that provide exactly the amount of energy required to keep the body in optimal balance; however, we waste a good deal of energy trying to disarm those alien and often toxic chemicals, some of which cannot be eliminated and end up accumulating in our bodies, particularly in fatty tissue. As we have seen, some of the synthetic chemicals used as pesticides in non-organically grown vegetables and fruit leave residues that disrupt the functioning of our hormones. It is now impossible to avoid all toxic chemicals in the environment, as there is nowhere on this planet that is not contaminated in some way from the by-products of our modern chemical age. So choosing organic foods whenever possible is the nearest we can get to eating a pure diet today. By supporting the movement to return to the foods produced as naturally as possible we help to minimise the damage of chemical pollution, which appears to pose a genuine threat to the future of humanity.

Raw, organic food is the most natural and beneficial way to take food into the body. Many foods contain enzymes that help to digest them once the food is chewed. Raw food is full of vital phytochemicals whose effect on our health may prove as important as vitamins and minerals. Cooking food destroys enzymes and reduces the activity of phytochemicals; therefore, I recommend including some raw food in your diet every day.

Organic produce tends to be nutritionally superior to non-organic, although one of the critical factors is how mineral rich the soil is. Some artificial fertilisers bind minerals and make them less available to plants. Also, pesticides and herbicides interfere with the plant's ability to make its own phytonutrients. The salvestrol story on page 238 gives some insight into why phytonutrient availability in fruit and vegetables that are intensively farmed is likely to be less. (Organic berries are particularly good sources of salvestrols.) We also know that nutrients are used by the body to detoxify hormone-disrupting chemicals and so it seems logical that eating organic produce will be less toxic and therefore require fewer nutrients, which can be used to nourish the body instead.

The basic principles of a good diet

Following a few simple 'rules' will help you to achieve maximum nourishment from your food.

1. Reduce the amount of dairy foods and red meat you eat. This will reduce your saturated fat intake, and keep oestrogen lower. If you do eat dairy, vary the sources; for example, eat dairy foods from cows, sheep and goats, not just from cows.

2. Eat organic foods when you can or peel your fruit and vegetables to remove pesticide residues.

3. Eat deep-sea fish in preference to farmed (avoid the larger fish such as marlin and swordfish which may accumulate more mercury and pollutants).

4. Cook from fresh whenever possible, and choose simple but nutrient-rich dishes.

5. Use organic butter and extra-virgin cold-pressed coconut or olive oil. Avoid cooking with polyunsaturated oils. Cook with minimal amounts of butter, coconut oil or olive oil.

6. Eat wild game, oily and white fish, nuts, seeds, berries, fresh fruits, pulses and root vegetables. Eat vegetables in a variety of colours – choose green and red or yellow foods with every meal.

7. Make two days a week completely vegetarian. Learn how to use protein-rich vegetarian foods such as quinoa, beans and lentils.

8. Avoid alcohol, cigarettes and refined carbohydrates/sugar and confectionery, which can lessen your intake of the good nutrients. Limit caffeine and avoid after 3.00 p.m. if possible. Use a little xylitol to sweeten food if needed.

9. Are any foods upsetting your digestion? If you suspect one food, then try excluding it to see if it makes a difference to the way you feel (see Chapter 6). Introduce suitable alternative foods if avoiding a food that you know you react to.

10. Variety is the spice of life! Try to eat many different foods each day; this way you will take in more nutrients. Expand your range of foods and cooking methods.

11. Minimise your intake of burned, fried or barbecued food.

12. Limit dried fruit, as it is a concentrated source of sugar.

13. Minimise, or avoid where possible, your intake of hydrogenated or trans fats.

Keep fit

Exercise helps to reduce oestrogen, so walk, swim, practise yoga, Pilates, and so on. A body mass index (BMI) between 21 and 25 is best for fertility (you can check your BMI on the Internet).

What kind of activity is best?

The two main forms of exercise that boost the health of your bones and increase bone mass are weight-bearing exercise and resistance exercise:

A weight-bearing exercise is one where bones and muscles work against the force of gravity. This is any exercise in which your feet and legs carry your weight. Examples are walking, jogging, dancing and climbing stairs.

Resistance exercise involves moving your body weight or objects to create resistance. This type of exercise uses the body areas individually, which also strengthens the bone in that particular area.

For women before the menopause
You can either do all the following suggestions or a combination of them based on your level of fitness:

- Jumping or skipping on the spot (50 jumps daily).
- Jogging or walking for 30 minutes (5–7 days per week).
- Resistance weight training (2–3 days per week).
- High-impact circuit or aerobic-style class (1 or 2 times per week).

For post-menopausal women
You can either do all of the following suggestions or a combination of them based on your level of fitness:

- Weight training (one set of 8–12 repetitions using maximum effort. If 12 can be reached on a regular basis then the weight is slightly too light).
- Jogging/walking for 10–20 minutes (5–7 days per week).
- Stair climbing (10 flights of 10 steps per day).
- Exercise classes such as yoga or aqua aerobics (1 or 2 per week).

Quantities to aim for

1. Two to three portions of different coloured fresh fruit daily (but not overly ripe).

2. Five to seven portions of different coloured vegetables daily.

3. One to two portions of red meat (beef, pork and lamb) weekly.

4. One to two portions of poultry weekly.

5. One to two portions of white fish weekly.

6. Two to four portions of oily fish weekly.

7. Six to eight eggs weekly.

8. Eat pulse and whole-grain meals two to three times a week.

9. Eat nuts and seeds daily or 1 tablespoon of omega-3 and 6 oils daily.

10. Add lots of herbs and spices to food.

11. Use minimal amounts of salt. Don't add it at the table and add only very small amounts while cooking, if at all.

12. Choose meals that provide a good balance of alkaline-forming foods in preference to acid-forming foods (see Appendix 3).

13. Drink 1–2 litres (1¾–3½ pints) of fluid daily. Home filtered water or natural mineral water is best. Dilute fruit juice by at least one-third juice to two-thirds water, as it is a concentrated source of sugar.

Recommended portion sizes

1. A portion of fruit or vegetable is equal to 80g (3oz) or enough to fill a cup (not a mug).

2. A portion of meat, poultry, fish or game is equal to the size of a deck of playing cards.

3. A portion of cooked starchy carbohydrate is equal to a cupful, and no more than a mugful.

4. A handful is based on your handful and no one else's.

5. A non-alcoholic drink, such as juice, is based on a 150–200ml (¼–⅓ pint) measure.

Meal plans

The following meal plans take the above basic principles into account and provide good hormonal support. If you are vegan, vegetarian or avoid any specific food then you will need to refer to the special guidelines section below.

Whether a meat-eater, vegan or vegetarian, I believe that the most important concept for health is to ensure that your food intake has a good protein–carbohydrate balance, and acid–alkaline food balance; also that it contains a good intake of beneficial fats, vitamins, minerals and phytonutrients, as well as drinking adequate fluids from appropriate sources.

There are many good cookery books now available that you can use to create great-tasting main meals based on the principles given in the following menu plans. See my *Optimum Nutrition Cookbook*, *Food GLorious Food* and *The Low-GL Diet Cookbook* for lots of hormone-friendly recipes. (This last book is the best if you also want to lose weight.) There is nothing wrong with having a healthy dessert at weekends or special occasions but not every day.

Special guidelines

If you are avoiding wheat, include as many of the following as possible in the quantities indicated in the meal plans below: rye, oats, barley, rice, corn, millet, quinoa and buckwheat.

If you are avoiding gluten/gliadin, include as many of the following as possible in the quantities indicated in the meal plans below: oats, rice, corn, millet, quinoa and buckwheat.

Oats contain gluten but not gliadin, which is what most coeliacs react to, but oats can be contaminated during processing and some people will avoid oats when following a gluten-free diet. Some oats – for example, certain products made by Nairns – say 'uncontaminated oats'. See Menu 2 for a gluten-free meal plan and use this to adapt for meals throughout the week. Those following a wheat-free diet can include rye and barley as options.

If you are avoiding dairy, regularly include the following foods to gain a good supply of calcium: nuts, seeds, dark green leafy vegetables (broccoli, cabbage, kale), calcium-enriched soya, oat or rice milk, and eat the small bones when you eat fish such as sardines.

If you are a vegetarian, include the following as sources of protein: eggs, dairy products, soya, nuts, seeds, mushrooms, a combination of pulses and whole grains (see Menus 3 and 4 for vegetarian menu plans and use these to adapt for other meals throughout the week).

If you are vegan, include the following as sources of protein: soya, quinoa, nuts, seeds, mushrooms, a combination of pulses and whole grains (see Menu 4 for a vegan menu plan and use this to adapt for other meals throughout the week).

If you are a regular meat-eater, include one vegan or vegetarian main meal each day and have at least one completely vegetarian day a week, and vary your breakfasts and snacks from any of the menu options given below.

If you are a migraine sufferer, see Menu 5 for a low-amine diet and use this to adapt for meals throughout the week based on the list of foods to restrict on page 334.

Menu 1

On rising Drink water flavoured with lemon or lime, if you like.

Breakfast Eat 1–2 eggs (poached, boiled or scrambled) with 1 slice of rye or wholemeal bread, followed by one portion of fresh fruit for speed, otherwise grill some tomatoes and mushrooms and/or lightly toss some cabbage in coconut oil for a few minutes. If opting for 1 egg for breakfast, also have 25g (1oz) smoked salmon or 1–2 rashers of bacon with your egg. This option works well at weekends for those without time for food preparation in the week. Drink 1 mug of green or black tea, herbal tea or coffee alternative, or coffee if you like.

Mid-morning Eat a handful of nuts and seeds with a piece of fruit or a piece of raw vegetable. (Taking a couple of washed raw carrots with you to work or when out and about is as easy as taking an apple.) Drink 1 mug of green or black tea, herbal tea or coffee alternative, or real coffee if you have to – but no more than 1.

Lunch/dinner A portion of meat, fish, poultry or game with three portions of different coloured vegetables (as a salad or steamed, baked, in soup or a stir-fry). Add 1 tablespoon of omega-3 and 6 oil over salad or vegetables once cooked. Accompany with one portion of potato, pasta, rice, quinoa or other starchy carbohydrate. Drink a glass of water or diluted juice. If you like, have 1 unit of red wine with 4 squares of dark chocolate after dinner. Or choose a green tea in the evening.

Mid-afternoon Eat 25g (1oz) hard cheese and an apple or other fruit. Drink 1 mug of green or herbal tea, or water.

Evening Drink a hot or cold cherry juice (use CherryActive concentrate, see Resources) particularly if you have difficulty getting to sleep. Or choose a green tea.

Menu 2

On rising Drink water flavoured with lemon or lime, if you like.

Breakfast Prepare ⅓ mug of oats, or ⅓ mug of rice, buckwheat or quinoa flakes, or a mixture, to make a porridge. Combine with 1 mug of half-water/half-dairy, soya or oat milk to cook, or cook with only water. Then sprinkle 1 tablespoon of ground mixed seeds over the porridge and add some fresh berries. If using only water to cook the porridge, add 3 tablespoons of yoghurt on top. Alternatively, add 10–15g (¼–½oz) of protein powder to the porridge as it cooks. Drink 1 mug of green or black tea, herbal tea or coffee alternative, or real coffee, if you like.

Mid-morning Eat 1–2 oatcakes with 1 tablespoon of hummus on each. Combine with a fresh piece of fruit or raw vegetable such as a tomato or carrot. Drink 1 mug of green or black tea, herbal tea or coffee alternative, or real coffee, if you like.

Lunch Eat a small jacket potato with a topping of meat, poultry, fish or 1 cup of cottage cheese plus a large soup or salad. If buying your meal out, take some fruit or extra vegetables with you that you can use to bump up the salad or eat in addition to the soup. Aim for a minimum of 2 vegetable portions and 1 fruit portion. Drink a glass of water or diluted juice.

Mid-afternoon Eat a commercial gluten-free nut/seed bar that has a minimum of 10g (¼oz) protein indicated on the label, and look for one that has the lowest carbohydrate content. Drink green or herbal tea or water.

Dinner Eat gluten-free pasta or 1 portion of cooked rice with 1 portion of chicken, fish or meat. Accompany with a large side salad or cooked vegetables in various colours equal to eating three vegetable portions. Add 1 tablespoon of cold-pressed oil rich in omega-3 and 6 fats over the salad or vegetables once cooked. Drink a glass of water. If you like, drink 1 unit of gluten-free alcohol (some wines contain grain, so purchase from known gluten-free sources) and a few squares of dark chocolate. Or choose a green tea.

Evening Drink a hot or cold cherry juice (use CherryActive concentrate, see Resources), particularly if you have difficulty getting to sleep. Or choose a green tea.

Menu 3

On rising Drink water flavoured with lemon or lime, if you like.

Breakfast Eat 1 cup of dairy or soya yoghurt with 1 tablespoon of ground nuts and seeds topped with 1 portion of fruit. Drink 1 mug of green or black tea, herbal tea or coffee alternative, or real coffee, if you like.

Mid-morning Eat 2 tablespoons hummus with raw vegetable sticks and half a handful of nuts and seeds. Drink 1 mug of green or black tea, herbal tea or coffee alternative, or real coffee, if you like.

Lunch Eat a 2-egg plain omelette or fill it with mushrooms, courgettes or other vegetables. Accompany with a large side salad, soup or cooked vegetables of varying colours equal to eating three vegetable portions. Add 1 tablespoon of omega-3 and 6 oil over the salad or vegetables once cooked. Drink a glass of water or diluted juice.

Mid-afternoon Eat a slice of rye or wholemeal bread with 1 tablespoon of cashew, hazelnut, walnut or Brazil nut butter, or sunflower or sesame spread. Drink green or herbal tea or water.

Dinner Eat 1 cup of cooked pulses (beans or lentils) with 1 cup of cooked rice, quinoa or pasta. Combine the pulses with the equivalent of three vegetable portions and add 1 tablespoon of omega-3 and 6 oil over salad or vegetables once cooked. If you like, have 1 unit of red wine, or green tea, with 4 squares of dark chocolate after dinner.

Evening Drink hot or cold cherry juice (use CherryActive concentrate, see Resources), particularly if you have difficulty getting to sleep. Or choose a green tea.

Menu 4

On rising Drink water flavoured with lemon or lime, if you like.

Breakfast Mix 1 cup of sugar-free, raisin-free muesli and 1 mug of soya, oat or rice milk. Alternatively, try a shake made with Get Up & Go (see Resources), berries and milk. If making your own muesli, limit the amount of dried fruit and add extra nuts and seeds, and chop a fresh portion of fruit to go on top. Drink 1 mug of green or black tea, herbal tea or coffee alternative, or real coffee, if you like.

Mid-morning Eat a small pot of plain soya yoghurt and add 1 tablespoon of almond, hazelnut, Brazil or cashew nut butter, or 1 fruit, and blend thoroughly. Drink 1 mug of green or black tea, herbal tea or coffee alternative, or real coffee, if you like.

Lunch Eat 1 cup of cooked pasta with pine nuts or other nuts, mushrooms and tomato sauce plus a large salad equal to 2–3 vegetable portions. Drink a glass of water or diluted juice.

Mid-afternoon Eat tahini as a dip with carrot, apple and celery sticks. Drink a green or herbal tea, or water.

Dinner Stir-fry 125g (4½oz) plain tofu, with the equivalent of three portions of colourful vegetables, plus 1 cup of cooked rice or a small jacket potato; sprinkle over 2 teaspoonfuls of soy sauce (tamari) and a teaspoon of nori flakes once cooked. If you like, have 1 unit of red wine, or a green tea, with 4 squares of dark chocolate after dinner.

Evening Drink hot or cold cherry juice (use CherryActive concentrate, see Resources), particularly if you have difficulty getting to sleep. Or choose a green tea.

Menu 5

Following a low-amine diet

Restricting amines in the diet is not the same as avoiding a food because of an allergy. You do not have to totally exclude foods containing amines or high-amine foods. If you suffer with migraines, restricting the amine load may well help. Typical foods that are regularly consumed include spinach, tomatoes, berry fruits, fish, chocolate, curry, beer and wine (see Appendix 4). If your diet is high in these foods then you might start by restricting them and choosing lower-amine options. It will be a case of trial and error. If your migraines lessen or disappear on a low-amine diet then, after a period of time, gradually trial some of the high-amine foods, many of which are healthy foods, and aim to build up to an intake that you can tolerate. You may also find that, for example, you can tolerate some tomatoes with a salad as long as you do not also include spinach leaves and fish. So be mindful of the total amine load of a meal or snack and you may find you can include some of your favourites in small quantities. Drinking more water is encouraged when following a low-amine diet, as it should help the detoxification of amines.

On rising Drink water flavoured with lemon or lime, if you like.

Breakfast Eat 1–2 eggs (poached, boiled or scrambled) with 1 slice of rye or wholemeal bread, toasted. Follow with some cabbage lightly cooked in coconut oil for a few minutes or a crisp green apple if there's limited time to cook cabbage. Alternatively, have homemade muesli made with a mixture of wholegrain wheat, rye, barley or oat flakes, and a small handful of nuts and seeds (not pecan nuts or walnuts) and 1 mug of cow's, goat's or sheep's milk. Add a piece of fresh fruit (not those listed on the high-amine list). Drink 1 glass of water or a mug of coffee with either option.

Mid-morning Eat a handful of nuts and seeds and a piece of fresh fruit (avoiding nuts and fruit high in amines). Drink 1 glass of water or a mug of coffee with either option.

Lunch Eat a small pot of hummus with a large salad equal to three portions of vegetables (excluding those from the high-amine list). Add 1 tablespoon of omega-3 and 6 oil over the salad, and serve with 1 slice of wholegrain wheat or rye bread. Drink 1 glass of water or diluted juice (from allowed fruits). Or bean salad (not soya or red kidney beans) with a cup of cooked rice and three portions of vegetables. Add omega-3 and 6 oil over the bean salad. Drink a glass of water or diluted juice.

Mid-afternoon Eat a high-protein nut/seed bar or any options from Menus 1 to 4 that are not high in amines.

Dinner Have freshly cooked meat, poultry or game with three portions of vegetables (excluding those in the high-amine list), plus a cup of cooked pasta, rice or potato. Drink 1 glass of water.

Treats An occasional spirit from the allowed alcoholic drinks. Cashew cream (grind cashew nuts finely then whiz in a blender with water to make a thin cream), add a portion of fruit from the allowed list and sprinkle with extra flax or chia seeds.

CHAPTER 27

Phytonutrients – The Hormone Helpers

Hormone-like substances abound in natural foods. This is hardly surprising since hormones are, after all, made from food components; however, the extent to which foods that are rich in certain phytonutrients influence hormone balance and health has only recently been recognised.

Phytoestrogens – friend or foe?

Oestrogen-like plant compounds are often called phytoestrogens ('phyto' = plant). At first glance, given the health problems associated with oestrogen dominance, one might think that eating foods rich in phytoestrogens might be bad news. If anything, however, the reverse seems to be true. Soya products, rich in the isoflavones genistein and diadzein, are reputed to protect against breast and prostate cancer, which are notably low among communities with a soya-based diet.

Two possible explanations may explain this apparent contradiction. The first is that phytoestrogens may lock onto and block the body's oestrogen receptors, making it harder for the body's own potent oestrogen to lock onto the receptor. The second is that these phytonutrients may act more like hormone regulators by regulating the amount of SHBG rather than simply mimicking oestrogen or progesterone (see Chapters 19 and 22 for more about SHBG). Since mankind has been exposed to these plant chemicals for millennia, it is highly likely that we have adapted to deal with these compounds in the kind of quantities we are exposed to from eating natural foods.

While the general consensus is in favour of eating foods rich in these phytonutrients in moderate amounts, there are also grounds for caution; that is, not eating vast amounts of phytoestrogen-rich foods, especially at key phases of development, such as during pregnancy or early infancy. Also, if you suffer from endometriosis it is important to limit soya and other very phytoestrogen-rich foods (see Chapter 19).

Nature's hormone helpers

Soya products are a rich source of isoflavones, which are powerful phytoestrogens. Two particular isoflavones have been identified – genistein and diadzein. Unlike conventional HRT, isoflavones have also been shown to protect against hormone-related cancers; for example, we know that people in Asia who consume a traditional diet rich in phytoestrogens have much lower rates of breast, prostate and colon cancer than we do in the UK, elsewhere in Europe or the US. The majority of research into the effects of one of the richest sources of phytoestrogens, soya beans or their products such as tofu, shows that they reduce breast cancer.[2] (Furthermore, an American study involving more than 12,000 men showed that frequent consumption – more than once a day – of soya milk was associated with a 70 per cent reduction in prostate cancer risk.[3])

To help people understand how to boost levels of phytoestrogens in their diet, Dr Margaret Ritchie, an expert in phytoestrogens from the Bute Medical School at the University of St Andrews has spent three years measuring levels of the isoflavone family of phytoestrogens in commonly eaten foods. She's created a database that's a world first, as it assesses levels based not only on the actual food content but that are also corroborated with what's absorbed and excreted after human consumption.

311

For the best results, she recommends having some phytoestrogen-rich foods at least once a day, as blood levels of the beneficial compounds they contain start to decline six hours after eating. 'Asians eat small quantities of soya and other plant-based foods regularly throughout the day and this seems to be the most beneficial,' she says.

Based on her research, I recommend you aim for around 15,000mcg of phytoestrogens a day (see Appendix 5). This is easily achieved by having a small portion of tofu (a 100g/3½oz serving provides 78,000mcg), or a 100ml/3½fl oz glass of soya milk or soya yoghurt (11,000mcg) and a portion of chickpeas, perhaps as hummus (2,000mcg). Eating rye bread, beansprouts, beans, lentils, nuts and seeds also helps to boost your levels – these are the very foods that are staples in the East. Fermented sources, such as natto and tempeh, are considered the most healthy, as fermenting the soya reduces those digestive issues that are associated with it.

Food sources

Other good sources of phytoestrogens include:

- Lignans – found richly in linseeds, black/green tea, coffee, fruits and vegetables, split peas, lentils and beans

- Flavones – found richly in fruits, nuts and green vegetables

- Coumarins – in cabbage, peas and liquorice

- Acyclics – in hops

- Triterpenoids – in liquorice and hops

- Coumestans – found in alfalfa, beans, split peas and lentils

Citrus fruits, wheat, alfalfa, hops, oats, fennel, celery and rhubarb all contain phytoestrogens. There is a small amount of evidence that these foods may help to balance hormones and could play a part in helping to reduce symptoms associated with hormonal imbalance.[4]

For a list showing the phytoestrogen content of food see Appendix 5.

Isoflavone supplements, either soya or red clover, are an alternative, although I favour food as the best source. The effective amount is the equivalent of 80mg of isoflavones a day, as instructed on the supplements. Isoflavones take time to work, so try these for a couple of months.

If you have endometriosis or polycystic breasts you will need to limit even phytoestrogens until you get better (see Chapters 18 and 19).

Phytonutrient herbal remedies

Many herbal remedies are now available as supplements on the basis of their beneficial effects on balancing hormones. These include:

Agnus castus The plant Vitex agnus castus (chasteberry) has a long history as a herb for women's problems. Traditionally, it has been used to relieve premenstrual and menopausal problems. One study of 1,542 women found that 90 per cent reported a significant reduction in PMS symptoms.[5] This was supported by a randomised, double-blind, placebo-controlled study, which showed that a particular dry extract of agnus castus extract is an effective and well tolerated treatment for the relief of PMS symptoms.[6] Agnus castus has an action on the pituitary gland, mimicking the action of the corpus luteum, which produces progesterone. By stimulating the release of LH, and inhibiting the release of FSH, progesterone levels would tend to be increased in relation to oestrogen.[7]

Chasteberry's therapeutic powers were also proven in a series of double-blind trials, attributed to its indirect effects on decreasing oestrogen levels while increasing progesterone and prolactin.[8] Raised prolactin is known to lower oestrogen levels. In most trials, 4mg a day of a standardised extract (containing 6 per cent agnusides – one of the active ingredients) was used.

Black cohosh, dong quai and wild yam These all have progesterone-favourable effects on the body. Yams are especially rich in diosgenin, from which progesterone can be made in the laboratory. We cannot, however, turn these phytonutrients into progesterone itself, so while these plants may help to balance the hormones, they do not replace the need for progesterone in a person who is progesterone deficient. Fennel also has a progesterone-favourable effect on hormone balance.

The most promising of the herbs used to treat the symptoms of menopause is black cohosh, which can help to reduce hot flushes, sweating, insomnia and anxiety. Three double-blind trials have been published.[9] One showed no effect, the other was beneficial and the third showed reduced sweating but no reduction in the number of hot flushes. Also encouraging is new research that seems to indicate that black cohosh neither increases cancer risk nor is anti-oestrogenic.[10] It also helps relieve depression by raising serotonin levels. Even so, I'd recommend that you take black cohosh three months on, one month off. Take 50mg twice a day. Avoid black cohosh if you are taking liver-toxic drugs or have a damaged liver or if you suffer from endometriosis or polycystic ovaries, unless otherwise advised by your nutritional therapist.

The other 'hot' herb for hot flushes is dong quai, whose scientific name is *Angelica sinensis*. In one placebo-controlled study, 55 post-menopausal women who were given dong quai and chamomile instead of HRT had an 80 per cent reduction in hot flushes. These results became apparent after one month.[11] An earlier study didn't find this effect, however.[12] If you want to try dong quai, which doesn't appear to have oestrogenic or cancer-promoting properties, I recommend 600mg a day for relief from hot flushes.

DIM Broccoli is especially rich in diindolylmethane (DIM), which assists the healthy metabolism of oestrogen, mopping up excess oestrogens and helping to metabolise it into a form that has little activity. It also helps DNA repair. This is associated with lower risk for certain cancers and positive effects on a wide variety of hormonal health problems.[13] All the cruciferous vegetables, which contain glucosinolates (containing DIM) – including kale, cabbage, cauliflower and Brussels sprouts – are good sources of this and help to protect against oestrogen dominance. You can also buy supplements of DIM. I recommend 100–300mg a day for anyone with suspected oestrogen dominance.

Ginseng and liquorice are considered to contain quite powerful 'adaptogens' – substances that help restore hormonal balance; for example, liquorice appears to potentiate oestrogen when levels are too low and inhibit oestrogen when levels are too high. Both liquorice and ginseng influence adrenal hormones, responsible for stress. Ginseng is a classic herbal remedy for increasing one's ability to deal with stress. Both have widespread uses for a number of hormone-related conditions probably because adrenal hormones and sex hormones are very closely related, with the adrenal glands producing small amounts of sex hormones.

St John's wort, a herb renowned for its antidepressant effects, has been demonstrated to relieve other menopausal symptoms, including headaches, palpitations, lack of concentration and decreased libido. In fact, a German study found that 80 per cent of women felt their symptoms had gone or had substantially improved at the end of 12 weeks.[14] The combination of black cohosh and St John's wort (300mg a day) can be particularly effective for women who are experiencing menopause-related depression, irritability and fatigue.[15]

Side effects

There are no known serious adverse effects from black cohosh. Dong quai may thin the blood and is therefore contraindicated for women on the drug warfarin. St John's wort, at the dosage given above, has no reported serious adverse effects, but be aware that it is best to consult your doctor if you are on an antidepressant.

Summary

The inclusion of the correct phytonutrient foods and herbs may help your body to adapt, thus restoring and maintaining its hormonal balance. Many supplements that are designed to support female health contain combinations of these herbs and are likely to be beneficial; however, I advise that if you are considering taking large amounts of the herbs individually you do so under the guidance of a qualified herbal practitioner.

CHAPTER 28

Supplementary Benefit

The wealth of evidence supporting the value of nutritional supplements is substantial and I certainly recommend taking them on a daily basis to support hormonal, and overall, health. There is, of course, a lot of anti-supplement propaganda but that is hardly surprising since an optimum-nutrition approach to health largely eradicates the need for pharmaceutical drugs. With sales close to 1 trillion dollars, this is an industry that can afford to fight its turf.

Supplements, as the name indicates, are supplementary to a sound nutritionally rich diet. Avoid falling into the trap of believing that supplements are more important than what we eat and the balance of our meals. It is impossible to emulate in a supplement what is in good, wholesome food. In my experience the best results are found with a combination of a healthy diet and supplements.

Relative to our ancestors, we consume considerably fewer calories; many of our food choices are also depleted of nutrients – for example, the use of refined grains – and many other foods contain chemical pollutants that require valuable nutrients to detoxify them. Many soils used for intensive farming are also depleted in minerals compared to the way they were in the mid twentieth century.

All in all it is difficult, even with the best of diets, to gain enough micronutrients (vitamins and minerals) and phytonutrients to support optimal health. Don't settle for mediocrity; alongside the best diet you can achieve, add a daily multivitamin and mineral, plus extra vitamin C and essential fats. These are the basics of a good daily supplement programme.

Ideal levels vary from person to person. For maximum hormonal health, especially if you have a particular health problem, I recommend you work with a nutritional therapist who will take many factors into account before recommending nutritional supplements, and this could include results from laboratory tests. If you don't have a disease as such, my online 100% Health Programme works out the best diet and supplements for you based on a comprehensive online questionnaire, which you can fill out for free (see www.patrick holford.com).

As indicated in Chapter 2, digestive health is fundamental for hormonal balance, and the health of the gut membrane is critical for the absorption of nutrients.

If you are generally well and not suffering from any diagnosed hormonal problems, I recommend you look for a good multivitamin and mineral to supplement your diet, as well as taking extra vitamin C and essential fats. Levels of nutrients that I consider worthwhile supplementing for each individual nutrient are listed below.

These levels are also appropriate if you are pregnant. Do, however, make sure you don't supplement more than 2,250mcg (7,500iu) of retinol (the animal form of vitamin A) if you are pregnant. Beta-carotene, the vegetable form of vitamin A, has no associated risk.

If in doubt, consult a nutritional therapist (see Resources to find one in your area).

Supplementary nutrient intake for hormonal support

Nutrient	For maintenance	For correction	For extra bone building
Vitamins			
Vitamin A	5,000mcg	8,000mcg	
as retinol	2,000mcg	3,000mcg	
as beta-carotene	3,000mcg	5,000mcg	
Vitamin C	1,000–2,000mg	2,000–4,000mg	2,000–4,000mg

Nutrient	For maintenance	For correction	For extra bone building
Vitamin D	15mcg	20mcg	30mcg
Vitamin E	150mg (200iu)	500mg (600iu)	
Vitamin K	40mcg		250mcg
Vitamin B₁ (Thiamine)	25mg		
Vitamin B₂ (Riboflavin)	25mg		
Vitamin B₃ (Niacin)	50mg		
Vitamin B₅ (Pantothenic acid)	50mg		
Vitamin B₆ (Pyridoxine)	20mg	50–100mg	
Vitamin B₁₂	10mcg	20mcg	250mcg
Folic acid	200mcg	400–800mcg	
Biotin	50mcg		
Minerals			
Calcium	350mg	500mg	600mg
Magnesium	150mg	300mg	300mg
Zinc	15mg	25mg	25mg
Iron	10mg	20–30mg	
Manganese	2.4mg		4mg
Chromium	50mcg	100mcg	
Selenium	30mcg	100mcg	
Boron	1mg		3mg

cont ▶

Nutrient	For maintenance	For correction	For extra bone building
Copper	0.5mg		2mg
Beneficial Fats			
GLA	50mg	250mg	
EPA/DPA/DHA (fish oil)	600mg	1,200mg	
Flax/chia oil (for vegans)	2,000mg	3,000mg	

Easy supplementing

In practical terms, the easiest way to achieve these levels is to supplement:

- A good, all-round multivitamin and multimineral, taken twice a day.

- Extra vitamin C, taken twice a day (to achieve 2,000mg a day total).

- An essential omega-3 and 6 capsule, using fish oils and GLA from borage oil or evening primrose oil.

Plus, for those with special needs:

- A female phytonutrient supplement with at least extra B_6, zinc, phytonutrients, such as DIM, I3C and isoflavones.

- A bone mineral complex for extra calcium, magnesium, zinc, and so on.

Choose quality

Like most things in life, you tend to get what you pay for. There are many supplements available and I recommend that you resist buying cheap, potentially low-quality products. Look for products that tell you the form and amount of vitamin and mineral included in the product. Dosage and form are important criteria for the bioavailability of the nutrient. The more expensive products are more likely to have the levels I suggest and in the best forms for the body to absorb and use.

Good supplement companies provide preparations that can meet these needs (see Resources). Take your supplements with food, unless otherwise stated. Many vitamins help to boost your energy levels so are best taken with breakfast or lunch. Calcium and magnesium, if taken separately to a multinutrient – for example in a bone-building formula – can be worth taking in the evening as they have a calming effect and may aid a good night's sleep. Be consistent – take your multinutrients every day.

Iron deficiency is the most common mineral deficiency worldwide. Many menstruating women are short of iron, particularly if suffering from heavy periods. Although a good multi gives 10mg, which is fine for most women, after a heavy period or if you are anaemic, you'll need 20 to 30mg a day for a couple of weeks to restore iron levels. Post-menopausally, extra iron is rarely necessary. Some people are genetically more prone to absorbing iron extra-efficiently and an excess can lead to widespread tissue damage. The only way to identify such a problem is through testing. If your ferritin levels are high, don't supplement extra iron.

Follow a three-month period of daily supplementation, which will help to build the practice of taking a supplement into your lifestyle. It can take some time before you notice beneficial effects, however. Ideally, water-soluble nutrients like vitamin C and the B vitamins are best taken in divided doses two to three times a day, because after four hours or so what the body hasn't used will be passed out in the urine.

The Hormonal Health Questionnaire

The questionnaire below can help you identify which underlying factors may be affecting your overall health and contributing to hormonal imbalances. It isn't diagnostic as such but it can help you focus in on key areas if you are unsure where to start. If you answer 'yes' to a question, tick the box or boxes shaded in grey. You'll see that each of these falls under a particular column: 'A' is for allergy, 'C' is for candida, 'D' is for digestion, 'G' is for glucose balance, and 'H' is for hormone imbalances. Add up your scores: if you score 5 or less it's unlikely you have a problem; if you score 6 or more there's a possibility that this issue is contributing to your health problems – and obviously the higher the score the more likely this is. Please see the relevant chapter (outlined above), though I do advise everyone to read Part 1 and undertake the Action Plan in Part 5. If you score highly for hormonal balance in general you will benefit from the advice given in many parts of this book, but I recommend that you also seek the guidance of a nutritional therapist (see Resources), who can advise you about testing for hormone imbalances and, if any are present, whether you need to correct it with natural hormone supplements. These are only available on prescription, but your nutritional therapist can liaise with your GP.

Question	A	C	D	G	H
Have you ever used the contraceptive pill, or been prescribed HRT or IVF treatment?		■			■
Have you ever taken antibiotics for a month, or for several times in a year?		■	■		
Have you ever been prescribed any type of steroid treatment, e.g. for eczema or asthma?		■			
Have you been diagnosed with Irritable Bowel Syndrome, or do you suffer from either constipation or diarrhoea?	■	■	■		■
Do you have difficulty losing weight?		■		■	■
Do you suffer from lack of energy or unexplained tiredness (including a diagnosis of CFS/ME)?	■	■		■	
Do you experience numbness or burning or tingling sensations?					■
Do you suffer from joint pains or muscle aches (including a diagnosis of arthritis or fibromyalgia)?	■	■			■
Do you experience water retention?	■				■
Is it cyclical?					■
Do you ever suffer from headaches?	■			■	
Do they happen after eating?			■		
Are they often cyclical?					
Do you have excess hair on your body or thinning hair on your scalp?					
Have you gained weight on your upper body?				■	
Have you gained weight on your thighs and hips?					■
Do you suffer from bad breath?		■	■		
Do you suffer from heartburn, get a burning sensation in your stomach or regularly use indigestion or antacid tablets?			■		

Question	A	C	D	G	H
Do you often feel nauseous, suffer from indigestion or have an uncomfortable feeling of fullness in your stomach after eating?			■		
Do you suffer from abdominal bloating or wind?	■	■	■		■
Do you often have very loose stools or diarrhoea?		■	■		
Do you suffer from constipation or strain when having a bowel movement?		■	■		
Do you have less than one bowel movement per day?			■		
Have you suffered from food poisoning or gastric infection in the last six months?			■		
Do you suffer from breast tenderness or lumpy breasts?					■
Do you have a bad reaction to perfumes, odours or chemicals?		■			
Do you have athlete's foot, anal irritation or any skin problems such as acne, psoriasis or eczema?		■			
Have you had a hysterectomy or have you been sterilised?					■
Do you often suffer from vaginal soreness, dryness or irritation, or from thrush in your mouth?		■			■
Do you have any hormonal problems, including heavy or irregular periods, cramps, PMS or hot flushes?		■			■
Have you at any time been bothered with problems affecting your reproductive organs?		■			■
Do you have trouble conceiving or a history of miscarriage?					■

Question	A	C	D	G	H
Do you fail to chew your food thoroughly?			■		
Do you eat wheat products (such as bread, rolls, pasta or cereal) at least twice a day?			■		
Is your diet high in stimulants such as sugar, alcohol, tea, coffee, or coke, or has it been in the past?		■		■	
Do you suffer from food cravings, such as sweet foods, bread, salt, cheese, alcohol?	■			■	
Do you especially crave foods premenstrually?					■
Are you addicted to sweet foods?		■		■	
Do you experience excessive thirst?	■			■	
Do you become irritable without food?	■	■			
Do you have any known allergies?	■				
Do you feel worse, or excessively sleepy, after meals?			■		
Do you suffer from poor memory or have difficulty concentrating?	■	■		■	■
Have you experienced prolonged stress at any time in your life?		■			
Do you often suffer from mood swings?	■			■	■
Are they often cyclical?					■
Do you suffer from fatigue or drowsiness during the day?	■	■		■	
Are you slow to wake up in the morning?	■			■	
Do you suffer from insomnia?		■			
Do you easily become irritable?	■	■		■	
Do you suffer from depression or anxiety?	■				■
Is it often cyclical?					■
Do you suffer from reduced libido?	■				
Do any of your symptoms get worse premenstrually?		■			■

Question

Are your symptoms worse on damp days or in mouldy places?

Count up the number of highlighted A's, C's, D's, G's and H's you have ticked

A	C	D	G	H

The GL Scores of Common Foods

The following chart gives the GL score of an average serving of a range of common foods. Foods with a GL of less than 10 (shown in bold) are good and should be the staple foods of your diet. A GL of 11–14 (shown in regular type) can be eaten in moderation. A GL higher than 15 (shown in italics) are to be avoided.

Glycemic load (GL) scores of common foods

Food	Serving size in grams	Serving	GLs per serving
Bakery products .			
low-carb muffin	**60**	**1 muffin**	**5**
muffin – apple, made without sugar	**60**	**1 muffin**	**9**
muffin – apple, made with sugar	60	1 muffin	13
crumpet	50	1 crumpet	13
croissant	*57*	*1 croissant*	*17*
doughnut, plain	*47*	*1 doughnut*	*17*
sponge cake, plain	*63*	*1 slice*	*17*

Food	Serving size in grams	Serving	GLs per serving
Breads			
wholemeal rye or pumpernickel-style rye bread	20	1 thin slice	5
wheat tortilla (Mexican)	30	1 tortilla	5
wholemeal wheat-flour bread	30	1 thick slice	9
pitta bread, white	30	1 pitta bread	10
baguette, white, plain	30	*1/9 baton*	15
bagel, white	70	*1 bagel*	25
Crispbreads and crackers			
rough oatcakes (Nairn's)	10	1 oatcake	2
fine oatcakes (Nairn's)	9	1 oatcake	3
cream cracker	25	2 biscuits	11
rye crispbread	25	2 biscuits	11
water cracker	25	*3 biscuits*	17
puffed rice cakes	25	*3 biscuits*	17
Dairy products and alternatives			
yoghurt (plain, no sugar)	200	1 small pot	3
non-fat yoghurt (plain, no sugar)	200	1 small pot	3
soya yoghurt (Provamel)	200	1 large bowl	7
soya milk (no sugar)	250ml	1 glass	7
low-fat yoghurt, fruit, sugar (Ski)	150	1 small pot	7.5
Fruit and fruit products			
blackberries, raw	120	1 medium bowl	1
blueberries, raw	120	1 medium bowl	1
raspberries, raw	120	1 medium bowl	1
strawberries, raw	120	1 medium bowl	1
cherries, raw	120	1 medium bowl	3
grapefruit, raw	120	½ medium	3
pear, raw	120	1 medium	4
melon/cantaloupe, raw	120	½ small	4
watermelon, raw	120	1 medium slice	4

cont ▶

Food	Serving size in grams	Serving	GLs per serving
apricots, raw	120	4	5
oranges, raw	120	1 large	5
plum, raw	120	4	5
apple, raw	120	1 small	6
kiwi fruit, raw	120	1	6
pineapple, raw	120	1 medium slice	7
grapes, raw	120	16	8
mango, raw	120	1½ slices	8
apricots, dried	60	6	9
fruit cocktail, canned (Del Monte)	120	small can	9
papaya, raw	120	½ small papaya	10
prunes, pitted	60	6	10
apple, dried	60	6 rings	10
banana, raw	120	1 small	12
apricots, canned in light syrup	120	1 small can	12
lychees, canned in syrup and drained	*120*	*1 small can*	*16*
figs, dried, tenderised (Dessert Maid)	*60*	*3*	*16*
sultanas	*60*	*30*	*25*
raisins	*60*	*30*	*28*
dates, dried	*60*	*8*	*42*

Jams/spreads

pumpkin seed butter	16	1 tbsp	1
peanut butter (no sugar)	16	1 tbsp	1
blueberry spread (no sugar)	10	2 tsp	1
orange marmalade	10	2 tsp	3
strawberry jam	10	2 tsp	3

Snack foods (savoury)

eggs (boiled)	–	2 medium	0
cottage cheese	120	½ medium tub	2
hummus	200	1 small tub	6
olives, in brine	50	7	1
peanuts	50	2 medium handfuls	1
cashew nuts, salted	50	2 medium handfuls	3

Food	Serving size in grams	Serving	GLs per serving
potato crisps, plain, salted	**30**	**1 small packet**	**7**
popcorn, salted	**25**	**1 small packet**	**10**
pretzels, oven-baked, traditional			
wheat flavour	*30*	*15*	*16*
corn chips, plain, salted	*50*	*18*	*17*
Snack foods (sweet)			
Fruitus apple cereal bar	**35**	**1**	**5**
Euroviva Rebar fruit and veg bar	**50**	**1**	**8**
muesli bar with dried fruit	30	1	13
chocolate bar, milk, plain			
(Mars/Cadbury/Nestlé)	50	1	14
Twix biscuit and caramel bar (Mars)	*60*	*1 bar (2 fingers)*	*17*
Snickers bar (Mars)	*60*	*1*	*19*
Polos, peppermint sweets (Nestlé)	*30*	*16*	*21*
Jelly beans, assorted colours	*30*	*9*	*22*
Kellogg's Pop-Tarts, double choc	*50*	*1*	*24*
Mars Bar	*60*	*1*	*26*

A comprehensive list of the GL values of foods is also available online at www.holforddiet.com. This allows you to 'build a menu' and also work out your total GL intake for the day.

The Acid and Alkaline Levels of Foods

An alkaline-forming diet, as explained in Chapter 26, is best for health. The following chart shows the acid and alkaline levels of a selection of foods. Choose more of the alkaline foods – fresh fruit and vegetables – in your diet every day.

Acid, neutral and alkaline foods

High acid	Medium acid	Neutral	Medium alkaline	High alkaline
	Brazil nuts			Almonds
	Walnuts			Coconut
Edam	Cheddar cheese	Butter		Milk
Eggs	Stilton cheese	Margarine		
			Avocados	
Mayonnaise			Beetroot	Beans
		Coffee	Carrots	Cabbage
Fish	Herrings	Tea	Potatoes	Celery
Shellfish	Mackerel	Sugar	Spinach	Lentils
				Lettuce
Bacon	Rye			Mushrooms

High acid	Medium acid	Neutral	Medium alkaline	High alkaline
Beef	Oats			Onions
Chicken	Wheat			Root vegetables
Liver	Rice			Tomatoes
Lamb			Dried fruit	
Veal	Plums		Rhubarb	Apricots
	Cranberries			Apples
	Olives			Bananas
				Berries
				Cherries
				Figs
				Grapefruit
				Grapes
				Lemons
				Melons
				Oranges
				Peaches
				Pears
				Raspberries
				Tangerines
				Prunes

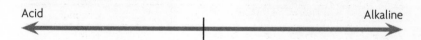

Acid   Alkaline

High-amine Foods

Foods high in amines can trigger migraines in susceptible people. You do not have to totally exclude all high-amine foods though, but restricting the load may help. See Menu 5 on page 308 for details.

High-amine foods to restrict, and their alternatives

	Food to restrict *	Foods allowed
Vegetables	Aubergine	All other vegetables
	Avocado	
	Broad beans	
	Green peas	
	Over-ripe vegetables	
	Pickled vegetables	
	Potato	
	Sauerkraut	
	Spinach	
	Sweet potato	
	Tomato	
	Pumpkin	
	Dishes that include restricted vegetables	

	Food to restrict *	Foods allowed
Fruit	Banana Over-ripe fruit Plums Prunes Raisins Raspberries Apricot Cherry Cranberry Currant Date Loganberry Nectarine Orange Papaya Peach Pineapple Strawberries Dishes that include restricted fruits	All other fruit
Meat, fish and poultry	Dry fermented sausages: Bologna, pepperoni, salami Caviar All leftover meat, fish and poultry Oysters Pickled herring Smoked or pickled fish or fish roe (eggs) Smoked salmon All shellfish All processed meat	All other meat, fish and poultry

cont ▶

	Food to restrict *	Foods allowed
Milk and dairy	All dairy products other than those listed as allowed	Plain cream cheese Plain pasteurised milk Ricotta cheese
Eggs	Dishes that include another restricted ingredient	Plain eggs
Cereals	Dishes that include another restricted ingredient	Plain cereals
Pulses	Soya beans, tofu, fermented soya products: soy sauce, tofu, miso, soybean paste Red kidney beans	All other pulses
Nuts and Seeds	Pecans Walnuts Dishes that include another restricted ingredient	All other nuts
Fats and oils	Dishes that include another restricted ingredient	All plain fats and oils
Herbs and spices	Dishes that include another restricted ingredient Anise Cinnamon Cloves Curry powder Hot paprika Nutmeg	All fresh, frozen or dried herbs All other fresh, frozen or dried spices
Drinks	Cider Cola drinks Beer, including non-alcoholic Vermouth Wine, particularly red wine All other alcoholic drinks if they contain another restricted ingredient All tea	All unless they contain another restricted ingredient Coffee Gin Vodka White rum

	Food to restrict *	Foods allowed
Other	All vinegars and foods containing vinegar Chocolate Cocoa beans Cocoa Yeast and meat extracts Mincemeat Soy sauce Dishes that include another restricted ingredient	All unless containing another restricted ingredient

* The three main amines most likely to elicit symptoms are tyramine, histamine and phenylethylamine and these foods contain the highest levels; however, as explained above it is not a case of excluding all these foods, just be mindful of the quantity you are eating and when.

Phytoestrogens in Food

I recommend you aim for around 15,000mcg of phytoestrogens a day, unless you have endometriosis or polycystic breasts. See Chapter 27.

The phytoestrogen content of food

Mcg per 100g

Soya flour, full fat	166,700	Frankfurter sausages	676
Soya beans	142,100	Premium sausages	620
Miso	126,500	Currant bread	547
Soya mince	121,100	Granary bread	370
Tofu	78,700	Pitta bread	321
Soya cheese	33,000	Malt loaf	293
Vegetarian sausages	26,300	Currants	250
Vegeburger	26,200	Runner beans	222
Tofu burger	24,200	Mung beans	212
Soya milk, plain	11,815	Nut and seed roast	162
Soya yoghurt, plain	11,815	Brown rice	133
Chickpea channa dahl	1,960	Chickpeas	124
Soy sauce	1,800	Mixed nuts and raisins	100
Multigrain crispbread	1,187	Fruit cake, wholemeal	96
Wholemeal bread	830	Fruit loaf	94
Beansprouts	758	Ice cream, dairy	91
Rye bread	757	Sage and onion stuffing	90

Sausage and bean hotpot	85	New potatoes	8
Nut cutlets	62	Waldorf salad	8
Muesli, Swiss-style	52	Mangoes	7
Red kidney beans	40	Dates, dried	7
Turkey burgers, breaded	40	Okra	7
Green beans/French beans	38	Mixed bean salad	5
Blackeyed beans	32	Sesame seeds	5
Hazelnuts	24	Strawberries	5
Haricot beans	24	Mixed nuts	5
Peanuts, plain	24	Sun-dried tomatoes	5
Noodles, wheat	23	Apricots, dried	4
Lentils, green and brown	22	Tomatoes, stuffed with rice	4
Mung bean dhal	21	Cranberries	4
Aubergine, stuffed with lentils and vegetables	19	Tomatoes	3
Passion fruit	17	Sweetcorn	3
Prunes, ready-to-eat	13	Tuna pasta	2
Apples	12	Curly kale	2
Brown rice and red kidney beans	12	Lentil soup	2
Hummus	11	Peppers, stuffed with rice	2

Adapted from the Phytoestrogen Database 2004, compiled by Dr Margaret Ritchie, Bute Medical School at the University of St Andrews.

Diakath Breathing

One way to deal with stress is to learn a breathing technique. This breathing exercise (reproduced with the kind permission of Oscar Ichazo), connects the Kath Point – the body's centre of equilibrium – with the diaphragm muscle so that deep breathing becomes natural and effortless. You can practise this exercise at any time, while sitting, standing or lying down, and for as long as you like. You can also do it unobtrusively during moments of stress. It is an excellent natural relaxant and energy booster, helping you to feel more connected and in tune.

The diaphragm is a dome-shaped muscle attached to the bottom of the rib cage. The Kath is not an anatomical point like the navel, but is located in the lower belly, about three finger-widths below the navel. When you remember this point, you become aware of your entire body.

Find somewhere quiet first thing in the morning to do this exercise. As you inhale, you will expand your lower belly from the Kath point and your diaphragm muscle. This allows the lungs to fill with air from the bottom to the top. As you exhale, the belly and the diaphragm muscle relax, allowing the lungs to empty from top to bottom. Inhale and exhale through your nose.

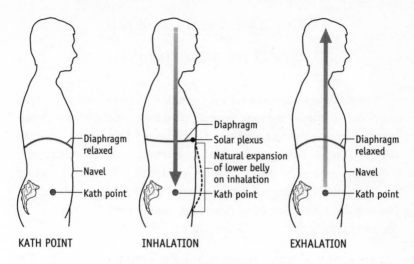

Diakath breathing

How to do it

Every morning, sit down in a quiet place before breakfast and practise Diakath Breathing for a few minutes.

Whenever you are stressed throughout the day, check your breathing. Practise Diakath breathing for nine breaths. This is great to do before an important meeting or when something has upset you.

1. Sit comfortably, in a quiet place with your spine straight.

2. Focus your attention in your Kath point.

3. Let your belly expand from the Kath point as you inhale slowly, deeply and effortlessly. Feel your diaphragm being pulled down towards the Kath point as your lungs fill with air from the bottom to the top. On the exhale, relax both your belly and your diaphragm, emptying your lungs from top to bottom.

4. Repeat at your own pace.

© 2002 Oscar Ichazo. Diakath breathing is the service mark and Kath the trademark of Oscar Ichazo. Used by permission.

Vital energy exercise is good for your health

This awareness, taught as Diakath Breathing, is also a vital part of the excellent 16-minute exercise system called Psychocalisthenics, developed by Ichazo for the purposes of generating vital energy – a way of helping you feel more grounded, alive, energised and in control, with a delicate sense of vitality. I have been practising Psychocalisthenics for 30 years. This form of exercise keeps you fit, strong and supple, but has the added benefit of generating vital energy. (See Resources for more details on Psychocalisthenics.)

Recommended Reading

Dr James Braly and Patrick Holford, *The H-Factor: Homocysteine – the Biggest Health Breakthrough of the Century*, Piatkus (2003)

Donna Gates and Linda Schatz, *Body Ecology Diet: Recovering your Health and Rebuilding your Immunity*, Body Ecology (2006)

Marilyn Glenville, *Getting Pregnant Faster*, Kyle Cathie (2008)

Dr Marion Gluck and Vicki Edgson, *It Must Be My Hormones: Getting Your Life on Track with the Help of Natural Bio-Identical Hormone Therapy and Nutrition*, Penguin Books (2010)

Dr Richard Halvorsen, *The Truth about Vaccines*, Gibson Square Publishing (2007)

Colette Harris and Dr Adam Carey, *PCOS: A Woman's Guide to Dealing with Polycystic Ovary Syndrome*, Thorsons (2000)

Colette Harris and Theresa Francis-Cheung, *PCOS Diet Book: How You Can Use the Nutritional Approach to Deal with Polycystic Ovary Syndrome*, Thorsons (2002)

Patrick Holford, *The Low-GL Diet Bible*, Piatkus (2005)

Patrick Holford, *The Low-GL Diet Cookbook*, Piatkus (2005)

Patrick Holford and Susannah Lawson, *Optimum Nutrition Before, During and After Pregnancy*, Piatkus (2004)

Patrick Holford, *Say No to Arthritis, Piatkus* (2010)

Patrick Holford, *Say No to Cancer*, Piatkus (2010)

Patrick Holford and Dr James Braly, *Hidden Food Allergies*, Piatkus (2006)

Patrick Holford, Shane Heaton and Deborah Colson, *The Alzheimer's Prevention Plan*, Piatkus (2005)

Patrick Holford, Susannah Lawson and Fiona McDonald Joyce, *The Perfect Pregnancy Cookbook*, Piatkus (2010)

Patrick Holford and Fiona McDonald Joyce, *Food GLorious Food*, Piatkus (2008)

Patrick Holford, David Miller and Dr James Braly, *How to Quit Without Feeling S**t*, Piatkus (2008)

Dr John Lee, *Natural Progesterone: The Multiple Roles of a Remarkable Hormone*, BLL (1993)

Dr John Lee and Virginia Hopkins, *Hormone Balance Made Simple: The Essential How-to Guide to Symptoms, Dosage, Timing, and More*, BLL (1999)

Dr John Lee and Virginia Hopkins, *What Your Doctor May Not Tell You About Menopause*, BLL (1999)

Dian Shepperson Mills and Michael Vernon, *Endometriosis: A Key to Healing and Fertility Through Nutrition*, Thorsons (2007)

Jane Plant, *Your Life in Your Hands*, Virgin Books (2003)

Erica White, *Beat Candida Cookbook*, Thorsons (1999)

Resources

Bioidentical Hormone Health www.bio-hormone-health.com is a site dedicated to offering women information, news and expert opinion from doctors and experienced professionals working in the field of women's health and natural bio-identical hormones. Millions of women around the world are looking for safe, natural alternatives for the symptoms of hormone imbalance but without the health risks associated with synthetic hormones and HRT. Bioidentical Hormone Health brings together practitioners from various disciplines, including doctors, therapists and healthcare commentators to bring women information and expert opinion on natural hormones and their use. The website also provides a forum where women can exchange views and share their experiences on any aspect of hormonal health.

Dr John Lee's website, www.johnleemd.com, is a source of information on natural progesterone, bio-identical hormone replacement therapy and information on balancing hormones.

Dr Richard Halvorsen founded www.babyjabs.co.uk, the Children's Immunisation Service that provides information on the pros and cons of children's vaccinations.

Foresight provides information and personal advice on the importance of pre-conceptual care and nutrition. Visit www.foresight-preconception.org.uk or write to: Foresight, 78 Hawthorn Road, Bognor Regis, West Sussex PO21 2UY.

The Institute for Optimum Nutrition (ION) offers a three-year foundation degree course in nutritional therapy. There is a clinic, a list of nutrition practitioners across the UK, an information service and a quarterly journal, *Optimum Nutrition*. Visit www.ion.ac.uk, address: Avalon House, 72 Lower Mortlake Road, Richmond TW9 2JY, UK, tel: 020 8614 7800.

The Natural Progesterone Information Service (NPIS) provides women and their doctors with information on natural progesterone and details of how to obtain information packs as well as books and other resources relating to natural hormone health, including all the works of Dr John Lee. Visit www.npis.info/ for more information; tel: 07000 784849, address: NPIS, PO Box 41, Robertsbridge TN32 5XG.

Nutritional therapy and consultations To find a nutritional therapist near you, visit www.patrickholford.com. This service gives details on whom to see in the UK as well as internationally. If there is no one available near by, you can always take an on-line assessment – see below.

On-line 100% Health Programme Are you 100 per cent healthy? Find out with my FREE health check and comprehensive 100% Health Programme giving you a personalised action plan, including diet and supplements. Visit www.patrickholford.com.

Psychocalisthenics is an excellent exercise system that takes less than 20 minutes a day. It develops strength, suppleness and stamina as well as generating vital energy, which brings peace of mind, mental vitality and well-being. The best way to learn it is to do the Psychocalisthenics Training. See www.patrickholford.com (events) for details. Also available is the book *Master Level Exercise: Psychocalisthenics* and the Psychocalisthenics CD and DVD, available from www.patrickholford.com (shop). For further information please see www.pcals.com.

Zest4Life is a health and nutrition club, based on low-GL principles, that provides advice, coaching and support for losing weight and gaining health through a series of weekly meetings. For more information, visit www.zest4life.eu.

Clinics

Dian Shepperson Mills can be contacted at The Endometriosis and Fertility Clinic, 56 London Road, Hailsham, East Sussex BN27 3DD, tel: +44 (0)1323 846888. Dian also holds consultations at The Hale Clinic, 7 Park Crescent, London W1B 1PF, tel: 020 7631 0156. Visit: www.endometriosis.co.uk; www.makingbabies.com; email: dian@ endometriosis.co.uk.

Dr Barry Peatfield runs a complementary therapy clinic, The Peatfield Clinic for Metabolic Health (tel: 01883 623125).

Laboratory tests

Adrenal Stress Index A person's levels of cortisol and another key stress hormone called DHEA (both of which are good measures of adrenal stress) are best measured in saliva, and this standard stress test involves providing four saliva samples at different intervals over a 24-hour period. These are then sent for analysis. Such tests, available through nutritional therapists (see 'Nutritional therapy and consultations' above), can determine whether a person needs to pursue a nutritional or hormonal strategy, or perhaps other therapies such as meditation, to restore the body so that it can respond to stress in a healthy way.

BioCard Celiac Test A home-test kit which provides results in less than 10 minutes. Available through Totally Nourish (www.totally nourish.com) and Boots, or call freephone (UK) 0800 085 7749.

Food allergy, homocysteine and GL tests Food allergy (IgG ELISA), homocysteine and GLCheck (measures your level of glycosylated haemoglobin, also called HbA1C) tests are available through YorkTest Laboratories, using a home-test kit where you can take your own pinprick blood sample and return it to the lab for analysis. Visit www. yorktest.com, or call freephone (UK) 0800 074 6185. These test kits are also available from www.totallynourish.com.

Intestinal permeability (leaky gut) test is available from the following labs through qualified nutritional therapists and doctors:

- Biolab Medical Unit (doctor's referral only): visit www.biolab. co.uk or call +44 (0)20 7636 5959/5905.

- Genova Diagnostics: visit www.gdx.uk.net or call +44 (0)20 8336 7750.

Bone Resorption Assessment and Oestrogen Metabolism Assessment are non-invasive urine tests available from Genova Diagnostics. The 1-Day Progesterone/Oestradiol (a saliva test) and Total Thyroid Screen, which requires a blood sample are also available from Genova Diagnostics (www.gdx.uk.net, tel: +44 (0)20 8336 7750) and can be arranged by your nutritional therapist or doctor.

Patient support groups

Breast Cancer Care, for anyone affected by breast cancer, www. breastcancercare.org.uk.

Breast Cancer, for active online discussion, www.breastcancer.org.

The Daisy Network supports women experiencing a premature menopause, www.daisynetwork.org.uk.

Endometriosis.org provides information on endometriosis support groups worldwide, www.endometriosis.org.

The **Endometriosis and Fertility Clinic** information website www. endometriosis.co.uk run by nutritional expert Dian Shepperson Mills, who is also available for consultation in East Sussex, tel: 01323 846888, and the Hale Clinic, London W1, tel: 020 7631 0156.

National Osteoporosis Society, a UK-based site that will help you find local support groups, www.nos.org.uk or tel: 0845 450 0230.

Natural Menopause Advice Service, a UK-based site, www.patient. co.uk/leaflets/natural_menopause_advice_service.htm.

Natural Progesterone Advisory Network, an Australian-based information site, www.natural-progesterone-advisory-network.com.

Polycystic Ovarian Syndrome Association, Inc., www.pcosupport. org/.

Thyroid Patient Advocacy-UK, provides education and support for patients and their families, www.tpa-uk.org.uk.

Thyroid UK, the leading charitable organisation providing clear advice on thyroid issues, www.thyroiduk.org.

Women's Health Concern for unbiased information on all health concerns, www.womens-health-concern.org.

Health products

Cervagyn is a vaginal/probiotic cream that contains *Lactobacillus acidophilus*, blended with naturally derived vegetable emollients to help maintain the normal balance of vaginal flora. *L. acidophilus* is a friendly bacteria that occurs naturally on the epithelial tissue of the mouth, throat, gastrointestinal tract and vagina. Lactic acid bacteria acidify the tissues and reduce the potential proliferation of opportunistic yeasts such as *Candida albicans*.

CherryActive is sold in a highly concentrated juice format. Mix a 2 tbsp (30ml) serving with 250ml (9fl oz) water to make a deliciously healthy, low-GL cherry juice. Each 946ml bottle contains the juice from over 3,000 cherries – that's half a tree's worth – and contains a month's supply. CherryActive is also available as a dried cherry snack and in capsules. For more information and to order, visit www.totallynourish.com (see below).

Get Up & Go is a delicious low-GL breakfast shake powder. It contains a range of vitamins and minerals, one-third of your daily protein requirements, and relevant levels of essential fatty acids and is made from the best-quality whole foods, ground into a powder.

Organic food delivered to your door: www.soilassociation.org, www.riverford.co.uk, www.abelandcole.co.uk, www.organicdelivery.co.uk.

Silence of Peace **CD**, specifically designed to put you into the 'alpha' brain wave state that is the prerequisite of sleep. Available from The Alpha Music Shop. Order online from www.patrickholford.com or, in the US (+ 1 (347) 408 0457) and Australia (+61 (02) 8003 3132).

Sugar alternative, xylitol, is a low-GL natural sugar alternative, available from high-street health-food shops. Also available by mail order from www.totally nourish.com (see below), sold as XyloBrit.

Transdermal skin cream This form of 'natural progesterone' HRT, called Projuven, is only available on prescription in the UK, so you should consult a doctor who is trained in its use (see NPIS above). Although it is available over the counter in other countries, I do not recommend that you use it without supervision.

Waterfall D-Mannose Single sachets and tubs can be purchased from www.waterfall-d-mannose.com or phone +44(0)1904 789559.

Water filters There are many water filters on the market. One of the best is offered by The Fresh Water Filter Company, who produce mains-attached water-filtering units using gravity rather than reverse osmosis (which can filter out some useful minerals as well). You can buy a whole-house filter or an under-sink version. Visit www.totally nourish.com or www.freshwaterfilter.com.

Skincare, personal care and household products

Environ products were developed by the cosmetic surgeon Dr Des Fernandes to prevent skin cancer and address the damaging effects of the environment on our skin. Formulated with scientifically proven active ingredients, including vitamin A and antioxidant vitamins C, E and beta-carotene, which are used in progressively higher concentrations, Environ will maintain a normal healthy skin or effectively treat and prevent the signs of ageing, pigmentation, problem skin and scarring. Environ products are available from www.totallynourish. com or direct from an Environ skincare therapist. See www.iiaa.eu (Institute for Anti-Ageing) to find one near you in the EU. For international enquiries call +27 21 671 1467 or email factory@environ. co.za or visit www.environ.co.za.

RAD is a revolutionary sunscreen containing sun filters and sun reflectants that give an SPF 16 to provide protection from both UVA and UVB irradiation. Also contains antioxidant vitamins to combat the effects of the sun and pollution on the skin. Suitable for all skin types and ages, including babies.

Supplements

Nutritional supplements are available from a wide variety of companies. Two companies that provide an extensive range, between them covering the speciality supplements referred to in this book, are Solgar and BioCare (see 'Supplement suppliers' on page 355).

Finding your own perfect supplement programme can be confusing, but my website, www.patrickholford.com, offers useful guidance. The backbone of a good supplement programme is:

- A high-strength multivitamin and mineral

- Additional vitamin C

- An essential fat supplement containing omega-3 and omega-6 oils

In this section are examples of supplements that provide the herbs and nutrients at the levels discussed in this book. The addresses of the companies whose products I've referred to are given at the end.

Antioxidants

A good all-round antioxidant complex should provide vitamin A (beta-carotene and/or retinol), vitamins C and E, zinc, selenium, glutathione or cysteine, anthocyanidins of berry extracts, lipoic acid and co-enzyme Q_{10}. Two products that fulfil these criteria are BioCare's AGE Antioxidant and Solgar's Advanced Antioxidant Nutrients. Complexes of bioflavonoids, often found together with vitamin C, are available from both companies.

Bone health

It takes more than just calcium to support bone health. A good formulation should include magnesium, calcium and boron as well as vitamins A, D and K. BioCare's Osteoplex combines magnesium and calcium in a ratio of 2:1.

352

Digestive enzymes and support

A good digestive enzyme combination should contain protease, amylase and lipase, which digest protein, carbohydrate and fat respectively. Some also contain amyloglucosidase (helps to digest glucosides found in certain beans and vegetables) and lactase (helps to digest milk sugars). If you get bloated after lentils or beans, such as soya products, choose an enzyme that contains alpha-galactosidase. Try Solgar's Vegan Digestive Enzymes. You can also buy digestive enzymes *with* probiotics – BioCare's DigestPro contains all these enzymes and probiotics.

Essential fats and fish oil supplements

The most important omega-3 fats are DHA, DPA and EPA, found both in oily fish and in cod liver oil. The most important omega-6 fat is GLA, the richest source being borage (also known as starflower) oil. Try BioCare's Essential Omegas, which provide a highly concentrated mix of EPA, DHA, DPA and GLA. They also produce Mega-EPA, a high potency omega-3 fish oil supplement. Seven Seas produce Extra High Strength Cod Liver Oil. A good essential oil blend is Udo's Choice, distributed by Savant and available in health-food shops.

Homocysteine-lowering nutrients

A good methyl nutrient complex should contain at least B_6, B_{12} and folic acid. Some formulas also contain vitamin B_2, trimethylglycine (TMG), zinc and N-acetyl-cysteine. Three products that fulfil these criteria are BioCare's Connect, which contains them all; Solgar's Gold Specifics Homocysteine Modulators, which contain TMG, vitamins B_6 and B_{12} and folic acid; and Higher Nature's H Factors, which contains vitamins B_2, B_6, B_{12}, folic acid and zinc, plus TMG (see www.highernature.co.uk).

Hormone balancing herbs and nutrients

BioCare (see page 356) supply Female Balance, a specially formulated blend of B vitamins, vitamin C, zinc and magnesium with isoflavones and the herbs black cohosh, agnus castus, wild yam and fennel. They also supply a number of single herbal preparations such as Agnus Castus Plus and Red Clover Extract. Other herbs such as dong quai and black cohosh are available through Solgar.

Diindolymethane (DIM) is available through your nutritional therapist from Allergy Research (www.allergyresearchgroup.com). Choose from DIM Vitex PMS Formula (DIM combined with Vitex and Green Tea Extract) or the simple high-potency formulation DIM Enhanced Delivery System.

Festuca arundina is available in a supplement formula called Asphalia, a high anti-oxidant formulation that also contains red clover and white clover. Available from www.asphalia.co.uk.

Multivitamin and mineral supplements

Supplementing the right multivitamin is the most important supplement decision you make. Most multis are based on RDA levels of nutrients, which are not the same as optimum nutrition levels. A good multivitamin based on optimum nutrition levels is BioCare's Advanced Optimum Nutrition Formula. Another is Solgar's VM2000. Both of these recommend taking two tablets a day. Advanced Optimum Nutrition Formula has higher mineral levels, especially for calcium and magnesium. Ideally, take a multivitamin and mineral with an extra 1g of vitamin C. BioCare's Optimum Nutrition Pack contains the Optimum Nutrition Formula, ImmuneC and Essential Omegas all in a convenient daily strip.

Probiotics

Probiotics are supplements of beneficial bacteria, the two main strains being *Lactobacillus acidophilus* and *Bifidobacterium bifidus*. There are various types of strains within these two, some more important in children, others in adults. There is quite some variability in quantities of bacteria (some labels say things like 'a billion viable organisms per capsule') and quality. A very good product is BioCare's Bio-Acidophilus and also DigestPro, which also contains digestive enzymes.

Salvestrols

Available from BioCare (see below). For higher, therapeutic dosage levels, contact: Nature's Defence (UK) Ltd, Charnwood Science Centre, 103 High Street, Syston, Leicester LE7 1GQ; email: info@ naturesdefence.com; tel: 01162 602963, to find a practitioner near you who is knowledgeable in the use of salvestrols. Also see www.1880life.com.

Sugar balance

Look for a product that contains 200mcg of chromium, either as chromium polynicotinate or chromium picolinate, ideally with a cinnamon high in MCHP (Cinnulin PF® is the name of a concentrated extract of cinnamon that is especially high in MCHP).

Supplement suppliers

The following companies produce good-quality supplements that are widely available in the UK.

BioCare offers an extensive range of nutritional and herbal supplements, including daily 'packs', which are especially convenient for travelling/when you are away from home. Their products are stocked by most good health-food shops. Visit www.biocare.co.uk, tel: +44 (0)121 433 3727. They are also available by mail order from Totally Nourish (www.totallynourish.com) – see below.

Higher Nature, available in many good health-food shops or visit www.highernature.co.uk, tel: 0800 458 4747 (freephone within the UK).

Solgar, available in most independent health-food shops or visit www.solgar.com, tel: +44 (0) 1442 890355.

Totally Nourish is an 'e'-health shop that stocks many high-quality health products, including home-test kits and supplements. Visit www.totallynourish.com, tel: 0800 085 7749 (freephone within the UK).

And in other regions

South Africa

The original Patrick Holford vitamin and supplement brand from the UK is now available in South Africa through leading health-food shops, Dis-Chem and Clicks retail pharmacies. They are also available online direct from www.holforddirect.co.za by post or by courier direct to your door. Patrick Holford supplements, books and CDs can also be ordered by phone on 011 2654 554.

Australia

Solgar supplements are available in Australia. Visit www.solgar.com, tel: 1800 029 871 (free call) for your nearest supplier. Another good brand is Blackmores.

New Zealand

BioCare products (see above) are available in New Zealand through Pacific Health, PO Box 56248, Dominion Road, Auckland 1446, New Zealand, tel: 0064 9815 0707. Visit www.pachealth.co.nz.

Singapore

BioCare (see above) and Solgar products are available in Singapore through Essential Living. Visit www.essliv.com, tel: 6276 1380.

UAE

BioCare supplements (see page 356) are available in Dubai from Organic Foods & Café, PO Box 117629, Dubai, United Arab Emirates; tel: +971 4338 4822; fax: +971 4338 2449.

References

Part 1

1. Dr M. Herman-Giddens, University of North Carolina. Article in *Daily Mail* by Gaby Hinscliff, medical reporter. Originally published in *Journal of Paediatrics* (9 April 1997)
2. I. Rogers, et al., 'Diet throughout childhood and age at menarche in a contemporary cohort of British girls', *Public Health Nutrition*, 2009 Aug, Published online by Cambridge University Press
3. Women's Nutritional Advisory Service, 'Social implications of premenstrual syndrome – 11 years on' (1996)
4. P. Holford, et al., '100% Health Survey', 2010, see www.patrickholford.com/100healthsurvey
5. E. Coutinho, 'Progress in management of endometriosis', *Proceedings of the Fourth World Congress on Endometriosis 25–28 May 1994*, Salvador, Bahia, Brazil, Parthenon Publishing Press
6. M. Carruthers, *The Male Menopause*, HarperCollins (1996)
7. D. Cadbury, *The Feminisation of Nature*, Hamish Hamilton (1997)
8. A. Anderson, et al., 'Adverse trends in male reproductive health: We may have reached a crucial "tipping point"', *International Journal of Andrology*, 2008;31:74–80
9. Comment in relation to his paper BMJ 2004;328:447 doi: 10.1136/bmj.328.7437.447 R.M. Sharpe and D. Stewart Irvine, 'How strong is the evidence of a link between environmental chemicals and adverse effects on human reproductive health?', *Clinical Review*, 2004 Feb. 19
10. R. Sharpe and D. Irvine, 'How strong is the evidence of a link between environmental chemicals and adverse effects on human reproductive health?', *British Medical Journal*, 2004 Feb. 21;328(7437):447–51

11. See http://consumerreports.org/cro/magazine-archive/december-2009/food/ bpa/overview/bisphenol-a-ov.htm

12. A. Herbst, et al., 'Adenocarcinoma of the vagina. Association of maternal stilbestrol therapy with tumor appearance in young women', *New England Journal of Medicine*, 1971 Apr. 15;284(15):878–81

13. W. Gill, 'Effects on human males of in-utero exposure to exogenous sex hormones', in T. Mori and H. Nagasawa, eds, *Toxicity of Hormones in Perinatal Life*, CRC Press Inc. (1988). See also: W. Gill, et al., 'Structural and functional abnormalities in the sex organs of male offspring of mothers treated with diethylstilbestrol (DES)', *Journal of Reproductive Medicine*, 1976 Apr;16(4):147–53

14. J. Lee, 'Viewpoint – an interview with Dr John Lee', *Optimum Nutrition*, 1997;10(1):12–13

15. L. Bergkvist, et al., 'The risk of breast cancer after estrogen and estrogen-progestin replacement', *New England Journal of Medicine*, 1989 Aug. 3;321(5):293–7

16. G. Colditz, et al., 'The use of estrogens and progestins and the risk of breast cancer in postmenopausal women', *New England Journal of Medicine*, 1995 June 15;332(24):1589–93

17. K. Chang, et al., 'Influences of percutaneous administration of estradiol and progesterone on human breast epithelial cell cycle in vivo', *Fertility and Sterility*, 1995 Apr.;63(4):785–91

18. C. Antunes, et al., 'Endometrial cancer and estrogen use. Report of a large case-control study', *New England Journal of Medicine*, 1979 Jan. 4;300(1):9–13; A. Paganini-Hill, et al., 'Endometrial cancer and patterns of use of oestrogen replacement therapy: a cohort study', *British Journal of Cancer*, 1989 Mar.;59(3):445–7; P. Green, et al., 'Risk of endometrial cancer following cessation of menopausal hormone use (Washington, United States)', *Cancer Causes and Control*, 1996 Nov.;7(6):575–80

19. S. Beresford, et al., 'Risk of endometrial cancer in relation to use of oestrogen combined with cyclic progestagen therapy in postmenopausal women', *Lancet*, 1997 Feb. 5;349(9050):458–61; E. Weiderpass, et al., 'Risk of endometrial cancer following estrogen replacement with and without progestins', *Journal of the National Cancer Institute*, 1999 July 7;91(13):1131–7

20. C. Rodriguez, et al., 'Estrogen replacement therapy and fatal ovarian cancer', *American Journal of Epidemiology*, 1995 May 1;141(9):828–35

21. V. Beral, 'Breast cancer and hormone-replacement therapy in the Million Women Study', *Lancet*, 2003 Aug. 9;362(9382):419–27

22. R. Chlebowski, et al., 'Breast cancer after use of estrogen plus progestin in postmenopausal women', *New England Journal of Medicine*, 2009 Feb. 5;360(6):573–87

23. B. Melnik, 'Permanent impairment of insulin resistance from pregnancy to adulthood: The primary basic risk factor of chronic Western diseases', *Medical Hypotheses*, 2009 Nov.;73(5):670–81

24. H. Koponen, et al., 'Metabolic syndrome predisposes to depressive symptoms: A population-based 7-year follow-up study', *Journal of Clinical Psychiatry*, 2008 Feb.;69(2):178–82

25. K. Yaffe, et al., 'The metabolic syndrome and development of cognitive impairment among older women', *Archives of Neurology*, 2009 Mar.;66(3):324–8

26. E. Epel, 'Psychological and metabolic stress: a recipe for accelerated cellular aging?', *Hormones (Athens)*, 2009 Jan.;8(1):7–22

27. I. Kyrou and C. Tsigos, 'Chronic stress, visceral obesity and gonadal dysfunction', *Hormones (Athens)*, 2008 Oct.;7(4):287–93; G. Kabat, et al., 'Repeated measures of serum glucose and insulin in relation to postmenopausal breast cancer', *International Journal of Cancer*, 2009 Dec. 1;125(11):2704–10

28. A. Larnkjaer, et al., 'Early programming of the IGF-I axis: negative association between IGF-I in infancy and late adolescence in a 17-year longitudinal follow-up study of healthy subjects', *Growth Hormone IG. Resources*, 2009 Feb.;19(1):82–6

29. E. Giovannucci, et al., 'Nutritional predictors of insulin-like growth factor I and their relationships to cancer in men', *Cancer Epidemiology, Biomarkers and Prevention*, 2003 Feb.;12(2):84–9; M. Holmes, et al., 'Dietary correlates of plasma insulin-like growth factor I and insulin-like growth factor binding protein 3 concentrations', *Cancer Epidemiology, Biomarkers and Prevention*, 2002 Sept.;11(9):852–61; J. Cadogan, et al., 'Milk intake and bone mineral acquisition in adolescent girls: randomised, controlled intervention trial', *British Medical Journal*, 1997 Nov. 15;315(7118):1255–60; J. Ma, et al., 'Milk intake, circulating levels of insulin-like growth factor-I, and risk of colorectal cancer in men', *Journal of the National Cancer Institute*, 2001 Sept. 5;93(17):1330–6; C. Hoppe, et al., 'Animal protein intake, serum insulin-like growth factor I, and growth in healthy 2.5-y-old Danish children', *American Journal of Clinical Nutrition*, 2004 Aug.;80(2):447–52; C. Hoppe, et al., 'High intakes of milk, but not meat, increase s-insulin and insulin resistance in 8-year-old boys', *European Journal of Clinical Nutrition*, 2005 Mar.;59(3):393–8; C. Hoppe, et al., 'High intakes of skimmed milk, but not meat, increase serum IGF-I and IGFBP-3 in eight-year-old boys', *European Journal of Clinical Nutrition*, 2004 Sept.;58(9):1211–6; I.S. Rogers, et al., 'Cross-sectional associations of diet and insulin-like growth factor levels in 7- to 8-year-old children', *Cancer Epidemiology, Biomarkers and Prevention*, 2005 Jan.;14(1):204–12; R. Heaney, et al., 'Dietary changes favorably affect bone remodeling in older adults', *Journal of the American Dietetic Association*, 1999 Oct.;99(10):1228–33; L. Esterle, et al., 'Milk, rather than other foods, is associated with vertebral bone mass and circulating IGF-1 in female adolescents', *Osteoporosis International*, 2009 Apr.;20(4):567–75

30. E. Ostman, et al., 'Inconsistency between glycemic and insulinemic responses to regular and fermented milk products', *American Journal of Clinical Nutrition*, 2001 July;74(1):96–100

31. E. Liljeberg and I. Bjorck, 'Milk as a supplement to mixed meals may elevate postprandial insulinaemia', *European Journal of Clinical Nutrition*, 2001 Nov.;55(11):994–9

32. L. Moisey, et al., 'Caffeinated coffee consumption impairs blood glucose homeostasis in response to high and low glycemic index meals in healthy men', *American Journal of Clinical Nutrition*, 2008 May;87(5):1254–61

33. F. Danby, 'Acne and milk, the diet myth, and beyond', *Journal of the American Academy of Dermatology*, 2005 Feb.;52(2):360–2; F. Danby, 'Acne, dairy and cancer: The 5α-P link,' *Dermato-Endocrinology*, 2009;1(1):12–16; D. Ganmaa and A. Sato, 'The possible role of female sex hormones in milk from pregnant cows in the development of breast, ovarian and corpus uteri cancers', *Medical Hypotheses*, 2005;65(6):1028–37

34. C. Hoppe, et al., 'Cow's milk and linear growth in industrialized and developing countries', *Annual Review of Nutrition*, 2006;26:131–73; C. Hoppe, et al., 'The effect of seven-day supplementation with milk protein fractions and milk minerals on IGFs and glucose–insulin metabolism in Danish prepubertal boys', 2008; Poster Presentation; Department of Human Nutrition Faculty of Life Sciences, University of Copenhagen

35. S. Lee, et al., 'Adolescent and adult soy food intake and breast cancer risk: results from the Shanghai Women's Health Study', *American Journal of Clinical Nutrition*, 2009 June;89(6):1920–6

36. M. Messina and S. Barnes, 'The role of soy products in reducing risk of cancer', *Journal of the National Cancer Institute*, 1991 Apr. 17;83(8):541–6; W. Troll, et al., 'Soybean diet lowers breast tumor incidence in irradiated rats', *Carcinogenesis*, 1980 June;1(6):469–72

37. S. Barnes, 'Soybeans inhibit mammary tumor growth in models of breast cancer', in M. Pariza, ed., *Mutagens and Carcinogens in Diet*, Wiley, (1990); see also: S. Barnes, et al., 'Soybeans inhibit mammary tumors in models of breast cancer', *Progress in Clinical and Biological Research*, 1990;347:239–53

38. C. Kirk, et al., 'Do dietary phytoestrogens influence susceptibility to hormone-dependent cancer by disrupting the metabolism of endogenous oestrogens?', *Biochemical Society Transactions*, 2001 May;29(Pt 2):209–16

Part 2

1. L. Högberg, et al., 'Oats to children with newly diagnosed celiac disease: A randomised double blind study', *Gut*, 2004 May;53(5):649–54.

2. G. Hardman and G. Hart, 'Dietary advice based on food-specific IgG results', *Nutrition and Food Science*, 2007;37:16–23

3. J. Ahn, et al., 'Adiposity, adult weight change, and postmenopausal breast cancer risk', *Archives of Internal Medicine*, 2007 Oct. 22;167(19):2091–102

4. D. Royall, et al., 'Clinical significance of colonic fermentation', *American Journal of Gastroenterology*, 1990 Oct.;85(10):1307–12; G. Latella and R. Caprilli, 'Metabolism of large bowel mucosa in health and disease', *International Journal of Colorectal Disease*, 1991 May;6(2):127–32; R. Hoverstad, 'The normal microflora and short-chain fatty acids', *Proceedings of the Fifth Bengt E. Gustafsson Symposium, Stockholm* (1–4 June 1988)

5. G. Abraham and M. Lubran, 'Serum and red cell magnesium levels in patients with premenstrual tension', *American Journal of Clinical Nutrition*, 1981 Nov.;34(11):2364–6

6. P. O'Brien and H. Massil, 'Premenstrual syndrome: Clinical studies on essential fatty acids', in D. Horrobin, ed., *Omega-6 Essential Fatty Acids: Pathophysiology and Roles in Clinical Medicine*, Wiley-Liss, (1990), 523–45

7. J. Wurtman, 'The involvement of brain serotonin in excessive carbohydrate snacking by obese carbohydrate cravers', *Journal of the American Dietetic Association*, 1984 Sept.;84(9):1004–7

8. J. Wurtman, 'Depression and weight gain: the serotonin connection', *Journal of Affective Disorders*, 1993 Oct.;29(2–3):183–92; R. Wurtman and J. Wurtman, 'Carbohydrate craving, obesity and brain serotonin', *Appetite*, 1986;7 Suppl:99–103; R. Wurtman and J. Wurtman, 'Brain serotonin, carbohydrate-craving, obesity and depression', *Obesity Research*, 1995 Nov.;3 Suppl 4:477S–80S

9. M. Glenville, *The Nutritional Health Handbook for Women*, Piatkus (2001)

10. M. Bryant, et al., 'Effect of consumption of soy isoflavones on behavioural, somatic and affective symptoms in women with premenstrual syndrome', *British Journal of Nutrition*, 2005 May;93(5):731–9

11. D. Berger, et al., 'Efficacy of Vitex agnus castus L. extract Ze 440 in patients with pre-menstrual syndrome (PMS)', *Archives of Gynecology and Obstetrics*, 2000 Nov.;264(3):150–3

12. D. Lithgow and V. Politzer, 'Vitamin A in the treatment of menorrhagia', *South African Medical Journal*, 1977 Feb.;51:191–3

13. I. Gal, et al., 'Effects of oral contraceptives on human plasma vitamin-A levels', *British Medical Journal*, 1971 May 22;2(5759):436–8; see also F. Cumming and M. Briggs, 'Changes in plasma vitamin A in lactating and non-lactating oral contraceptive users', *British Journal of Obstetrics and Gynaecology*, 1983 Jan.;90(1):73–7

14. C. Kalamis and S. Brennan, *Women Without Sex*, Self Help Direct (2007); also see E. Laumann, et al., 'Sexual dysfunction in the United States: Prevalence and predictors', *Journal of the American Medical Association*, 1999 Feb. 10;281(6):537–44

15. J. Simons and M. Carey, 'Prevalence of sexual dysfunctions: Results from a decade of research', *Archives of Sexual Behavior*, 2001 Apr.;30(2):177–219

16. K. Dunn, et al., 'Sexual problems: A study of the prevalence and need for health care in the general population', *Family Practice*, 1998 Dec.;15(6):519–24

17. D. Ferguson, et al., 'Randomized, placebo-controlled, double-blind, cross-over design trial of the efficacy and safety of Zestra for women in women

with and without female sexual arousal disorder', *Journal of Sex and Marital Therapy*, 2003;29 Suppl 1:33–44

18. C. Meston and M. Worcel, 'The effects of yohimbine plus L-arginine gluta-mate on sexual arousal in postmenopausal women with sexual arousal disor-der', *Archives of Sexual Behavior*, 2002 Aug.;31(4):323–32; also see T. Ito, et al., 'The enhancement of female sexual function with ArginMax, a nutritional supplement, among women differing in menopausal status', *Journal of Sex and Marital Therapy*, 2006 Oct.;32(5):369–78

19. R. Estrada-Reyes, et al., 'Turnera diffusa Wild (Turneraceae) recovers sexual behavior in sexually exhausted males', *Journal of Ethnopharmacology*, 2009 June 25;123(3):423–9

20. T. Ito, et al., 'The enhancement of female sexual function with ArginMax, a nutritional supplement, among women differing in menopausal status', *Journal of Sex and Marital Therapy*, 2006 Oct.;32(5):369–78

21. T. Zenico, et al., 'Subjective effects of Lepidium meyenii (Maca) extract on well-being and sexual performances in patients with mild erectile dysfunction: A randomised, double-blind clinical trial', *Andrologia*, 2009 Apr.;41(2):95–9

22. N. Brooks, et al., 'Beneficial effects of Lepidium meyenii (Maca) on psycho-logical symptoms and measures of sexual dysfunction in postmenopausal women are not related to estrogen or androgen content', *Menopause*, 2008 Nov.;15(6):1157–62

23. C. Dording, et al., 'A double-blind, randomized, pilot dose-finding study of maca root (L. meyenii) for the management of SSRI-induced sexual dysfunc-tion', *CNS Neuroscience & Therapeutics*, 2008;14(3):182–91

24. H. Nakhai-Pour, et al., 'Use of antidepressants during pregnancy and the risk of spontaneous abortion', *Canadian Medical Association Journal*, 2010 May; [Epub ahead of print]; S. Gentile, 'On categorizing gestational, birth, and neonatal complications following late pregnancy exposure to antidepres-sants: the prenatal antidepressant exposure syndrome', *CNS Spectrums*, 2010 Mar.;15(3):167–85

25. Dr E. Grant, *Sexual Chemistry, Understanding our Hormones, the Pill and HRT*, Cedar Books (1994)

26. Dr E. Grant, *Sexual Chemistry, Understanding our Hormones, the Pill and HRT*, Cedar Books (1994)

27. B. Barnes and S.G. Bradley, *Planning for a Healthy Baby*, Vermilion, 2nd edn (1992)

28. B. Pickard, 'Nausea and Vomiting in Early Pregnancy', *Nutrition & Food Science*, 83(1):20–2

29. Annual Meeting of the American Psychiatric Association, San Francisco, USA, 20 May 2003

30. P. Komesaroff, et al., 'Effects of wild yam extract on menopausal symptoms, lipids and sex hormones in healthy menopausal women', *Climacteric*, 2001 June;4(2):144–50

31. J. Tice, et al., 'Phytoestrogen supplements for the treatment of hot flashes: The Isoflavone Clover Extract (ICE) Study: A randomized controlled trial', *Journal of the American Medical Association*, 2003 July 9;290(2):207–14

32. No authors listed, 'Treatment of menopause-associated vasomotor symptoms: Position statement of The North American Menopause Society', *Menopause*, 2004 Jan.;11(1):11–33

33. S. Dormire and N. Reame, 'Menopausal hot flash frequency changes in response to experimental manipulation of blood glucose', *Nursing Research*, 2003 Sept.;52(5):338–43

34. P. McSorley, et al., 'Vitamin C improves endothelial function in healthy estrogen-deficient postmenopausal women', *Climacteric*, 2003 Sept.;6(3): 238–47

35. W. Wuttke, et al., 'The Cimicifuga preparation BNO 1055 vs. conjugated estrogens in a double-blind placebo-controlled study: Effects on menopause symptoms and bone markers', *Maturitas*, 2003 Mar. 14;44 Suppl 1:S67–S77; J. Jacobson, et al., 'Randomized trial of black cohosh for the treatment of hot flashes among women with a history of breast cancer', *Journal of Clinical Oncology*, 2001 May 15;19(10):2739–45; W. Stoll, 'Cimifuga vz Estrogenis Substances', *Mediziische Welt*, 1985;36:871–4

36. R. Lupu, et al., 'Black cohosh, a menopausal remedy, does not have estrogenic activity and does not promote breast cancer cell growth', *International Journal of Oncology*, 2003 Nov.;23(5):1407–12

37. C. Kupfersztain, et al., 'The immediate effect of natural plant extract, Angelica sinensis and Matricaria chamomilla (Climex) for the treatment of hot flushes during menopause: A preliminary report', *Clinical and Experimental Obstetrics and Gynecology*, 2003;30(4):203–6

38. J. Hirata, et al., 'Does dong quai have estrogenic effects in postmenopausal women? A double-blind, placebo-controlled trial', *Fertility and Sterility*, 1997 Dec.;68(6):981–6

39. B. Roemheld-Hamm, 'Chasteberry', *American Family Physician*, 2005 Sept. 1;72(5):821–4

40. C. Li, et al., 'Menopause-related symptoms: what are the background factors? A prospective population-based cohort study of Swedish women (The Women's Health in Lund Area study)', *American Journal of Obstetrics and Gynecology*, 2003 Dec.;189(6):1646–53

41. L. Germaine and R. Freedman, 'Behavioral treatment of menopausal hot flashes: evaluation by objective methods', *Journal of Consulting and Clinical Psychology*, 1984 Dec.;52(6):1072–9; R. Freedman and S. Woodward, 'Behavioral treatment of menopausal hot flashes: evaluation by ambulatory monitoring', *American Journal of Obstetrics and Gynecology*, 1992 Aug.;167(2):436–9; R. Freedman, et al., 'Biochemical and thermoregulatory effects of behavioural treatment for menopausal hot flashes', *Menopause*, 1995;2:211–18

42. T. Lien, et al., 'Supplementary health benefits of soy aglycons of isoflavone by improvement of serum biochemical attributes, enhancement of liver

antioxidative capacities and protection of vaginal epithelium of ovariect-omized rats', *Nutrition & Metabolism (Lond.)*, 2009;6:15

43. B. Grube, et al., 'St. John's Wort extract: Efficacy for menopausal symptoms of psychological origin', *Advances in Therapy*, 1999 July;16(4):177–86

44. R. Uebelhack, et al., 'Black cohosh and St. John's wort for climacteric com-plaints: A randomized trial', *Obstetrics and Gynecology*, 2006 Feb.;107(2 Pt 1):247–55

Part 3

1. See the website of The American Association of Clinical Endocrinologists http://media.aace.com/article_display.cfm?article_id=4584

2. A. Jabbar, et al., 'Vitamin B_{12} deficiency common in primary hypothyroidism', *Journal of the Pakistan Medical Association*, 2008 May; 58(5):258–61

3. R. Premont, et al., 'Following the trace of elusive amines', *Proceedings of the National Academy of Sciences*, 2001;98:9474–5

4. J. Joneja, *Dietary Management of Food Allergies & Intolerances: A Comprehensive Guide*, J.A. Hall Publications Ltd, 2nd edn (2003)

5. V. Glover, et al., 'Biochemical predisposition to dietary migraine: the role of phenolsulphotransferase', *Headache: The Journal of Head and Face Pain*, 1983 Mar.; 23(2):53–8; see also A. Jones, et al., 'Reduced platelet phenolsulpho-transferase activity towards dopamine and 5-hydroxytryptamine in migraine', *European Journal of Clinical Pharmacology*, 1995 Nov.;49(1–2):109–14

6. K. Abu-Elteen, 'The influence of dietary carbohydrates on *in vitro* adherence of four *Candida* species to human buccal epithelial cells', *Microbial Ecology in Health and Disease*, 2005;17(3):156–62

7. O. Lee and B. Lee, 'Antioxidant and antimicrobial activities of individual and combined phenolics in Olea europaea leaf extract', *Bioresource Technology*, 2010 May;101(10):3751–4

8. J. Cizmárik and J. Trupl, 'Action of propolis on dermatophytes', *Pharmazie*, 1976;31(1):55

9. T. Tang, et al., 'Insulin-sensitising drugs (metformin, rosiglitazone, piogli-tazone, D-chiro-inositol) for women with polycystic ovary syndrome, oligo amenorrhoea and subfertility', *Cochrane Database of Systematic Reviews*, 2009, Issue 4. Art. No.: CD003053

10. P. Essah, et al., 'The metabolic syndrome in polycystic ovary syndrome', *Clinical Obstetrics and Gynecology*, 2007 Mar.;50(1):205–25; J. Vrbikova, et al., 'Insulin sensitivity in women with polycystic ovary syndrome', *Journal of Clinical Endocrinology and Metabolism*, 2004 June;89(6):2942–5; J. Nestler and D. Jakubowicz, 'Lean women with polycystic ovary syndrome respond to insulin reduction with decreases in ovarian P450c17 alpha activity and serum androgens', *Journal of Clinical Endocrinology and Metabolism*, 1997

Dec.;82(12):4075–9; J. Nestler, 'Role of hyperinsulinemia in the pathogenesis of the polycystic ovary syndrome, and its clinical implications', *Seminars in Reproductive Endocrinology*, 1997 May;15(2):111–22

11. D. Cibula, 'Is insulin resistance an essential component of PCOS? The influence of confounding factors', *Human Reproduction*, 2004 Apr.;19(4):757–9

12. J. Nestler, 'Obesity, insulin, sex steroids and ovulation', *International Journal of Obesity and Related Metabolic Disorders*, 2000 June;24 Suppl 2:S71–S73

13. M. La, et al., 'Metformin treatment of PCOS during adolescence and the reproductive period', *European Journal of Obstetrics, Gynecology, and Reproductive Biology*, 2005 July 1;121(1):3–7; T. Tang, et al., 'Combined lifestyle modification and metformin in obese patients with polycystic ovary syndrome. A randomized, placebo-controlled, double-blind multi-centre study', *Human Reproduction*, 2006 Jan.;21(1):80–9; J. Nestler, 'Should patients with polycystic ovarian syndrome be treated with metformin? An enthusiastic endorsement', *Human Reproduction*, 2002 Aug.;17(8):1950–3; J. Nestler, et al., 'Strategies for the use of insulin-sensitizing drugs to treat infertility in women with polycystic ovary syndrome', *Fertility and Sterility*, 2002 Feb.;77(2):209–15

14. R. Homburg, 'Should patients with polycystic ovarian syndrome be treated with metformin? A note of cautious optimism', *Human Reproduction*, 2002 Apr.;17(4):853–6

15. J. Lord, et al., 'Metformin in polycystic ovary syndrome: Systematic review and meta-analysis', *British Medical Journal*, 2003 Oct. 25;327(7421):951–3

16. J. Lord, et al., 'Metformin in polycystic ovary syndrome: Systematic review and meta-analysis', *British Medical Journal*, 2003 Oct. 25;327(7421):951–3

17. C. McCartney, et al., 'Obesity and sex steroid changes across puberty: Evidence for marked hyperandrogenemia in pre- and early pubertal obese girls', *Journal of Clinical Endocrinology and Metabolism*, 2007 Feb. 92(2):430–6

18. J. Lord, et al., 'Metformin in polycystic ovary syndrome: Systematic review and meta-analysis', *British Medical Journal*, 2003 Oct. 25;327(7421):951–3

19. T. Tang, et al., 'Insulin-sensitising drugs (metformin, rosiglitazone, pioglitazone, D-chiro-inositol) for women with polycystic ovary syndrome, oligo amenorrhoea and subfertility', *Cochrane Database of Systematic Reviews* 2009, Issue 4. Art. No.: CD003053

20. B. Eskenazi and M. Warner, 'Epidemiology of endometriosis', *Obstetrics and Gynecology Clinics of North America*, 1997 June;24(2):235–58

21. T. D'Hooghe, et al., 'Health economics of endometriosis', *Endometriosis*, Luk Rombauts, Jim Tsaltas, Peter Maher and David Healy, eds, Blackwell Publishing (2008), Chapter 1, p. 3

22. S. Simoens, et al., 'Endometriosis: Cost estimates and methodological perspective', *Human Reproduction Update*, 2007 July;13(4):395–404

23. R. Galeo, 'La Dysmenorrhea, syndrome multiforme [Dysmenorrhea, a multiple syndrome]', *Gynecologie*, 1974;25(2):125–7 (in French)

24. T. D'Hooghe and L. Hummelshoj, 'Multi-disciplinary centres/networks of excellence for endometriosis management and research: A proposal', *Human Reproduction*, 2006;21(11):2743–8

25. A. Shanti, et al., 'Autoantibodies to markers of oxidative stress are elevated in women with endometriosis', *Fertility and Sterility*, 1999 June;71(6):1115–18; E. Schisterman, et al., 'TBARS and cardiovascular disease in a population-based sample', *Journal of Cardiovascular Risk*, 2001 Aug.;8(4):219–25

26. N. Foyouzi, et al., 'Effects of oxidants and antioxidants on proliferation of endometrial stromal cells', *Fertility and Sterility*, 2004 Oct.;82 Suppl 3:1019–22

27. L. Jackson, et al., 'Oxidative stress and endometriosis', *Human Reproduction*, 2005 July;20(7):2014–20

28. C. Hernandez Guerrero, et al., 'Endometriosis and deficient intake of antioxidants molecules related to peripheral and peritoneal oxidative stress', *Ginecologia y Obstetricia de Mexico*, 2006 Jan.;74(1):20–8

29. P.R. Konincks, et al., 'Dioxin pollution and endometriosis in Belgium', *Human Reproduction*, 1994;9:1001–2

30. S. Rier, et al., 'Serum levels of TCDD and dioxin-like chemicals in Rhesus monkeys chronically exposed to dioxin: Correlation of increased serum PCB levels with endometriosis', *Toxicological Sciences*, 2001 Jan.;59(1):147–59

31. C. Nagata, et al., 'Total and monounsaturated fat intake and serum estrogen concentrations in premenopausal Japanese women', *Nutrition and Cancer*, 2000;38(1):37–9

32. M. Ballweg, 'Selected food intake and risk of endometriosis', *Human Reproduction*, 2005 Jan.;20(1):312–13

33. K. Miyazawa, 'Incidence of endometriosis among Japanese women', *Obstetrics and Gynecology*, 1976;48:407–9

34. S. Stock, 'Nutrition and Hormones', *Nutrition Therapy Today*, 1995;3–4, Society for the Promotion of Nutritional Therapy (no page number available)

35. L. Cowan, et al., 'Breast cancer incidence in women with a history of progesterone deficiency', *American Journal of Epidemiology*, 1981 Aug.;114(2):209–17

36. N. Barnards, et al., 'Diet and sex-hormone binding globulin, dysmenorrhea, and premenstrual symptoms', *Obstetrics and Gynecology*, 2000 Feb;95(2):245–50

37. J. Spallholz, et al., 'Immunologic responses of mice fed diets supplemented with selenite selenium', *Proceedings of the Society for Experimental Biology and Medicine*, 1973 July;143(3):685–9

38. J. Halme, 'Role of peritoneal inflammation in endometriosis associated with infertility. Endometriosis Today: Advances in research and practice', *The Proceedings of the Vth World Congress on Endometriosis, Yokahama*, Japan, October 1996, Parthenon Publishing: 132–5

39. P. Koninckx, et al., 'Diagnosis of the luteinized unruptured follicle syndrome by steroid hormone assays on peritoneal fluid', *British Journal of Obstetrics and Gynaecology*, 1980 Nov.;87(11):929–34

40. V. Kassis, 'The prostaglandin system in human skin', *Danish Medical Bulletin*, 1983 Sept.;30(5):320–43

41. A. Covens, et al., 'The effect of dietary supplementation with fish oil fatty acids on surgically induced endometriosis in the rabbit', *Fertility and Sterility*, 1988 Apr.;49(4):698–703

42. B. Deutch, 'Menstrual pain in Danish women correlated with low n-3 poly-unsaturated fatty acid intake', *European Journal of Clinical Nutrition*, 1995 July;49(7):508–16

43. H. Fontana-Klaiber and B. Hogg, 'Therapeutic effects of magnesium in dysmenorrhea', *Schweizerische Rundschau fur Medizin Praxis*, 1990 Apr. 17;79(16):491–4

44. S. Ziaei, et al., 'A randomised controlled trial of vitamin E in the treatment of primary dysmenorrhoea', *BJOG : an International Journal of Obstetrics and Gynaecology*, 2005 Apr.;112(4):466–9

45. H. Hieber, 'Treatment of vertebragenous pain and sensitivity disorders using high doses of hydroxocobalamin', *Medizinische Monatsschrift*, 1974 Dec.;28(12):545–8

46. M.A. Mibielli, et al., 'Diclofenac plus B vitamins versus diclofenac mono-therapy in lumbago: the DOLOR study', *Current Medical Research & Opinion*, 2009 November; 25(11):2589–99

47. A. Misra, et al., 'Differential effects of opiates on the incorporation of [14C] thiamine in the central nervous system of the rat', *Experientia*, 1977 Mar. 15;33(3):372–4

48. L. Gokhale, 'Curative treatment of primary (spasmodic) dysmenorrhoea', *Indian Journal of Medical Research*, 1996 Apr.;103:227–31

49. J. Chavarro, et al., 'Use of multivitamins, intake of B vitamins, and risk of ovulatory infertility', *Fertility and Sterility*, 2008 Mar.;89(3):668–76

50. W. Willett and M. Stampfer, 'Rebuilding the Food Pyramid', *Scientific American reports: Special Edition on Diet and Health*, 2003 Jan;288(1):64–71

51. A. Czeizel, et al., 'The effect of preconceptional multivitamin supplementation on fertility', *International Journal for Vitamin and Nutrition Research*, 1996;66(1):55–8

52. 'Nutritional Therapy Provides an Effective Method of Improving Fertility Rates and Reducing Abdominal Pain in Women with Endometriosis', 'What is One Man's Meat is Another Man's Poison, May Presumably Have a Chemical Basis', 'Integrated Medicine at the Point of Diagnosis May Enhance Treatment of Women with Compromised Fertility and Abdominal Pain', D. Shepperson Mills. *Fertility and Sterility*, September 2006, Suppl 2;86:S270

53. P. Band, et al., 'Treatment of benign breast disease with vitamin A', *Preventive Medicine*, 1984 Sep.;13(5):549–54

54. K. Lockwood, et al., 'Apparent partial remission of breast cancer in "High Risk" patients supplemented with nutritional antioxidants, essential fatty acids and Coenzyme Q_{10}', *Molecular Aspects of Medicine*, 1994;15(1):s231–s240

55. S. Qureshi and N. Sultan, 'Topical nonsteroidal anti-inflammatory drugs versus oil of evening primrose in the treatment of mastalgia', *Surgeon*, 2005 Feb.;3(1):7–10

56. World Cancer Research Fund/American Institute for Cancer Research, *Food, Nutrition, Physical Activity, and the Prevention of Cancer: a Global Perspective.* AICR (2007)

57. M. Rookus, et al., 'Oral contraceptives and risk of breast cancer in women aged 20–54 years', *Lancet*, 1994 Sep.;344 (8926):844–51

58. G. Colditz, et al., 'The use of estrogens and progestins and the risk of breast cancer in postmenopausal women', *New England Journal of Medicine*, 1995 June;333(20):1355

59. P. Lichtenstein, et al., 'Environmental and heritable factors in the causation of cancer – analyses of cohorts of twins from Sweden, Denmark, and Finland', *New England Journal of Medicine*, 2000 July 13;343(2):78–85

60. J. Lee with Virginia Hopkins, *What Your Doctor May Not Tell You About Menopause*, Warner Books (1996)

61. J. Lee with Virginia Hopkins, *What Your Doctor May Not Tell You About Menopause*, Warner Books (1996)

62. N. Boyd, et al., 'Dietary fat and breast cancer risk revisited: A meta-analysis of the published literature', *British Journal of Cancer*, 2003 June;89:1672–85

63. M. Gunter, et al., 'Insulin, insulin-like growth factor-I, and risk of breast cancer in postmenopausal women', *Journal of the National Cancer Institute*, 2009 Dec.;101(1):48–60

64. A. Barclay, et al., 'Glycemic index, glycemic load, and chronic disease risk: A meta-analysis of observational studies', *American Journal of Clinical Nutrition*, 2008 Mar.;87(3):627–37; see also A. Tavani, et al., 'Consumption of sweet foods and breast cancer risk in Italy', *Annals of Oncology*, 2006 Feb.;17(2):341–5; see also C. Krone and J. Ely, 'Controlling hyperglycemia as an adjunct to cancer therapy', *Integrative Cancer Therapies*, 2005 Mar.;4(1):25–31

65. P. Boffetta, et al., 'Fruit and vegetable intake and overall cancer risk in the European Prospective Investigation into Cancer and Nutrition (EPIC)', *Journal of the National Cancer Institute*, 2010 Apr. 21;102(8):510–11

66. K. Ng, et al., 'Circulating 25-hydroxyvitamin D levels and survival in patients with colorectal cancer', *Journal of Clinical Oncology*, 2008 June 20;26(18):2984–91

67. N. Buyru, et al., 'Vitamin D receptor gene polymorphisms in breast cancer', *Experimental and Molecular Medicine*, 2003 Dec. 31;35(6):550–5

68. J. Lin, et al., 'Intakes of calcium and vitamin D and breast cancer risk in women', *Archives of Internal Medicine*, 2007 May 28;167(10):1050–9

69. M. Saunders, et al., 'A novel cyclic adenosine monophosphate analo induces hypercalcemia via production of 1,25-dihydroxyvitamin D in patients with solid tumors', *Journal of Clinical Endocrinology and Metabolism*, 1997 Dec.;82(12):4044–8

70. C. Garland, et al., 'Vitamin D and prevention of breast cancer: Pooled analysis', *Journal of Steroid Biochemistry and Molecular Biology*, 2007 Mar.;103(3–5):708–11

71. C. Garland, et al., 'What is the dose-response relationship between vitamin D and cancer risk?', *Nutrition Reviews*, 2007 Aug.;65(8 Pt 2):S91–S95

72. J. Rossouw, et al., 'Risks and benefits of estrogen plus progestin in healthy postmenopausal women: principal results from the Women's Health Initiative randomized controlled trial', *Journal of the American Medical Association*, 2002 July 17;288(3):321–33

73. D. Felson, et al., 'The effect of postmenopausal estrogen therapy on bone density in elderly women', *New England Journal of Medicine*, 1993 Oct. 14;329(16):1141–6; J. Rossouw, et al., 'Risks and benefits of estrogen plus progestin in healthy postmenopausal women: principal results from the Women's Health Initiative randomized controlled trial', *Journal of the American Medical Association*, 2002 July 17;288(3):321–33

74. Medicines and Healthcare Products Regulatory Agency (MHRA), 'Further advice on safety of hormone replacement therapy (HRT)', press release, 3 December 2003, see: http://mhra.gov.uk/NewsCentre/Pressreleases/CON002044

75. D. Felson, et al., 'The effect of postmenopausal estrogen therapy on bone density in elderly women', *New England Journal of Medicine*, 1993 Oct. 14;329(16):1141–6

76. Report of the European Expert Working Group on HRT, for the Committee on Safety of Medicines in the UK, 2003

77. J. Prior, 'Progesterone as bone-trophic hormone', *Endocrine Reviews*, 1990;11(2):386–98

78. J. Prior, et al., 'Spinal bone loss and ovulatory disturbances', *New England Journal of Medicine*, 1990;323(18):1221–7

79. J. Lee, 'Osteoporosis reversal: The role of progesterone', *International Clinical Nutritional Review*, 1990;10:384–91; J. Lee, 'Osteoporosis reversal with transdermal progesterone', *Lancet*, 1990 Nov. 24;336(8726):1327

80. A. Cooper, et al., 'Systemic absorption of progesterone from Progest cream in postmenopausal women', *Lancet*, 1998 April;351:1255–6

81. No author, 'Milk increases osteoporosis risk', *Optimum Nutrition*, 1998;1(1):15

82. K. Neil, 'Osteoporosis', *Optimum Nutrition*, 1996;9(1)

83. D. Feskanich, et al., 'Protein consumption and bone fractures in women', *American Journal of Epidemiology*, 1996;143(5):472–9

84. L. Allen, et al., 'Protein-induced hypercalcuria: A longer-term study', *American Journal of Clinical Nutrition*, 1979;32(4):741–9; C. R. Anand and H. Linkswiler, 'Effect of protein intake on calcium balance of young men given 500mg calcium daily', *Journal of Nutrition*, 1974;104(6):695–700

85. R. Cumming, et al., 'Calcium intake and fracture risk: results from the study of osteoporotic fractures', *American Journal of Epidemiology*, 1997;145(10):926–34

86. S. Reddy, et al., 'Effect of low-carbohydrate high-protein diets on acid-base balance, stone-forming propensity, and calcium metabolism', *American Journal of Kidney Diseases*, 2002;40(2):265–74

87. L. Allen, et al., 'Protein-induced hypercalcuria: A longer-term study', *American Journal of Clinical Nutrition*, 1979;32(4):741–9

88. A. Wachman and D. Bernstein, 'Diet and osteoporosis', *Lancet*, 1968;1(7549):958–9

89. J. Homik, et al., 'Calcium and vitamin D for corticosteroid-induced osteoporosis', *Cochrane Database of Systematic Reviews*, 1998, Issue 1. Art. No.: CD000952

90. J. Porthouse, et al., 'Randomised controlled trial of calcium and supplementation with cholecalciferol (vitamin D3) for prevention of fractures in primary care', *British Medical Journal*, 2005 Apr. 30;330(7498):1003

91. R. Jackson, et al., 'Calcium plus vitamin D supplementation and the risk of fractures', *New England Journal of Medicine*, 2006 Feb. 16;354(7):669–83

92. D. Agnusdei, et al., 'A double-blind, placebo-controlled trial of ipriflavone for prevention of post-menopausal spinal bone loss', *Calcified Tissue International*, 1997;61(2):142–7; T. Ushiroyama, et al., 'Efficacy of ipriflavone and 1 alpha vitamin D therapy for the cessation of vertebral bone loss', *International Journal of Gynaecology and Obstetrics*, 1995;48(3):283–8; D. Agnusdei, et al., 'Prevention of early postmenopausal bone loss using low doses of conjugated estrogens and the non-hormonal, bone-active drug ipriflavone', *Osteoporosis International*, 1995;5(6):462–6

93. P. Lazzerini, et al., 'Homocysteine enhances cytokine production in cultured synoviocytes from rheumatoid arthritis patients', *Clinical and Experimental Rheumatology*, 2006;24(4):387–93

94. C. Gjesdal, et al., 'Plasma total homocysteine level and bone mineral density: The Hordaland Homocysteine Study', *Archives of Internal Medicine*, 2006;166(1):88–94; R. R. McLean, et al., 'Homocysteine as a predictive factor for hip fracture in older persons', *New England Journal of Medicine*, 2004 May 13;350(20):2042–9; J. B. van Meurs, et al., 'Homocysteine levels and the risk of osteoporotic fracture', *New England Journal of Medicine*, 2004 May 13; 350(20):2033–41

95. C. Gjesdal, et al., 'Plasma homocysteine, folate, and vitamin B_{12} and the risk of hip fracture: The Hordaland Homocysteine Study', *Journal of Bone and Mineral Research*, 2007;22(5):747–56

96. R.R. McLean, et al., 'Homocysteine as a predictive factor for hip fracture in older persons', *New England Journal of Medicine*, 2004 May 13;350(20):2042–9; J.B. van Meurs, et al., 'Homocysteine levels and the risk of osteoporotic fracture', *New England Journal of Medicine*, 2004 May 13;350(20):2033–41

97. M. Herrmann, et al., 'The role of hyperhomocysteinemia as well as folate, vitamin B(6) and B(12) deficiencies in osteoporosis: A systematic review', *Clinical Chemistry and Laboratory Medicine*, 2007;45(12):1621–32

98. L. Raisz, 'Homocysteine and osteoporotic fractures – culprit or bystander?' *New England Journal of Medicine*, 2004;350(20):2089–90

99. G. Ravaglia, et al., 'Folate, but not homocysteine, predicts the risk of fracture in elderly persons', *Journals of Gerontology. Series A, Biological Sciences and Medical Sciences*, 2005;60(11):1458–62; A. Cagnacci, et al., 'Relation of homocysteine, folate, and vitamin B_{12} to bone mineral density of postmenopausal women', *Bone*, 2003;33(6):956–9; J. Golbahar, et al., 'Association of plasma folate, plasma total homocysteine, but not methylenetetrahydrofolate reductase C667T polymorphism, with bone mineral density in postmenopausal Iranian women: A cross-sectional study', *Bone*, 2004;35(3):760–5

100. K. Tucker, et al., 'Low plasma vitamin B_{12} is associated with lower BMD: The Framingham Osteoporosis Study', *Journal of Bone and Mineral Research*, 2005;20(1):152–8; K. Stone, et al., 'Low serum vitamin B-12 levels are associated with increased hip bone loss in older women: A prospective study', *Journal of Clinical Endocrinology and Metabolism*, 2004;89(3):1217–21; M. Morris, et al., 'Relation between homocysteine and B-vitamin status indicators and bone mineral density in older Americans', *Bone*, 2005;37(2):234–42

101. R. McLean, et al., 'Homocysteine as a predictive factor for hip fracture in older persons', *New England Journal of Medicine*, 2004;350(20):2042–9

102. R. Dhonukshe-Rutten, et al., 'Vitamin B-12 status is associated with bone mineral content and bone mineral density in frail elderly women but not in men', *Journal of Nutrition*, 2003;133(3):801–7

103. R. Dhonukshe-Rutten, et al., 'Homocysteine and vitamin B_{12} status relate to bone turnover markers, broadband ultrasound attenuation, and fractures in healthy elderly people', *Journal of Bone and Mineral Research*, 2005;20(6):921–9

104. Y. Sato, et al., 'Effect of folate and mecobalamin on hip fractures in patients with stroke: A randomized controlled trial', *Journal of the American Medical Association*, 2005;293(9):1082–8

105. K. Dimitrova, et al., 'Estrogen and homocysteine', *Cardiovascular Research*, 2002;53(3):577–88

106. V. Mijatovic and M. J. van der Mooren, 'Homocysteine in postmenopausal women and the importance of hormone replacement therapy', *Clinical Chemistry and Laboratory Medicine*, 2001;39(8):764–7

107. G. Abraham, 'The importance of magnesium in the management of primary postmenopausal osteoporosis', *Journal of Nutritional Medicine*, 1991;2(2):165–78; A. Gaby and J. Wright, 'Nutrients and Osteoporosis', *Journal of Nutritional Medicine*, 1990;1(1):63–72

108. 'A Significant Advance in Bone Disease Management', Metra Biosystems Inc. (1994)

Part 4

1. V. Beral and Million Women Study Collaborators, 'Breast cancer and hormone-replacement therapy in the Million Women Study', *Lancet*, 2003 Aug. 9;362(9382):419–27

2. R.T. Chlebowski, et al., (WHI Investigators), 'Breast cancer after use of estrogen plus progestin in postmenopausal women', *New England Journal of Medicine*, 2009 Feb. 5;360(6):573–87

3. C. Dwivedi, et al., 'Effect of calcium glucarate on beta-glucuronidase activity and glucarate content of certain vegetables and fruits', *Biochemical Medicine and Metabolic Biology*, 1990 Apr.;43(2):83–92, and W.A. Nijhoff, et al., 'Effects of consumption of Brussels sprouts on plasma and urinary glutathione S-transferase class-alpha and -pi in humans', *Carcinogenesis*, 1995 Apr.;16(4):955–7

4. L. Carpenter, 'Heard the one about the Pill? It's a killer!' in K. Neil, *Balancing Hormones Naturally*, ION Press (1994)

5. I. Gal, et al., 'Effects of oral contraceptives on human plasma vitamin-A levels', *British Medical Journal*, 1971 May 22;2(5759):436–8; see also F.J. Cumming and M.H. Briggs, 'Changes in plasma vitamin A in lactating and non-lactating oral contraceptive users', *British Journal of Obstetrics and Gynaecology*, 1983 Jan.;90(1):73–7

6. W. Kuhnz, et al., 'Influences of high doses of vitamin C on the bio availability and the serum protein binding of levonorgestrel in women using a combination oral contraceptive', Elsevier Science Inc., New York, USA (1995)

7. D. Moskowitz, 'A comprehensive review of the safety and efficacy of bioidentical hormones for the management of menopause and related health risks', *Alternative Medicine Review*, 2006 Sept.;11(3):208–23

8. C.M. Antunes, et al., 'Endometrial cancer and estrogen use. Report of a large case-control study', *New England Journal of Medicine*, 1979 Jan. 4;300(1):9–13; A. Paganini-Hill, et al., 'Endometrial cancer and patterns of use of oestrogen replacement therapy: a cohort study', *British Journal of Cancer*, 1989 Mar.;59(3):445–7; P.K. Green, et al., 'Risk of endometrial cancer following cessation of menopausal hormone use (Washington, United States)', *Cancer Causes and Control*, 1996 Nov.;7(6):575–80; Kaiser-permanent Medical Centre study, in S. Batt, *Patients No More: The Politics of Breast Cancer*, Scarlet Press (1997)

9. J. Robbins, *Reclaiming Our Health: Exploring the Medical Myth and Embracing the Source of True Healing*, H. J. Kramer (1996)

10. T.W. McDonald, et al., 'Exogenous estrogen and endometrial carcinoma: case-control and incidence study', *American Journal of Obstetrics and Gynecology*, 1977 Mar. 15;127(6):572–80

11. S.A. Beresford, et al., 'Risk of endometrial cancer in relation to use of oestrogen combined with cyclic progestagen therapy in postmenopausal women', *Lancet*, 1997 Feb. 15;349(9050):458–61; E. Weiderpass, et al., 'Risk of endometrial cancer following estrogen replacement with and without progestins', *Journal of the National Cancer Institute*, 1999 July 7;91(13):1131–7

12. S.A. Beresford, et al., 'Risk of endometrial cancer in relation to use of oestrogen combined with cyclic progestagen therapy in postmenopausal women', *Lancet*, 1997 Feb. 15;349(9050):458–61; A. Cerin, et al., 'Adverse endometrial effects of long-cycle estrogen and progestogen replacement therapy. The

Scandinavian LongCycle Study Group', *New England Journal of Medicine*, 1996 Mar. 7;334(10):668–9; G.A. Colditz, et al., 'The use of estrogens and progestins and the risk of breast cancer in postmenopausal women', *New England Journal of Medicine*, 1995 June 15;332(24):1589–93; E. Daly, et al., 'Risk of venous thromboembolism in users of hormone replacement therapy', *Lancet*, 1996 Oct. 12;348(9033):977–80; F. Grodstein, et al., 'Postmenopausal estrogen and progestin use and the risk of cardiovascular disease', *New England Journal of Medicine*, 1996 Aug. 15;335(7):453–61; F. Grodstein, et al., 'Prospective study of exogenous hormones and risk of pulmonary embolism in women', *Lancet*, 1996 Oct. 12;348(9033):983–7; E. Hemminki and K. McPherson, 'Impact of postmenopausal hormone therapy on cardiovascular events and cancer: pooled data from clinical trials', *British Medical Journal*, 1997 July 19;315(7101):149–53; M.C. Pike, et al., 'Estrogen-progestin replacement therapy and endometrial cancer', *Journal of the National Cancer Institute*, 1997 Aug. 6;89(15):1110–16

13. www.cancer.gov/cancertopics/mothers-prescribed-des. The study detected a modest association between DES exposure and breast cancer risk, with a relative risk of about 1.3. In other words, 16 per cent of women prescribed DES during pregnancy developed breast cancer, in comparison with 13 per cent of women not prescribed DES. Therefore, it is estimated that one in six women who were prescribed DES will develop breast cancer, whereas one in eight women in the general population will develop the disease

14. K. Hunt, et al., 'Long-term surveillance of mortality and cancer incidence in women receiving hormone replacement therapy', *British Journal of Obstetrics and Gynaecology*, 1987 July;94(7):620–35; K. Hunt, et al., 'Mortality in a cohort of long-term users of hormone replacement therapy: an updated analysis', *British Journal of Obstetrics and Gynaecology*, 1990 Dec.;97(12):1080–6

15. L. Bergkvist, et al., 'The risk of breast cancer after estrogen and estrogen-progestin replacement', *New England Journal of Medicine*, 1989 Aug. 3;321(5):293–7

16. G.A. Colditz, et al., 'The use of estrogens and progestins and the risk of breast cancer in postmenopausal women', *New England Journal of Medicine*, 1995 June 15;332(24):1589–93

17. C. Rodriguez, et al., 'Estrogen replacement therapy and fatal ovarian cancer', *American Journal of Epidemiology*, 1995 May 1;141(9):828–35

18. No authors listed, 'Breast cancer and hormone replacement therapy: collaborative reanalysis of data from 51 epidemiological studies of 52,705 women with breast cancer and 108,411 women without breast cancer. Collaborative Group on Hormonal Factors in Breast Cancer', *Lancet*, 1997 Oct. 11;350(9084):1047–59

19. P.P. Garg, et al., 'Hormone replacement therapy and the risk of epithelial ovarian carcinoma: a meta-analysis', *Obstetrics and Gynecology*, 1998 Sept.;92(3):472–9

20. J.E. Rossouw, et al., 'Risks and benefits of estrogen plus progestin in healthy postmenopausal women: principal results from the Women's Health Initiative

randomized controlled trial', *Journal of the American Medical Association*, 2002 July 17;288(3):321–33

21. V. Beral, 'Breast cancer and hormone-replacement therapy in the Million Women Study', *Lancet*, 2003 Aug. 9;362(9382):419–27

22. M. Cushman, et al., 'Estrogen plus progestin and risk of venous thrombosis', *Journal of the American Medical Association*, 2004 Oct. 6;292(13):1573–80

23. Million Women Study collaborators, 'Breast cancer and hormone replacement therapy in the Million Women Study', *British Medical Journal*, 2003;362(9382):419–27

24. R.T. Chlebowski, et al., 'Breast cancer after use of estrogen plus progestin in postmenopausal women', *New England Journal of Medicine*, 2009 Feb. 5;360(6):573-87

25. P. Bach, et al., 'Hormone therapy use by postmenopausal women associated with increased incidence of more advanced breast cancer', *Journal of the American Medical Association*, 2010;304(15):1684–92

26. A. H. MacLennan, et al., 'Oral oestrogen and combined oestrogen/progestogen therapy versus placebo for hot flushes', *Cochrane Database of Systematic Reviews* 2004, Issue 3, Art. No.: CD002978

27. C. Minelli, et al., 'Benefits and harms associated with hormone replacement therapy: Clinical decision analysis', *British Medical Journal*, 2004 Feb. 14;328(7436):371

28. S. Somers, *Ageless: The Naked Truth About Bioidentical Hormones*, Crown Publishing Group (2006)

29. J. Szekeres-Bartho, et al., 'Progesterone in pregnancy: Receptor-ligand interaction and signaling pathways', *Journal of Reproductive Immunology*, 2009 Dec;83(1–2):60–4, Epub 31 Oct 2009

30. K. Holtorf of the Holtorf Medical Group, Torrance, California, in *Postgrad Med*, 2009 Jan.;121(1):73–85

31. M. Schumacher, et al., 'Novel perspectives for progesterone in hormone replacement therapy, with special reference to the nervous system', *Endocrine Reviews*, 2007 June;28(4):387–439

32. A. Fournier, et al., 'Unequal risks for breast cancer associated with different hormone replacement therapies: results from the E3N cohort study', *Breast Cancer Research and Treatment*, 2008 Jan.;107(1):103–11

33. K. Stephenson, et al., 'Transdermal progesterone: Effects on menopausal symptoms and on thrombotic, anticoagulant and inflammatory factors in post menopausal women', *International Journal of Pharmaceutical Compounding*, 2008;12(4)

34. K. Stephenson, American Heart Association Scientific Sessions, New Orleans, 8–12 November 2008

35. A.H. Follingstad, 'Estriol, the forgotten estrogen?', *Journal of the American Medical Association*, 1978 Jan. 2;239(1):29–30

36. T.F. Lien, et al., 'Supplementary health benefits of soy aglycons of isoflavone by improvement of serum biochemical attributes, enhancement of liver anti-

oxidative capacities and protection of vaginal epithelium of ovariectomized rats', *Nutrition & Metabolism (Lond.)*, 2009;6:15

37. H. Maia, Jr., et al., 'Testosterone replacement therapy in the climacteric: benefits beyond sexuality', *Gynecological Endocrinology*, 2009 Jan.;25(1):12–20; S.R. Davis, et al., 'Testosterone for low libido in postmenopausal women not taking estrogen', *New England Journal of Medicine*, 2008 Nov. 6;359(19):2005–17

38. P.A. Komesaroff, et al., 'Effects of wild yam extract on menopausal symptoms, lipids and sex hormones in healthy menopausal women', *Climacteric*, 2001 June;4(2):144–50

39. J. Lee, et al., *What Your Doctor May Not Tell You About Breast Cancer*, Thorsons (2002)

40. H.B. Leonetti, et al., 'Transdermal progesterone cream for vasomotor symptoms and postmenopausal bone loss', *Obstetrics and Gynecology*, 1999 Aug.;94(2):225–8

41. G. Holzer, et al., 'Effects and side effects of 2% progesterone cream on the skin of peri- and postmenopausal women: Results from a double-blind, vehicle-controlled, randomized study', *British Journal of Dermatology*, 2005 Sept.;153(3):626–34

42. J.T. Hargrove, et al., 'Menopausal hormone replacement therapy with continuous daily oral micronized estradiol and progesterone', *Obstetrics and Gynecology*, 1989 Apr.;73(4):606–12. Also see http://project-aware.org/Resource/Studies/warner.html

43. J.A. Chollet, et al., 'Efficacy and safety of vaginal estriol and progesterone in postmenopausal women with atrophic vaginitis', *Menopause*, 2009 Sep.–Oct.;16(5):978–83

44. 'Immunomodulation of the Mother during Pregnancy', *Medical Hypotheses*, Institute for Research and Reproduction, Parel, Bombay, India, 1991;35(2):159–164

45. P.E. Mohr, et al., 'Serum progesterone and prognosis in operable breast cancer', *British Journal of Cancer*, 1996 June;73(12):1552–5

Part 5

1. T. Remer and F. Manz, 'Potential renal acid load of foods and its influence on urine pH', *Journal of the American Dietetic Association*, 1995 July;95(7):791–7

2. FSA Committee on Toxicology (COT) report on Phytooestrogens and Health, May 2003, available from www.food.gov.uk/science/ouradvisors/toxicity/reports/phytooestrogensandhealthcot; S. Lee, et al., 'Adolescent and adult soy food intake and breast cancer risk: results from the Shanghai Women's Health Study', *American Journal of Clinical Nutrition*, 2009 Jun.;89(6):1920–6

3. B. Jacobsen, et al., 'Does high soy milk intake reduce prostate cancer incidence? The Adventist Health Study (United States)', *Cancer Causes and Control*, 1998 Dec.;9(6):553–7

4. N. Beckman, 'Phytoestrogens and compounds that affect estrogen metabolism – part 2', *Australian Journal of Medical Herbalism*, 1995;7(2):27–33

5. F. Dittmar, et al., 'Premenstrual syndrome: Treatment with a phytopharmaceutical', *TW Gynakologie*, 1992;5(1):60–8

6. R. Schellenberg, 'Treatment for the premenstrual syndrome with agnus castus fruit extract: Prospective, randomised, placebo controlled study', *British Medical Journal*, 2001 Jan. 20;322(7279):134–7

7. S. Mills, *Out of the Earth: The Science and Practice of Herbal Medicine*, Penguin (1991)

8. B. Roemheld-Hamm, 'Chasteberry', *American Family Physician*, 2005 Sept. 1;72(5):821–4

9. W. Wuttke, et al., 'The Cimicifuga preparation BNO 1055 vs. conjugated estrogens in a double-blind placebo-controlled study: effects on menopause symptoms and bone markers', *Maturitas*, 2003 Mar. 14;44 Suppl 1:S67–S77; J. Jacobson, et al., 'Randomized trial of black cohosh for the treatment of hot flashes among women with a history of breast cancer', *Journal of Clinical Oncology*, 2001 May 15;19(10):2739–45; W. Stoll, 'Cimifuga vz Estrogenis Substances', *Mediziische Welt*, 1985;36:871–4

10. R. Lupu, et al., 'Black cohosh, a menopausal remedy, does not have estrogenic activity and does not promote breast cancer cell growth', *International Journal of Oncology*, 2003 Nov.;23(5):1407–12

11. C. Kupfersztain, et al., 'The immediate effect of natural plant extract, Angelica sinensis and Matricaria chamomilla (Climex) for the treatment of hot flashes during menopause: A preliminary report', *Clinical and Experimental Obstetrics and Gynecology*, 2003;30(4):203–6

12. J. Hirata, et al., 'Does dong quai have estrogenic effects in postmenopausal women? A double-blind, placebo-controlled trial', *Fertility and Sterility*, 1997 Dec.;68(6):981–6

13. See www.dimfaq.com for a full list of research on DIM concentrates

14. B. Grube, et al., 'St. John's Wort extract: Efficacy for menopausal symptoms of psychological origin', *Advances in Therapy*, 1999 July;16(4):177–86

15. R. Uebelhack, et al., 'Black cohosh and St. John's wort for climacteric complaints: A randomized trial', *Obstetrics and Gynecology*, 2006 Feb.;107(2 Pt 1):247–55

Index

womb 5
   fibroids 13, 15–16, 89, 92
   lining 8, 11, 186
womb cancer *see* endometrial
   cancer
women's bodies 4–6
Women's Health Concern 349
Women's Health Initiative 208, 229, 261
Women's Nutritional Advisory Service 15
World Health Organization 64, 186, 213
Wright, Jonathan 255
Wylie, Kevan 94

xenoestrogens 20, 25, 27, 29, 41, 199, 233, 234, 239
   effect on men 95
xylitol 70, 159, 176, 299, 350

yam, wild 122, 219, 224, 253, 254, 266, 314

yeast (in diet) 156–7, 159, 161
yoghurt 161, 168
YorkTest 57, 348

Zest4Life 76, 347
Zestra 97–8
zinc 232, 295, 296, 319
   and bone health 218, 219
   and breast health 195, 203
   copper competes with 246
   for endometriosis 184, 185, 186, 189
   and fertility 106
   for gut health 50, 51, 58
   for menopause 125, 128
   for migraines 147, 148
   for PCOS 174
   for PMS 80, 81, 83
   and pregnancy 114
   for sex drive 97, 101–2
   for thyroid 144
   and vitamin A deficiency 90–1
   for weight control 66, 75

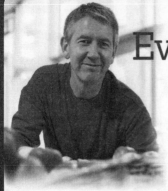

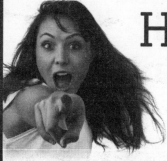